SALUD

SALUD

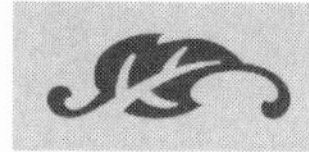

A Latina's Guide to Total Health

Revised Edition

Jane L. Delgado, Ph.D., M.S.

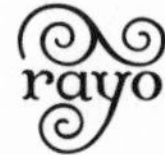

An Imprint of HarperCollins*Publishers*

The information contained in this book should not be substituted for the personal care and attention of a qualified health care provider but rather should be used in conjunction with your provider's care and advice. Before beginning any new health, diet, or exercise program, you should always consult with a health care provider or physician to be sure the new regimens are appropriate for your individual circumstances. The author and the publisher will not be responsible for any adverse effects resulting from the use or application of the information contained in this book.

Proceeds from this book will be donated to the National Alliance for Hispanic Health (the Alliance).

HarperCollins books may be purchased for educational, business, or sales promotional use. For information, please write: Special Markets Department, HarperCollins Publishers Inc., 10 East 53rd Street, New York, NY 10022.

SECOND EDITION

Originally published in 1997 as *Salud!* by Perennial, a division of HarperCollins Publishers Inc.

Library of Congress Cataloging-in-Publication Data is available upon request.

ISBN 0-06-000621-8

02 03 04 05 06 RRD 10 9 8 7 6 5 4 3 2 1

This book is dedicated to my mother,
Lucila Aurora Navarro Delgado (1926–1993)

National Hispanic Women's Health Initiative

CONTENTS

ACKNOWLEDGMENTS

Omayra Castro and countless other women I spoke to these last few years reaffirmed the need for *Salud*. This second edition was made possible through the vision of Rene Alegría, publisher and editor-in-chief of Rayo, and by the many people who gave generously of their time and expertise. All of them were motivated by knowing the major impact that this book has on the lives of Hispanic women and their families.

I was fortunate to be assisted by many of the same dedicated people that helped produce the first edition of *Salud*. The National Hispanic Women's Health Initiative provided comments on an ongoing basis. Ana Rojas reviewed, checked, and developed the resource lists, obtained web addresses wherever possible, and did whatever research was necessary while she worked from home, caring for her two delightful children, four year old Madeline and two year old Adam. Demitria Morrison, coordinated all of the communication and administrative tasks involved in the extensive collaborative and review process that makes *Salud* possible.

To include the latest in medical breakthroughs I relied on a broad spectrum of experts. Expert review for specific chapters was provided by Dr. Douglas E. Henley, Executive Vice President, American Academy of Family Physicians; Dr. John Seffrin, Executive Vice President, American Cancer Society; Cass Wheeler, Chief Executive Officer, and Dr. Kathryn Taubert, American Heart Association; Dr. Bernard Arons, Center for Mental Health Services; Dr. Jane Henney, former Commissioner, Food and Drug Administration (FDA) and Mary Wallace, FDA; Dr. Sandy Garfield, National Institute of Diabetes and Digestive and Kidney Diseases; and Debbie Delgado-Vega, President and CEO, Latino Organization for Liver Awareness. Thomas L. Sacks, MD, Professor of Medicine, Georgetown University Medical Center, an exceptional clinician, and gifted researcher, reviewed the updated manuscript and provided extensive comments based on his knowledge and experience as an internist.

There are others who through some combination of exceptional knowledge or life experiences provided additional guidance. These include: Adolph Falcón and Bill Starck (Taking Care of Your Families); Dr. Carmen Portillo (HIV/AIDS); Dr. Carolina Reyes

(Part II: Being Female); and Deborah Helvarg (commented on the entire book).

In addition to vision, Rene Alegría, provided the encouragement and support that are so rare and yet, essential. He gently prodded me to do major revisions and updates. His intellect couched in his disarming laughter and sensibility continue to be an inspiration.

At a spiritual level I want to thank Msgr. Thomas M. Duffy for the guidance and support he provides for me and my family. Through his guidance I continue to recognize the place that faith and prayer hold in the health of Latinas.

And finally, the two people who give the most of their time to make all I do possible, are my beloved husband, Mark A. Steo and my daughter, Elizabeth Ann Steo.

All these people and many others have worked to make *Salud* the most up-to-date resource possible. For this and so much more I remain very grateful.

FOREWORD

In a groundbreaking collaboration, Dr. Jane Delgado and the members of the National Hispanic Women's Health Initiative have put together a comprehensive "every woman should benefit from reading" guide to health and well-being for Hispanic women. Known for placing family needs above their own all their lives, Hispanic women need to become more aware that caring for themselves is as important as caring for others. Since it is well known that when the health of a woman collapses, the health of the family of which she is the center collapses as well, Hispanic women—through this book—should feel more inclined to care for themselves.

This guide to Latina wellness presents Hispanic women with much needed advice. Its well-written, common sense format, coupled with the most recent research advances and everyday life stories of Latina women, should make informed health choices an easier task. This guide offers hope, as it gives an understanding voice to those who for so long have heard what was needed but been unable to dictate when it could be achieved. Because this guide helps reaffirm the daily lives of so many, it has become an indispensable compendium of self-help, not only for the body, but for the spirit as well. This book represents what can be done when a dynamic group of women, with the best interests of Latinas at heart, dedicate their lives to helping their *hermanas.*

ANTONIA COELLO NOVELLO, M.D., M.P.H., DR.P.H.
Commissioner of Health, New York State Department of Health, and former U.S. Surgeon General

INTRODUCTION

I was fortunate—my mom was smart, and for most of my life I was relatively healthy.

Of course, there was some illness in my life. For instance, I knew from family lore that soon after I was born I developed some unnamed condition that caused me to vomit whenever I ate. When I was an adult, my mom often recounted to me with pain still in her voice how as a toddler I could not keep my food down even though I loved to eat. Fortunately, even though I knew I would have to leave the table to vomit, I would always come back and try to eat some more. What little food stayed with me must have provided some minimal nourishment. As a result, though, I was tiny in height, skinny, and had so little hair that rubber bands would slide off my much desired pony tail. But I was alive.

By the age of five I had somehow been cured or gotten over whatever was wrong with me, and I was able to eat and retain my food. I still do not know what was wrong with me. All I know is that as a result of that illness, throughout my life my mom was joyous whenever I ate, and I still love to eat.

As I continued to grow up, we had very little contact with health care providers. My mom worked in a variety of factories (boxing men's ties, assembling watches, keypunching cards), which rarely provided health benefits. When I became ill, whatever treatment I received was a result of my mom's wisdom and that shared by the ladies she worked with, who came to the United States from throughout the Americas. Somehow we survived.

When I went to college I was surprised at the different doctors my roommates had seen—they all seemed to have allergists, some still saw their pediatricians, and some even had a gynecologist. I thought the student health center was the state of the art in health care. While I do not remember when I went for my first gynecological exam, it must have been sometime in college.

My friends and I had little experience with health or "female problems." And even when we did, we were too embarrassed to talk about things that seemed "undainty." Somehow the frankness of the feminist movement seemed a little too harsh for us. Discharges, itchiness, and menstruation were not things we talked about.

With time, some of that changed as I found that health care providers were not able to answer my questions and that talking to other women was the best way to get information. I recall feeling awkward when I saw one gynecologist who thought the best way to examine my internal organs was to have me "get up on all fours like a dog." Although I was too embarrassed to talk about it at the time, after I had asked some of my friends about their experiences, I knew that was one gynecologist I would not see again.

As I continued my training as a clinical psychologist, I realized that much of what was known and taught about mental health did not seem to be integrated with what I had read about physical health. Moreover, the influence of culture, how it changes the way we interact with the world, was of interest only to medical anthropologists. My own issues of being a Latina in a non-Latina environment made it necessary for me to think about who I was and to understand my environment. Of course, all the religion and spirituality that I learned from my mom seemed to have no relevance to a society that valued only the material and technological.

My formal training was important in order to be properly credentialed and licensed, but listening to the stories of my friends and all our families made it essential that I look at health in a broader context.

Beginning in 1983 I worked for Secretary Margaret Heckler of the U.S. Department of Health and Human Services. Margaret was always a woman ahead of her time, and as a true visionary, her leadership gave birth to the Women's Health Initiative and the Black and Minority Health Task Force.

The work of the Black and Minority Health Task Force documented the lack of information on Hispanics. In 1985, when the final report was published, the U.S. government still did not include in its vital statistics information on the number of Hispanics who died in a given year. Since mortality data for Hispanics were not available, no one could say how many Hispanics died of heart disease, cancer, or any other disease. The assumption was that all minorities were the same, and what was true for the black community would be true for Hispanics.

As I read the research findings of these task forces, I recognized that only bits and pieces of each report applied to Hispanics and that even less described the Latina experience. It was my hope that one day the research results of those two initiatives would be integrated and lay the foundation for new avenues of research to understand the health of Hispanic women.

In 1985 the National Alliance for Hispanic Health (the Alliance) was twelve years old and looking for new leadership. When I was selected to take the helm of this network of health, mental health, and human service providers, I knew that the first and most important thing I had to do was to listen to the concerns and proposed recommendations of Hispanics throughout the nation.

I met with women throughout the country and talked to them about their views of life, themselves, and their health. I collected stories of their experiences and, most important, tried to listen to the lessons that each Hispanic woman had learned.

I could not help but resonate with the voices of other Latinas. In my own life and in the lives of my extended family, I also had to deal with a host of gynecological problems, depression, AIDS, heart disease, arthritis, diabetes, and all the illnesses that impact on our community more harshly than others. These topics touched me deeply, and when I lectured I used the objectivity of the data to shield the emotions I felt about how the health care system treated us.

Regardless of what part of the country I

happened to be in, the stories were very similar. Health care was changing. Our relationship with physicians was changing. And still we knew so little about the health of Latinas. I could not even list the major causes of death among Latinas or state the average life span of a Latina.

However, with much work and advocacy by the Alliance and its network, things changed. By the late 1980s there was such a widely recognized need for more information on the health of Hispanic women that the Alliance launched a series of projects, which eventually became the National Hispanic Women's Health Initiative (NHWHI).

In 1989 the U.S. Department of Health and Human Services recommended that a box be added to the national model death certificate to identify whether a person was Hispanic. While race data had been collected for decades, this little box meant that for the first time in the history of the United States it was going to be possible to collect and analyze data that documented the mortality of Hispanics.

Today the NHWHI national advisory committee and corresponding local groups represent the state of the art on the health of Latinas. It is a blending of science, our experiences, and our values with the goal of helping all Latinas take control of their lives.

What I learned through all of these experiences is reflected in this book. This book is intended for all Latinas who find that the general books on women's health seem to lack information relevant to their own experience and that often what is recommended does not work. We now know, for instance, that we Latinas differ in how we metabolize some drugs. Moreover, some Latinas may find that books geared to women in general, or to white, black, or minority women, lack a certain *sabor* (flavor) that resonates with their experience. *Salud* also recognizes that although we are diverse, there is a communal fountain of life, which we share.

And the experience of putting the book together often confirmed what I already knew. Our reluctance to know about or touch our vulva, for example, was mirrored in the uneasiness evidenced by those working on the book. Some of the younger Latinas were embarrassed to even talk about the drawing of the vulva; instead, the drawing was euphemistically referred to as the "little flower" picture.

At a more fundamental level, there were discussions with women throughout the country about use of the word *fetus* or *baby*. The concern was that using one word over the other would be perceived as reflecting a pro-life or pro-choice position. Our intent in this book is to present the Latina perspective and explain the medical and psychological ramifications of the various decisions a Latina could make. What we know about Latinas is complex. Latinas as a group are most likely to be Catholic and at the same time are more likely to have an abortion than non-Latina white women. Nevertheless, most Latinas who have had an abortion still refer to their experience in terms of the *baby* they did not have. For Latinas it seems that once they know they are pregnant, they do not use the words *embryo* or *fetus*—it is their *baby*.

The topic of sexuality brought up all sorts of experiences and comments. Some Latinas questioned whether the book should promote long-term monogamous relationships, while the discussion of masturbation produced both interest and distress. There was a concern by some that we include a separate section on lesbians, while others did not like that. Instead when we talked about our sexual partners, we used gender-neutral language whenever possible. The chapter on menopause was filled with experiences that were shared in private, and topics related to older Hispanic women were integrated throughout the book rather than placed in a stand-alone chapter.

For most of us, the days when our health care provider knew us and our family are gone. Our hope is that you will use this book to guide you and your family through this changing health care environment.

Increasingly, it is our responsibility to keep our own health history and understand some of the basics of how our body works and does not work. We also have to learn to recognize the complex relationship of our body with our mind and spirit. All three have to be addressed in a total manner, yet most health care providers and health care systems are barely able to take care of our bodies.

The stories of women throughout the book are included to give life to the facts presented. "*Consejos*" and "Warnings" have been highlighted throughout the book because of the critical information they provide. The resource section at the end of each chapter provides what we judged to be the best information available. Let us know what you think, and most of all let us know how you are doing.

We have a big job ahead, but we can do it. Keep in touch.

PART I

Being a Latina

1

Beyond *Aguantar*

Valuing Ourselves

I enjoy being a Latina.

When I talk about Hispanic women, I treasure the intimacy and warmth that the word *Latina* conveys, and I reserve the gender-neutral *Hispanic*, rather than the masculine *Latino*, for discussions that include males.

Latinas are unique. Each one of us is deeply affected by our collective cultural experiences, the languages many of us speak, and the complexity of relationships within our families. How we define ourselves sets us apart from non-Latinas.

Salud is an affirmation of who we are and recognizes what the scientific research clearly shows—that many of our health issues are unique and sometimes different from those of the majority population, and that to improve our health requires a new approach to wellness. This Latina approach is evident throughout the four major sections of the book: Being a Latina, Being Female, *Enfermedades* (Diseases), and *Para Vivir Bien* (Living Well).

"Being a Latina" explains why the mind and *espíritu* (spirit) are part of the health of Latinas. How we Latinas care for ourselves begins with the mind-set of where we place our individual needs within the priorities created by our relationships with our families.

For a Latina, a healthy self-esteem is the first step in the direction of taking care of her health. At the outset this means that we have to learn how to set limits. The steps involved in developing new attitudes and new behaviors help us to accept that we must take care of our own health.

At the same time, for Latinas, health is about more than just our body and mind. Our spirit is something Latinas experience and at the same time are reluctant to speak about. Many of the Latinas I spoke to were pleased and relieved to see that *espíritu* would be discussed throughout the book. Their view of other self-care books was that they were at the extremes—either too scientific or too spiritual. For Latinas, there needs to be a balance among the body, mind, and spirit.

Just as important for Latinas is to find a way to integrate conventional and traditional medicine within the context of the evolving health care environment. Where once we sought all the answers from our health care providers, increasingly those providers are expecting us to be able to make decisions about our own health. We need skills to help us monitor our own health in a systematic manner, be prepared for our visit to our health care provider, understand our health plans, and know our rights and responsibilities as consumers of health care.

"Being Female" covers all the available information on maintaining a healthy reproductive system throughout our lives. The facts on pregnancy, infertility, menopause, and sexuality are provided within a context that Latinas will find useful and constructive. Some of the stories will make you laugh, while others will help you understand that you are not alone in your pain.

"*Enfermedades* (Diseases)" focuses on the conditions that are of most concern to Latinas—alcoholism, arthritis, breast cancer, cervical cancer, depression, diabetes, heart disease, HIV/AIDS, liver disease, and sexually transmitted diseases. Each chapter shares the stories of Latinas and provides the most up-to-date information on diagnosis and treatment. At the end of each chapter is a discussion of how the condition affects the mind and the spirit.

"*Para Vivir Bien* (Living Well)" documents what we have to do in order to live healthy lives. The focus is on taking care of yourself by eating well, managing your weight, exercising, and using medicines properly. And, of course, no book for Latinas would be complete without a discussion of how we take care of our parents and other older family members. The final chapter on the environment helps us recognize threats to our clean water, clean air, and safe food supply that are not due to bioterrorism.

From the discussions of *espíritu* to the food we eat, the needs and experiences of Latinas frame the way information is presented. For Latinas, reading *Salud* is our first step toward taking care of ourselves.

I was talking to some of my friends about all the things I had to do now that I had to take care of my mother. She was getting older and could not live by herself. I had rearranged my schedule and worked it out so that I could take care of her daily needs. My friend Helga looked at me and said, "That is so nice that you take care of your mother."

I remember being surprised at her comment and thinking how being a Latina made me different. Nice *was not the word I had in mind to describe the reasons that motivated me to take care of my mother. I knew what was expected of me culturally, even though there were no support systems in the non-Latina environment where I worked and lived.*

Taking care of my mother was neither a matter of choice nor an obligation. It was like breathing—something I knew I would do as part of my life.

—Rosa, 56

Who We Are

When we look at ourselves in the mirror, we may see the differences. When we enter a room and make eye contact with one of our own, some of us affirm our cultural bonds while others make believe that they can blend in.

As Latinas, we are not surprised to find out that when information was finally available about some of our health problems it showed that we are often different from non-Hispanic white women and non-Hispanic black women. And sometimes this means that care and treatment may be different for us than it is for non-Latinas.

Our bodies come in an assortment of shapes, although they tend to be shorter and heavier than those of non-Latinas. Our emotions are often more pronounced and evident than they are for others. Our sense of *espíritu* (spirit) guides us through difficult times. When we look at other Latinas, it is easy to see that we are the product of the diverse communities that pulse through our veins.

We have much in common with each other.

At the same time, we are different from one another. Some of us prefer to be referred to as Hispanic women, Latinas, *Chicanas*, *Boricuas*, *Cubanas*, or any other word that has an *a* in its ending. Each one of us identifies with one or more of our ancestral roots: Spanish, Latin American, Native American, European, African, or Asian. Sometimes we identify so strongly with a specific subgroup that we lose sight of the combined strength that our common traits provide us with as a group.

The most compelling conclusion from the health research, however, is that even though there are differences among Latinas, and no matter what each one of us may choose to call herself, we are generally more alike than we are different and often have more in common with one another than we do with non-Latinas.

Hispanic woman, Latina, first generation, tenth generation, recent immigrant—there is much that we can learn from each other, and there is much that binds us.

What brings us closer is the immediate bond that comes to life when we gather together and laugh at the similarity of the messages that we have received throughout our lives. The cultural and—for some of us—linguistic glue is what binds us to each other.

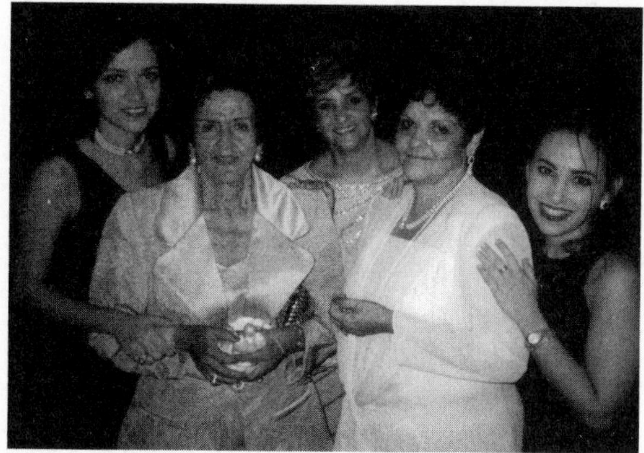

We need to share with each other our health histories.

The *dichos*, sayings, that were passed on to us by our mothers, *tías* (aunts), and *hermanas* (sisters) are what formed our understanding of how we should care for ourselves, how we should live our lives. These *dichos* provide us with a philosophy of existence, a pattern for living, that is our own.

Even what we know about health clearly shows that we, as Latinas, are different from non-Latinas. We tend to have lower rates of breast cancer, higher rates of cervical cancer, higher rates of diabetes, and lower rates of heart disease and stroke. The reasons for these differences are unclear because only now are health researchers beginning to explore who Latinas are and the reasons why our health differs from that of other women.

"Cuídate, Mi Hija"

Guiding messages are the axioms that language and culture give us as part of the building blocks of our lives. The struggle is to determine when to apply a message because it helps us and when not to apply it because it is destructive. This is difficult. Too often we think we have to use a rule all of the time when in fact we have to apply it only some of the time. The difficulty lies in knowing when that some of the time is, because life is dynamic and always changing. What may be the best option one day may be the worst on a different day. That a struggle exists in knowing when to apply it does not diminish the value of the message—it only celebrates the fluidity of life.

For some people it may be easier to have simple decision rules to guide them through life. But the complexity of life often requires that we learn not only what the rules are but also, through our experiences, when to apply them. And we learn different rules that apply in different contexts—rules that may at times be contradictory. Some may be very Latina in nature and may contradict values of the society in which we work and live. There are few easy answers. Life is a continuum, and, as Latinas, we have a wealth of guiding messages, which we must balance throughout our lives.

Besides the many *dichos* that we share, there are some words that convey concepts that guide us through our lives. One way or another, whether in Spanish or in English, these words and their impact on our behavior are very familiar to Latinas.

cuídate, mi hija	*(take care of yourself, my daughter)*
la familia primero	*(family first)*
hay que tener respeto	*(you must be respectful)*
hay que aguantar	*(you must tolerate, accept)*

The Spanish words are filled with meaning, while the English adaptations somehow miss the intensity that drives us. Think about each of those phrases.

Cuídate, mi hija literally means "take care of yourself, my daughter." Nevertheless, this is not a message that directs us to focus selfishly on "me first." Instead it creates a sense that each one of us is the person who is most responsible for watching out for herself. It is a message that is contrary to the narcissism and ego-centeredness that we see in other cultures. And yet the message of the words conveys even more.

It reminds us that the expectation for us, as Latinas, is that somehow, regardless of our resources, we must take care of ourselves and not allow *espíritus malos* (bad things, or evil) to come our way. We are expected to solve our own problems and to actively avoid getting into bad situations.

Cuídate is a very special message that Latinas receive. It is a message we learn early on—that we have to be careful. It is a message we hear throughout our lives. In many ways it drives us to take care of all of our problems ourselves. Sometimes that is good, and sometimes that is bad. Unfortunately, the directive *la familia primero* (family first) often makes it difficult for us to put ourselves first, as illustrated by Alicia in the following anecdote.

It had been four years since Alicia's grandparents had seen her, and now they were going to meet Alicia's beautiful daughter Camila. This would be a wonderful visit, and it would also be Camila's first plane trip. As they settled into their seats, Alicia fastened Camila's seat belt and then proceeded to lock her own seat belt into place.

As Alicia watched the safety video, she carefully followed the instructions and noted the exits in front of their row and behind their row. When the segment on how to use the oxygen mask was shown, Alicia was puzzled.

The video very emphatically instructed her to first put the oxygen mask on herself and then put it on her child. This did not make sense. After all, she had to take care of her family first.

But the safety message was clear, and Alicia concluded that sometimes to take care of your family you must take care of yourself first, so that you will be able to take care of your child in more dangerous situations.

It is not surprising that Alicia at first was reluctant to obey the safety message. *La familia primero* tells us that our families must come before anyone else. While many have said that this is true for all women, the cultural imperative is even stronger for Latinas. Somewhere along the way the message for Latinas became distorted, and some of us began to believe that caring for our families was separate from caring for ourselves.

Over time this changed even further, to the point where Latinas often put themselves last because they believe that they must first focus on taking care of their families. This means

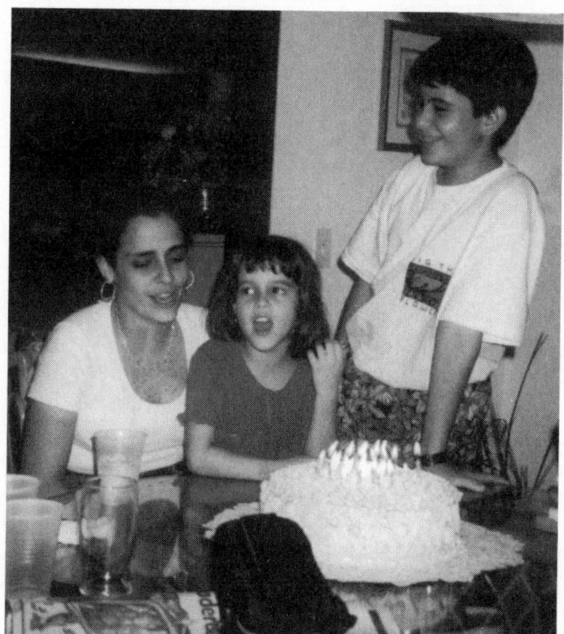

Families are about responsibility and celebration.

that a Latina will take care of herself only after she has taken care of her family.

This is evident when Latinas talk about their health. Very often their focus is on their family's health. It takes a Latina an extra effort to accept that taking care of her own health is the first step in insuring the health of her family.

When it comes to Hispanics, the imperative of *respeto* (respect) is a two-way concept, which needs to be fully understood. For Latinas it means deference based on age and on social, community, and professional standing. *Respeto* also means that we will not intrude in what we may identify as someone else's domain, and at the same time, they are not to intrude in what we have staked out as our domain. It means that I owe you respect, but you also owe me respect.

The problem is that *respeto* can lead to stalemate. For example, in the most common situation, two people have to find a solution to a problem but are unable to do so because each is concerned about not intruding in the other's territory. In order to resolve the impasse, what usually occurs is a slow approach to each other through a series of questions. This process insures that hierarchical relationships and personal domains are protected. It takes time.

The combined demands generated by the imperatives *cuídate*, *la familia primero*, and *respeto* leave Latinas with only one major coping strategy: *aguantar* (to tolerate, to bear, to suck it in with a smile of acceptance).

Aguántate is what we are often told, and it comes across in the story of Patricia. Although some of the details may change, the story of Patricia is not that uncommon. Too often we find, as Latinas, that even when we know we are in a situation that is beyond tolerance, we are nevertheless reluctant to make changes in our lives.

Patricia could not believe that after thirteen years of marriage her friend Juanita was still doing everything for Luis. Once again Luis was trying to start another business from home. He was so busy that he did not have time to help in the house. Juanita just kept on doing as she had always done—working, taking care of the family, and taking care of the house.

When Patricia asked Juanita if she was tired, Juanita just smiled and said no, life was good, and anyway she was doing well with all the things she was juggling. She knew she was a supportive wife. And things would get better over time—his drinking would stop one day.

Patricia sighed in disbelief. She did not know how Juanita could not see all the things in her life that she had put on hold for Luis. And what made it even worse was that she did not complain.

Aguantar is a common coping strategy among Latinas and is often a source of misinterpretation about who we are. We may be suffering, but we cannot complain. Life may be awful, but we cannot cry. We may be abandoned, but we cannot admit that we are alone. We do show our emotions—but not these and certainly not to an outsider.

To non-Latinas it appears that Latinas are demonstrative and very emotional. The assumption is that we reveal all of our feelings. The reality is that we do not. We may reveal more feelings than non-Latinas, but what we reveal is much less than what we feel. We are very guarded and thus also less likely to reveal our negative feelings. Too often the deeply ingrained notions of *respeto* and *la familia primero* silence our heavy hearts.

Because we do not complain and few of us cry in public, we are seen as doing well. Frequently I am told how well Latinas seem to tolerate the difficulties of life. But we know better. What outwardly looks like good coping skills inwardly means that we are *aguantando.*

Our lives have pain, harshness, and disappointments. We are not numb to any of it. The *angustia* (angst) of our lives is something we all recognize. We feel every torment throughout our bodies, minds, and spirits. And we feel and live those of our families.

Too often we do not fight these bad feelings, because for Latinas who believe that life is a series of trials, *aguantar* provides a method for accepting whatever life gives them. Some Latinas believe that if we do not complain and allow ourselves to just get through it, perhaps things will get better as each new day of our lives unfolds.

For many of us, *aguantar* enables us to cherish what there is in our lives. In our silence there is a strength that helps us see beyond today and the material world. The problem comes when *aguantar* becomes all we do. Then we fail to take care of ourselves, disregarding the signs that our bodies give us, the messages from our minds, or even the cries for sustenance from our *espíritu*. We know how to *aguantar*, but now, to take care of ourselves and our families, we have to learn when not to *aguantar*.

More Than *Aguantar*—Caring for Ourselves

There has been little to encourage Latinas to focus on themselves. Too often, the role assigned to Latinas has required that we care for the bodies and minds of our families and communities—and place our own needs last. Fortunately, the care of our own *espíritu* has always been one of the major areas which Latinas have been allowed and encouraged to develop. Our spiritual development has often been all that has nurtured us when we had few options but to neglect our bodies and minds.

Things are different now. Our experiences have brought us to the point where we know that to fulfill the diverse roles in our lives requires that sometimes we stop this *aguantar*. We need to develop a balance in the care of our body, mind, and spirit.

This has been a hard lesson to learn because Latinas are typically dismayed by images of self-centered women. In the early days of feminism in the United States, many Latinas were turned off by the suggestion that women should focus solely on their own needs and their own concerns. Latinas also didn't respond to the glorification of self-esteem and the major focus on the priorities of the individual, as opposed to the person in relationship to her family and other significant relationships.

Consequently, in the past, self-esteem was viewed as a negative characteristic because it was closely associated with self-centeredness and selfishness. Moreover, the concept of self-esteem was often presented in ways that seemed to devalue the family and community.

The focus was on *I* rather than *we*, and this created a problem that went beyond language.

Traditionally the concept of *I* versus *we* has been difficult for Latinas because we are often socialized to be more *we* or community oriented, as the *la familia primero* imperative shows. Thus Latinas often concluded somewhat derisively that non-Latinas were less likely to put their own needs aside for the greater good of the family or community. Latinas and non-Latinas today have learned to work with the values of our respective cultures to create a balance between *I* and *we*. Although some of us are going through a transition in the process of accepting the concept of *I*, the reality is that we are well on our way to a more balanced integration of the messages we receive.

The positive application of the messages of *cuídate*, *la familia primero*, *respeto*, and *aguantar* requires that we develop a healthy sense of who we are—a positive sense of self-esteem. This means that, as Latinas, we not only value who we are, we begin to talk about *I*. *I* begins to be real when each one of us knows that it is OK to say "I want," "I need," and "I feel."

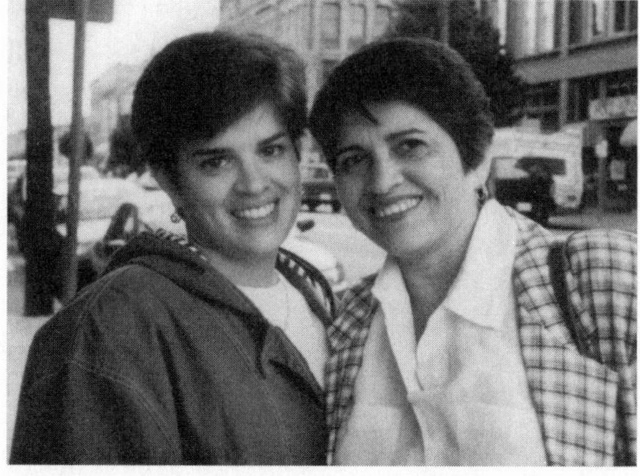

It's very special when a mother and daughter have a close and loving relationship.

Strategies for a Healthier Self-esteem

La familia primero and *respeto* create a double whammy of silence and acquiescence in our behavior. Following our guiding messages, our relationships with our families, friends, and lovers are our first priorities. The problem is that too often we put ourselves in last place, and we may end up as servants to everyone.

This means that in our day-to-day lives we are on call 24/7 (24 hours a day, seven days a week), every week of the year and especially on holidays—to everyone. Just thinking about where we place ourselves in the emotional food chain of our lives is exhausting. No wonder Latinas tend to have higher rates of depression than anyone else. With that sort of constant emotional demand on our lives, it is amazing that we are able to survive. But survive we have.

The fact that we have survived is often attributed to our sense of *espíritu*, which has buoyed us. Our *espíritu* may help us with the more spiritual aspects of our existence, but self-esteem focuses on our body and mind. It is exemplified by a more responsible version of *cuídate*, which urges us to take care of ourselves—body and mind—and not just others. It requires that we learn the skills to be good to others and to ourselves. This means that we must set limits to what we will and will not do.

Our relationships with other people are often a good indicator of our self-esteem. Regardless of income or education, some Latinas find themselves in relationships that are physically or emotionally abusive.

The issue of abuse is very complex. How we get into these relationships and how we are made to stay in them is more complicated than it appears to outsiders. To say "She should just leave" ignores the extraordinary psychological pull the abuser has created in the situation. And the abuser knows this.

Warning

Violence is never acceptable in a relationship.

Safety for the physical and emotional health of ourselves as well as our children is of the utmost concern and should be a primary reason for leaving a violent or abusive situation. Emotional abuse is just as scarring as physical abuse, and it is unacceptable.

Keep in mind that there is never an excuse for violence. Alcoholism, loss of a job, and a difficult childhood are not excuses for violence but factors used to explain what may have caused a person to become violent. Understanding why someone is abusive does not mean that it is OK or that you can fix it. The most important thing you can do is talk to your friends and family about the situation.

The abuser typically believes that you will be too embarrassed to talk to anyone about the situation. Although you may be embarrassed to discuss your situation, the support of friends and professionals will be very helpful for you when you are able to leave the situation. Make sure to use the resource list at the end of this chapter.

While it may be self-evident that it is important to set limits in abusive situations, it is also critical that Latinas learn to set limits in many other situations. To do so, we have to examine our knowledge of the need to set limits, our attitude about setting limits, and our behavior in actually setting limits.

Ramona finally had her own place. It was small but perfect for her needs. The two little bedrooms provided the privacy she had always longed for. One room was going to be her nest for cuddling under her covers and reading her favorite books. Her second room was going to be an office where she could do her work and have all her papers and files either organized or thrown about if that was how her mood moved her. She was so happy to finally be able to have her own space. And yet on this evening she was very unsettled.

Ramona had come home to find her mom cleaning the living room. Ramona knew that without any prompting from her mom, she had given her the keys so that she could visit whenever she wanted. It had felt good to do that, and there was no doubt in her mind that it was the right thing to do.

But there was no denying it—although she loved her little place, somehow it was starting to feel as if it was not her own anymore. And Ramona did not like that. She knew that she would have to do something with her mother that she had never done—set limits.

New Knowledge

We have an underlying belief that people know the socially acceptable limits of what they can expect and thus demand from someone else. Our unspoken belief is that we do not need to set limits because, in the context of *respeto*, people have the appropriate levels of expectation for each other and act accordingly. As Latinas, we bring these beliefs into our more intimate relationships. We assume that if we love and cherish someone, they will ask only what is reasonable from us and we will ask no more than what is reasonable from them. The reality is very different.

Sometimes people forget the appropriate or natural limits of the demands they can make on each other. At other times they might intentionally ignore these limits. Many of us have friends we care for and cherish but who are "high maintenance"—they need a lot of attention and support all the time. They call late at night and early in the morning; they always want us to be available to hear them bemoan the fate they have once again made for themselves. As Latinas, we are likely to have created the expectation that we will be available for them all the time, regardless of what may be going on in our lives and the demands of our families and jobs. We give ourselves to suit them *por que nos necesitan* (because they need us). This creates an imbalance.

In an ideal world this imbalance would not occur. We would recognize and respect each other's boundaries and know (because we were appropriately civilized) the limits of each other's desires. In those cases when we did not know the limits, we would negotiate with each other to set mutually acceptable ones.

Thus the major task for Latinas is to accept the fact that we need to set limits—both for ourselves and for the people we know. This will help us define the framework for our many relationships. People need to know our limits explicitly—what we will do and what we will not do.

The decision to set limits will not have much impact unless we recognize that making our needs explicit is not just something to add to our "To Do" list. Setting limits is a "Must Do." Remember to tell yourself: "I need limits, you need limits, we all need limits."

New Attitude

As Latinas, we are generally more formal in our behavior than non-Latinas in the United States. The important role of *respeto* in our culture establishes it as a key variable for setting limits. For example, when we say that someone is *informal*, we usually say so in a negative manner because it implies that someone behaved in a way that did not show knowledge of the proper respect due to others who were present. The Spanish language further reinforces the cultural value of *respeto* by having two different ways to say *you*, one that is more formal (*usted*), the other less formal (*tu*). Each form reflects a different combination of deference and intimacy.

Our sense of formality and expectation of proper behavior creates a mind-set that may undermine attempts to set our own limits. Although *la familia primero* establishes one dimension of the limits we set, a healthy attitude requires that sometimes, in order to meet our own needs, we set aside the demands of our family. If we focus on *cuídate*, then we can begin to create a positive attitude about setting limits.

As part of advancing our attitude about setting limits, we need to be clear about who has the responsibility for a given action. We must define whether something is mine, yours, or ours.

The concept "This is mine" is easiest for many of us to accept. With this attitude comes control over an activity from the beginning to the end.

Some of us avoid taking ownership because we may not want or like to take responsibility. While that may be the case, to set limits and have a healthy self-esteem we must begin to recognize what things we should not push off on someone else. We have to accept that some things are ours to handle alone. The needed attitude change in this direction must be to affirmatively admit, "This is mine."

"This is yours." In this situation we identify that a particular action is not ours to accept but rather resides within someone else's sphere of responsibility. For some of us, our families and friends may have become so accustomed to our acceptance of responsibility for a variety of tasks that they are reluctant to believe that someone besides ourselves should take action. They may also be hostile to the thought that they should do it themselves.

Some of us are caught up in our version of control or perfectionism. We feel that we are the only ones who can do something the right way. Our new attitude develops from our understanding that to be balanced, each indi-

> **Which of the Following Phrases Describes You?**
>
> 1. I am always available for my family.
> 2. My friends feel free to call me when they are in a crisis.
> 3. I usually solve all of my own problems.
> 4. To get it done right, I do it myself.
> 5. I feel good when I help others.
> 6. I never stay home sick.
> 7. My friends always count on getting birthday cards from me.
> 8. I have everything I need.
> 9. My coworkers know I am always loyal.
> 10. I am the best person to rely on.
>
> If you answered yes to more than half of these, you need to learn to set limits or you will burn out.

vidual must meet his or her respective set of responsibilities. That implies letting other people do their part. We have to learn to recognize when we are not the only responsible party and allow others to do their share.

"This is ours." We do not have to do it all ourselves. The message of *cuídate* means that we need to have a certain level of awareness of everything that is around us. Part of acknowledging the world around us is recognizing that we are not alone and that at times other persons share in responsibility. It is not our responsibility to fix everything. We have to learn that sometimes our goal is to allow ourselves to work with others.

That is when we say, "This is ours."

New Behavior: How to Set Limits

As Latinas, the major action we face in setting limits is to say what we mean and to do what we say. Be sure to speak at a moderate level, in a calm, caring way. Voice volume should never be used as a sign of whether you are sincere in what you say. Remember that loud voices are not conducive to improved communication.

Do not be surprised if when you start to set limits you have to repeat what you say several times. That is understandable because part of sharing your revised expectations with people requires them to unlearn their own patterns of interaction with you. Be patient and understand that while you may have decided to make changes, there are those around you who have benefited from the way you were before. Eventually they will understand.

To set limits means that you do one of three things: say yes, say maybe, or say no. When you give each of these answers, understand fully the ramification of your response.

Say Yes

This is often what is easiest for us to do. We may say yes actively, by the acquiescence communicated in our silence, or by our actions. Even if we grumble under our breath or make an angry comment before we do something we do not want to do or should not be doing, we are still saying yes.

To set limits requires that when you say yes, you do it with full awareness of what it means. To agree is more than just being pleasant—it means acceptance of responsibility. For Latinas, it is often easier to just say yes, and in that lies the danger.

Yes is not something we should say because it is the choice that creates the fewest problems. We should say yes because it is what we believe. As we work toward setting limits, we have to recognize when we support what is being said. When we want to show our support, our commitment, and the limit of what we will do by our actions and our words, we should say yes.

Say Maybe

Maybe is often frowned upon in a world that tends to be dichotomous. Too often, not saying yes or no is seen as a sign of being indecisive or wishy-washy. That is inaccurate. If we are going to be able to set meaningful limits, we need an option that provides additional time to develop a thoughtful response. For instance, sometimes you may not be sure about what limit to set. You may need to consult with others or get more information, or you may need to mull it over in your mind for a while longer. When you do not know or are unsure, you should say maybe.

Say No

As we sat around talking about our evening plans, María looked very glum. I asked her why she was so sad. And she offered that she was going out to dinner with Angel again.

"Angel? I thought you said you never wanted to go out with him again."

"I don't want to go out with him," María stated emphatically.

"Then why are you going to dinner with him?" I inquired.

María shook her head and said, "I told him I was busy. I don't return his calls, but he just keeps calling."

I was still surprised that she was going out with him and said, "María, just tell him no—that you do not want to go out with him."

She looked at me with her eyes opened wide and exclaimed, "I can't say no to him. That would be rude. I was not raised that way. I am just like my mother. I cannot say no."

Experience shows us that "No, thank you" and just plain no are the hardest words for many Latinas to say. No has been seen as an indelicate or unladylike response to a request. And yet no has to be something we feel comfortable saying. We need to learn how to say no in a way that allows us to maintain respect.

When we say no, it should be said thoughtfully, not emotionally. Often we have to say no because people have set limits that we do not accept. You may find that you have to repeat yourself several times (reminding yourself to maintain a moderate volume) or paraphrase what you want to say because those used to hearing yes may misinterpret your no as a yes or a maybe.

Remember that if it is hard for us to say no, it is even harder for many of those around us to hear it when we say it. Too often those closest to us have become accustomed to hearing us say yes. As part of strengthening our own self-esteem, we must acknowledge as acceptable that sometimes we will set limits that may not be consistent with what other people want us to do. Many of us have spent our lives responding affirmatively to the demands of our *familias.* But now we know that to take care of our loved ones means we have to take care of ourselves too, and to do so means that sometimes we say no. It is reasonable for you to draw a line and say, "*No. Basta. Hasta aquí y no más.*" ("No. Enough. No more.")

Three Steps Toward Setting Limits

1. *New Knowledge*
   I need limits.
   You need limits.
   We all need limits.
2. *New Attitude*
   This is mine.
   This is yours.
   This is ours.
3. *New Behavior*
   Say yes.
   Say no.
   Say maybe.

What Next?

The hardest consequence for Latinas to understand after they have set limits is that the limit may be either misheard, misinterpreted, or ignored. This occurs because the limit has not been accepted by others. Usually this is followed by increased demands in an attempt to determine whether you really did set a limit.

As Latinas, we know that emotional trespassing occurs on a regular basis. That is why, also as Latinas, we must communicate and enforce the emotional limits we establish. Redundancy becomes important as sometimes only through repetition will our new way of being be understood.

Summary

Our culture gives us many strengths: *cuídate*, *la familia primero*, *respeto*, and even *aguantar*. Reassessing and integrating these guiding words into a new mind-set helps us accept that by valuing ourselves, we value our families. The first step in valuing ourselves is to expand our knowledge, attitude, and behavior about setting limits. By doing this we will be making progress on the road that will take us beyond *aguantar*.

RESOURCES

GENERAL

Books

Alarcon, Norma, Rafaela Castro, Deena Gonzalez, Margarita Melville, Emma Perez, Tey Diana Rebolledo, Christine Sierra, and Adaliza Sosa Riddell. *Chicana Critical Issues*. Berkeley: Third Woman Press, 1993.

Estés, Clarissa Pinkola. *Women Who Run With the Wolves*. New York: Ballantine Books, 1992.

Gil, Rosa María, and Carmen Vazquez. *The María Paradox*. New York: Putnam, 1996.

VIOLENCE

Information Centers

Battered Women's Justice Project
4032 Chicago Avenue, South
Minneapolis, MN 55407
(800) 903-0111
www.vaw.umn.edu/bwjp

Health Resource Center on Domestic Violence
(888) 792-2873 (888-RX-ABUSE)

National Resource Center on Domestic Violence
6400 Flank Drive, Suite 1300
Harrisburg, PA 17112-2778
(800) 537-2238
www.fvpf.org

Resource Center on Domestic Violence, Child Protection and Custody
National Council of Juvenile and Family Court Judges (NCJFCHJ)
Family Violence Project
P.O. Box 8970
Reno, NV 89507
(800) 527-3223
(Resource for agencies *only*, not consumers)

Organizations

American Psychological Association
750 First Street NE
Washington, DC 20002
(800) 374-2721 or (202) 336-5500
www.apa.org

National Coalition Against Domestic Violence
P.O. Box 18749
Denver, CO 80218
(303) 839-1852
www.ncadv.org

Hotlines

National Child Abuse Hotline
(800) 422-4453
National Domestic Violence Hotline
(800) 799-SAFE (800-799-7233)

Books

Zambrano, Myrna M. *Mejor Sola Que Mal Acompañada: Para La Mujer Golpeada/For the Latina in An Abusive Relationship*. Bilingual English/Spanish. Seattle: Seal Press, 1985.

Zambrano, Myrna M. *No Mas! Guía para la mujer golpeada*. Seattle: Seal Press, 1994.

Publications and Pamphlets

"Violence Against Women: A Comprehensive Background Paper," March 1996. Compilation of articles describing abuse against women. The Commonwealth Fund, Commission on Women's Health, New York; (212) 666-3800/(888) 777-2744.

2

Body, Mind, and *Espíritu*

Lucy could not understand why she did not feel well. She had begun to exercise regularly and eat more thoughtfully. And her body felt OK. But at the same time she knew something was not right. She was not sleeping well, and she had even missed one of her periods.

Lucy bought several home-test pregnancy kits to see whether she was pregnant. They all came out negative. After her second missed period and more sleepless nights, she decided to see her gynecologist. Perhaps the home-test kits had missed something. The gynecologist did a highly sensitive test, which can tell if you are pregnant practically the first week after conception. Still her test results were negative.

Lucy talked to her friends about her symptoms, and the comadres *suggested that she might either have a thyroid problem or be going through an early menopause. Relieved at the thought of knowing what the problem was, Lucy went to see her internist. He confirmed what she knew in her soul—it was not her thyroid, she was not pregnant, and she was not premenopausal. He looked at her with concern and suggested that it was probably nothing.*

Lucy knew better. It was something. Work was wonderful, and she had a loving and supportive family and friends. Her mother's words echoed in her head: No puedes tapar el cielo con las manos *(You cannot cover the sky with your hands).*

Lucy understood. You can fool the mind, and sometimes you can fool the body, but your spirit will always reveal the truth. To heal her body, she had to regain her espíritu *(spirit). Lucy sighed as she accepted what she had tried to ignore—her sense of* espíritu *was depleted. What was missing was an internal sense of feeling complete and at peace with herself and with God.*

During the last century, health and illness were approached through a variety of treatments, each with its own philosophical base. Some were based purely on science (mainstream medicine), while others viewed the body as a machine (osteopaths). Still other schools of medicine developed treatments based on the relationship between physician and patient (homeopaths) or on a spiritual belief system (Christian Science). In addition, there was a rich practice of *curanderas* (folk healers), herbalists, and other practitioners.

Each school developed its method for diagnosis and treatment based on the underlying factors they had identified as defining the nature of health and illness. Practitioners were trained to look at either the body, the mind, or the spirit as the major culprit in illness and disease. Research continued in each of these areas, with little emphasis on studying the impact that possible interactions among these three aspects may have on health. From such a diversity of philosophies, conventional medicine, with its many successes, emerged as the most commonly taught and practiced.

Today conventional medicine continues focusing on the body, with little emphasis on the mind or spirit. Consequently, as consumers of health care, Latinas have become somewhat familiar with the language and procedures of mainstream medicine.

Latinas know that it is good to be told we have low blood glucose levels or low blood pressure. At the same time, we know that good blood levels do not mean that we feel healthy.

Sometimes, although all the results from our tests point to good health—"Everything is fine. Everything came out normal"—we are left very unconvinced by this knowledge. Typically the health care provider looks at us perplexed because we do not seem to be happy or satisfied at the news that we are in good shape. Our silence is based on the respect we have for the information shared with us and

Fact

Over 160 Latinas in Chicago were asked what being healthy means. After "Following a balanced diet," the next most common definition was "Being vigorous and happy," followed by "Exercising regularly" and "Being healthy emotionally and spiritually."

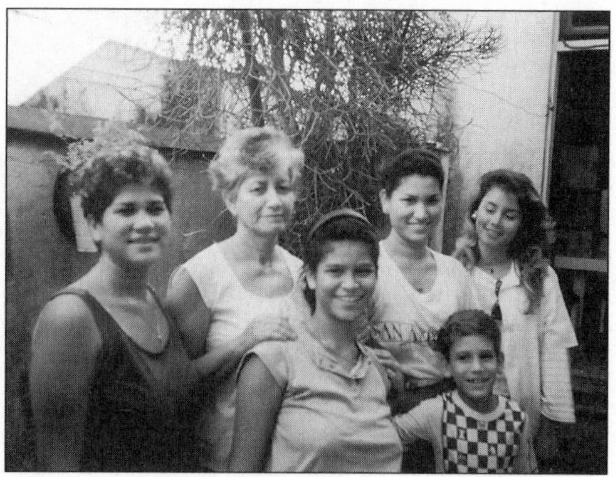

We are many generations. We are an extended family.

the conviction that physical test results do not tell us everything. Tests only convey information about what is measured, and in most cases these tests focus on our bodies. For Latinas, however, good health means more than the results from physical tests. To be complete, an assessment would have to include measurement of the mind and spirit too.

Unfortunately, the way that providers are trained and health care systems are structured, such an assessment would be beyond the scope of even a health care provider interested in such issues. Nevertheless, Latinas recognize that the state of our mind and spirit are crucial elements of our sense of well-being.

For Latinas, being healthy results from the integration of the state of the body, mind, and *espíritu*. It is this totality of health that makes us feel *sanas* (healthy). When we are *sanas*, we know that we are free of any type of illness—physical, mental, or spiritual.

Understanding what health means in relation to each of these components is a step in the right direction. As we explore each aspect, we have to remember that while the well-being of each component is important, it is the combined health of all three that is most powerful and beneficial.

Healthy Body

Much of what we perceive as a healthy body is based on what we are told by a variety of industries trying to sell us products rather than on any meaningful concept of what being healthy is. That is why some of us think that a healthy body is synonymous with a perfect body, while others believe that a healthy body is one that corresponds to a certain set of norms. Neither view is correct.

Marketing strategies aside, good science tells us that there is neither one standard for a perfect body nor one for what is normal. Specifically, there is no absolute measure of perfection, and the definition of normality varies as a function of age, body frame, genetics, and other factors. That is why, when it comes to defining good health, there is no such thing as "one size fits all." A healthy body is not one of a fixed size or weight. Neither is it a body that is free from all illness.

A healthy body is one that functions as well as is possible for each one of us. This means that while it is commendable that some of us can and do run in 10-kilometer races, the ability to do so, in and of itself, does not mean that we have healthy bodies. We should all, however, be able to do some moderate exercise on a regular basis (see Chapter 21).

For many of us, having a healthy body translates into managing our illnesses in a responsible manner. This means that we monitor our bodies on a regular basis, visit our health care providers as necessary, take our medications as prescribed, exercise, and eat a healthy diet.

There are five basic steps that lead toward having a healthy body.

Five Steps Toward a Healthy Body

1. Do not smoke.
2. Limit alcohol.
3. Eat healthy meals.
4. Exercise regularly.
5. Listen to your body.

1: Do not smoke. If you do smoke, please stop; if you do not smoke, please do not start. Over thirty years of scientific research clearly show that smoking is bad not just for your lungs, but for your heart, blood pressure, circulation—for your whole body and for those around you.

In 1965 the Surgeon General and institutions such as the Centers for Disease Control, the American Cancer Society, the American Lung Association, the American Heart Association, and numerous other governmental and nongovernmental agencies began to let us know that smoking is hazardous to our health. In the 1980s the message was expanded to point out that smoking is dangerous to our unborn babies, and in the 1990s the Environmental Protection Agency emphasized that smoking poses a threat to those around us.

2: Limit alcohol. This means that in one day you should have no more than one drink (5 ounces of wine or 12 ounces of beer or 1½ ounces of 80 proof hard liquor, either alone or in a mixed drink). If you do not drink for five days, on the sixth day your limit is still one drink.

As Latinas, we generally drink less than other women, but sadly, we are catching up to the bad drinking habits of non-Latinas. Chapter 10 details some of the problems that come with drinking too much.

3: Eat healthy meals. Eating habits can always use some improvement. To begin with, we should be aware of what we eat and how each food is used by our body. We also need to recognize that there are such things as "mood foods." For example, some Latinas report that chocolate not only tastes good but also lifts their spirits. Recognizing why we eat certain foods is as important as what we eat. In order to eat healthy meals, we need to learn to make better choices.

Eating healthy meals is not just about saying no to some of our favorite foods—it is also about saying yes to some of our traditional foods. The challenge is to get the nutrients and energy our bodies need from the foods that satisfy us. Chapter 19 provides details on how to do this.

4: Exercise regularly. Latinas need to exercise more. Some of us may feel that in our daily life, either at home or at our place of work, we get sufficient exercise. And we probably do get exercise in these settings. To have a healthy body, however, we need to exercise more than most of us typically have until now.

Exercising more does not necessarily mean that we have to join an expensive health club or buy special equipment. As a first step, we have to think of how we spend each day. How much does our body move? Most of us need to add at least 20 minutes of sustained movement to our daily routine. This is something we need to do for the rest of our lives. Chapter 21 gives us some good suggestions to follow in this area.

5: Listen to your body. Our bodies are constantly giving us information about our physical state and often about our mental and spiritual states too. The difficult part is to learn to notice and attend to the cues our bodies provide.

There are basic things we have to listen to if we are to satisfy the needs of our bodies. For example, at a primary level we have to learn to recognize when we are hungry and when we are tired. Too often we only focus on our bodily cues when we are at the extreme of depletion—when our bodies are starving or exhausted. At other times we let external cues (other people, the location, the time) direct us.

We have to learn to eat when we are hungry and sleep when we are tired. For some of us this may mean that a few large meals are replaced by several light snacks throughout the day. For others, it may mean that we need to sleep less than other people or plan more time for relaxation.

In a larger sense, Latinas must avoid the tendency toward *fatalismo* (fatalism) that inhibits us from seeking care for health problems. Listening to your body means that you acknowledge when some part of your body does not feel well and you seek care.

Many of the chapters in this book provide details on how to better understand the information your body is giving you. The task for each of us is to learn when we have to *aguantar* (tolerantly accept) and when we have to attend to our needs.

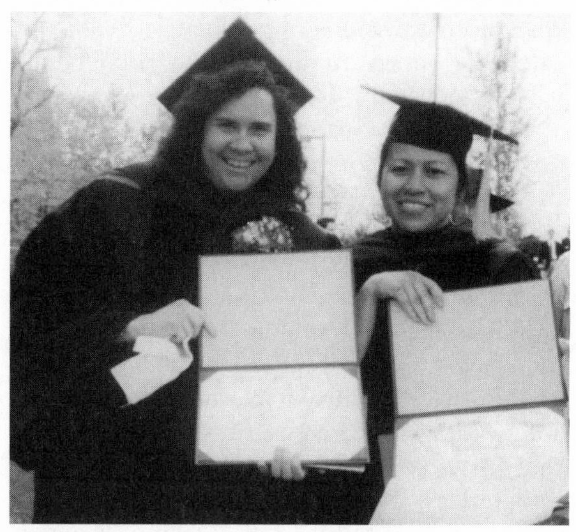

We learn and excel together.

Five Steps Toward a Healthy Mind

1. Set limits.
2. Learn to relax.
3. Worry less.
4. Give yourself time for pleasure.
5. Nurture healthy relationships.

Healthy Mind

A healthy mind requires that our mental and emotional states function to the best of our ability. To have a healthy mind means that we set realistic limits with ourselves and other people—especially with our *familia*—accurately evaluate situations, have healthy relationships with people around us, and have a generally positive outlook on life. If we have a chronic mental illness, to have a healthy mind means that we manage our illness in a way that maximizes our lives.

For Latinas, the cultural overlay, as manifested by our relationships with family and friends, needs careful consideration. That is why recent revisions of psychiatric diagnostic categories point to the need to understand what is culturally based behavior. Moreover, as Latinas, our struggle is to focus on ourselves as we incorporate into our daily lives the steps for a healthy mind.

1: Set limits. As Latinas, we are socialized to accept that our roles with respect to our families necessitate submission to the requests of others. Some of us acknowledge this by saying that "we are for others." Thus, for some Latinas, overtly setting limits is a task that may seem incompatible with cultural imperatives. Nevertheless, to have a healthy mind, we need to set limits. Chapter 1 details the steps for setting limits.

2: Learn to relax. Relaxation is one of the ways we nourish and heal our minds. It is an active process in which we give ourselves time to replenish our inner resources. When we relax, we give ourselves the "down time" that even computers need.

As Latinas, we are hardworking because we often believe that to do nothing is wrong. We often seem to believe that a body that is not alert, active, and doing work becomes a vacuum that is particularly vulnerable to be filled by illness. We accept the value that to be slothful is not only bad in itself but also leads to bad things occurring in our lives. For us to be slothful means that we will attract both physical and spiritual illness.

Latinas also have a heightened sense of responsibility about their work and about taking care of others. For some of us, the thought of relaxation seems incongruous, if not self-centered. Yet to have a healthy mind, we have to learn to relax, and that means rethinking our values about work.

The importance of work appears highlighted when we look at the role models in our lives. Our mothers, aunts, and friends were and continue to be always active. This tells us that we should always be doing something, and more often than not, it should be for the benefit of others.

Given this outlook, relaxation appears to be the opposite of what we should be doing. Relaxation seems to be an activity that entails doing nothing and benefits only the individual. That is why, for Latinas, learning to relax seems so self-indulgent. Many of us feel guilty even thinking about allowing ourselves to relax. Resting is something we must learn.

3: Worry less. Recent national surveys show that not only do Latinas worry a lot, but we worry more than other people do. It is unclear what need our worrying fulfills. Perhaps worrying is our way of preparing ourselves for the worst, or maybe it is a means of warding off the worst by thinking that it may happen. Regardless of the motivation, it is not a productive use of our mental resources.

Rather, when we are worried about something, instead of obsessing over the "what-ifs," we should choose either to do something about the problem or accept that it is out of our hands and move on. To simply worry with no creative outlet is a mental drain that produces nothing but an unhealthy mental environment.

Perhaps more important, over time, unresolved anxiety may result in depression. Chapter 13 discusses the problem of depression for Latinas.

Audrey knew that her relationship needed work. But she just did not have any energy left. All day long she took care of grumpy customers, and by the time she got home at night she was too exhausted to even smile. What was it she once said? "All my smiles were used up at work."

And then one day she came home and found a short note: "I needed more smiles." Audrey wept as she realized how she had neglected the one person who had always been good and loving to her.

4: Give yourself time for pleasure. To allocate time to ourselves is viewed as inconsistent with our focus on working and taking care of others. Just as relaxation is a means of replenishing our minds, however, allowing ourselves the opportunity to have pleasure balances our mental state.

Too often we get caught up in our day-to-day responsibilities and forget that we have to leave time for ourselves. This does not mean that we abandon our responsibilities. It means, rather, that to really respond to *cuídate, mi hija,* we need to give ourselves time to enjoy our lives. One Latina described how she takes bubble baths—they let her just enjoy the good feelings of the day, and it's good for her skin too.

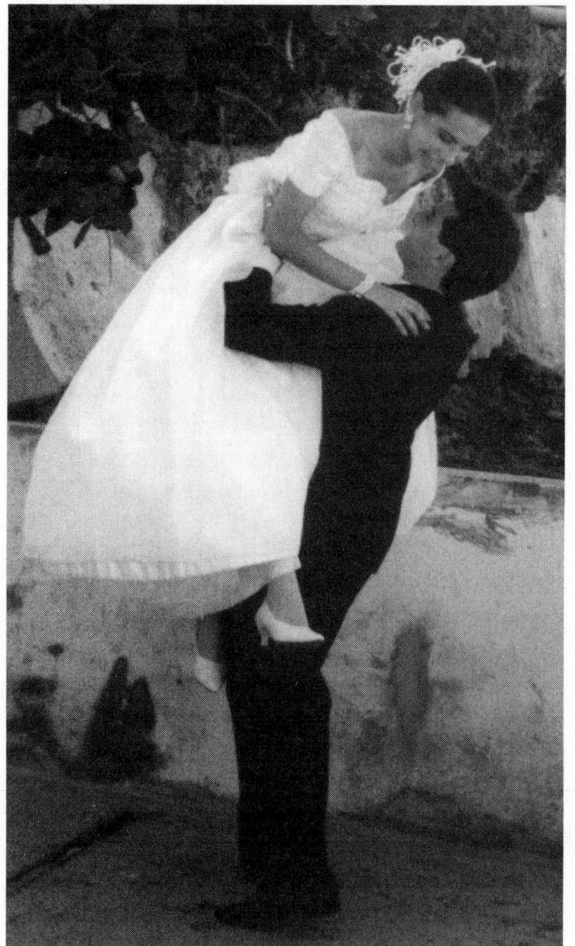

In marriage two become one—it is a joyous time.

5: Nurture healthy relationships. All relationships require work. Some Latinas have indicated that it is sometimes easier to maintain unhealthy relationships than healthy ones. By their very nature, unhealthy relationships are those in which the bonds we build are based on our weaknesses. Too often we get sucked into the abyss created by our own insecurities and doubts. The challenge is to disentangle ourselves from unhealthy relationships.

Latinas need to recognize that healthy relationships are based on our strengths and require work. Too often we take these relationships for granted as we focus on trying to make things better in some of our more troubled relationships. We have to remember to be vigilant and nurture the good relationships in our lives.

Our minds are a combination of our rational thinking, our intellect, and our sometimes not-so-rational emotions. Having a healthy mind requires that we create a framework within which giving is balanced with receiving, relaxation and pleasure are encouraged, and relationships build on our strengths.

Healthy *Espíritu*

Whether we acknowledge it or not, our *espíritu* is an essential part of each one of us, as Latinas, and has a major impact on our health. Our history and religion are intertwined in the development and nourishment of our *espíritu*. Whether we identify with our Spanish, Indigenous, African, European, or Asian heritage or a combination of those, who we are is the combined product of our past beliefs and creates our sense of *espíritu* and our sense of well-being.

Espíritu encompasses all that we know and do not know and integrates it into our own sense of being. *Espíritu* is neither body nor mind, and at the same time it is both and more. *Espíritu* refers to the totality of what sustains us. For some of us, it speaks as the voice of God within us; for others, it refers to our sense of oneness with the world. The recognition of our *espíritu* is a strength that makes us, Latinas, unique in how we care for and define our own health.

Organized Religion

Hispanics consider themselves either Catholic (77.3 percent), Pentecostal (4.5 percent), Baptist (2.1 percent), Presbyterian (1.0 percent), Lutheran (1.0 percent), Methodist (0.5 percent), or Other (i.e., Jews, Mormons, Episcopalians, Reformed, Churches of Christ, Islam, and Other Christians) (6.5 percent). The number of Hispanics without a religious preference (7.0 percent) is similar to that of the general population (8.0 percent).

Whether or not we are practicing Catholics, understanding who we are as Latinas necessitates a discussion of the Catholic church today because it is such a powerful force in our lives and health behaviors, even if we do not recognize it. Issues of sexuality, contraception, and even end-of-life care are all affected by organized religion.

Hispanics and Catholicism

- Hispanics are 37.7 percent of all U.S. Catholics.
- Of all Hispanics, 77.3 percent are Catholic.
- Only 7.4 percent of all bishops in the United States are Hispanic.

1: The Catholic Church. Our knowledge about the Catholic church is influenced by the experiences of our childhood. Good and bad, they are the memories that sculpted much of our current faith or lack of faith.

Latinas who received their religious education prior to Vatican II have a very different view of the Church than Latinas who are products of Vatican II. Since 1965 and the close of the Second Vatican Ecumenical Council, there have been significant changes in the Church. The changes made by Vatican II were meant to exemplify that the Holy Spirit is alive and responds to the realities of the day while still being consistent with key teachings. This belief is at the core of the Church as a living institution. It is this Grace from the Holy Spirit that is credited with maintaining the Church throughout the last 2,000 years. Nevertheless, change is never without its detractors.

After Vatican II, Latinas were able to be part of the mass and assist in the distribution of the Eucharist. In most dioceses there were altar girls. While some have applauded the use of laypersons during the Mass and the transition from a Latin mass, others have found these to be unacceptable changes.

It was not easy for Ana to go back to church—she had good and bad memories related to it. She remembered what it was like when she had to memorize the Catechism. She also remembered how soothing it had been to smell the incense and feel the Holy Spirit in the Latin words she did not understand. She also remembered confession.

Vatican II had changed many things. And she had heard that the 1994 Catholic Catechism was a new type of document that urged the reader not to memorize but to understand.

It had been a long time since Ana had gone to church. And yet at this point in her life, she felt it was necessary to go back to her church.

In 1985, after the twentieth anniversary of the close of Vatican II, Pope John Paul convened a special assembly to "celebrate the graces and spiritual fruits of Vatican II, to study its teaching in greater depth in order that all the Christian faithful might better adhere to it, and to promote knowledge and application of it." In 1986, as a follow-up to that meeting, a commission was set up to draft a new Catechism.

After six years of writing, review, and incorporation of comments, a unified document was produced. The document "is conceived as an organic presentation of the Catholic faith in its entirety." The 1994 release of the Catechism of the Catholic Church is a reference text to be used to "deepen the understanding of faith." The Catechism expands on the basic teachings of Catholicism.

This document provided clarification for some by making it clear that while wives were required to be obedient to their husbands, husbands were to be obedient to their wives too. Various clarifications such as these made it obvious that the role of women was changing. Women were no longer to think of themselves as last or as lesser beings.

In March of 1995, a decade since its last general meeting, the Society of Jesus developed a document at the Thirty-Fourth General Congregation to chart a course in preparation for the twenty-first century. To the surprise of many, the document contained landmark statements with respect to women's rights in the Church and society, such as the following:

> We Jesuits first ask God for the grace of conversion. We have been part of a civil and ecclesial tradition that has offended against women. And, like many men, we have a tendency to convince ourselves that there is no problem. However unwillingly, we have often been complicit in a form of clericalism which has reinforced male domination with an ostensibly divine sanction. We wish to . . . do what we can to change this regrettable situation.

Soon afterward, Pope John Paul announced that he would support the effort. Nevertheless, late in 1995 he made it clear that the Church would not allow the ordination of women.

Latinas have remained active in the Church throughout its changes and continue to be active parishioners. For many Latinas, the major women that they know from Scripture are Eve and the Virgin Mary.

Although the role of Eve is always associated with sin, Catholicism provides Latinas with the Virgin Mary, who is absent of all sin. For some Latinas, the Virgin Mary speaks to the universality of faith and is invoked in the Church under the titles of Advocate, Helper, Benefactress, and Mediatrix. The historical manifestations (*Virgen de Guadalupe*, *Virgen de la Caridad*) as well as the ongoing reports of apparitions of the Virgin Mary speak to her power.

These apparitions have been an important source of strength for some Latinas, who often turn to the Virgin Mary as the strongest woman in the Catholic Church. Some Latinas have expressed a heightened sense of their own *espíritu* based on the messages she brings. At an individual level, several Latinas have reported that the Virgin Mary served as their mother when they felt they had no one else to turn to and helped guide them to seek the help they needed.

2: Protestantism. The number of Latinas participating in Protestant churches has increased over the last twenty years. Many of the Latinas who have converted to a Protestant denomination indicate that they made the transition because they were looking for a church that was more consistent with their beliefs. Other Latinas mentioned that when they were young, their parents had been converted.

The decentralized nature of the Protestant churches makes it difficult to assess the number of Latinas who are active parishioners. What we do know is that soon after the year 2000, over half of all Protestant ministers were women. It is unclear whether this is something Latinas find appealing. Nevertheless, already Protestant churches have felt the impact of having women as ministers. For example, now the issue of women's rights is increasingly brought to the forefront of discussions.

3: Judaism. For Latinas who practice Judaism, there has always been an interest in the spiritual aspects of health. There are services for the healing of the spirit and the body. Moreover, in some congregations, prayers for healing are part of the weekly Shabbat (Sabbath) services.

The role of women in Judaism has also changed. Since the early 1900s, women's rights have been an important part of Judaism. Yet there were no female rabbis until 1972, when Sally Priesand was ordained in a Reform ceremony and became the first female rabbi. During the next decade, more women expressed their interest and qualified to become rabbis.

In 1983 Conservatives allowed ordination of women. Today over 50 percent of Reform and Reconstructionist rabbinical students are female. While Orthodox Judaism still holds women separate and apart from males, the bulk of Judaism has accepted women as rabbis.

Spirituality

Some Latinas have expressed feelings of alienation from most organized religions: they do not feel part of a religion in which all references to a God use a masculine pronoun. Others have indicated that the anomaly of language, which generally gives a nondescript entity a male pronoun, has had no effect on their belief about their God. Still other Latinas have found these musings irrelevant, pointing out that neither spirits nor angels have gender.

In the past decade, some Latinas have found their needs best met by belonging to nondenominational spiritual groups. They believe that within Christianity, as well as other faiths, theology and spirituality are male oriented. Other Latinas have found their answer within New Age groups. Latinas seeking a Deity who is more Latina in appearance

Five Steps Toward a Healthy *Espíritu*

1. Do good acts.
2. Think good thoughts.
3. Meditate.
4. Pray.
5. Listen.

and who espouses values more consistent with various aspects of their lives have joined Goddess groups.

Regardless of our faith, each Latina strives to have a cohesive sense of *espíritu*. Whether we look for intercession by angels or the Virgin Mary, we feel our faith deeply, and that changes our view of our own health. Fortifying one's spirit to help balance one's total health requires more than weekly attendance at a religious service or having good intentions. Regardless of where we worship, the five steps listed below are important to make our *espíritu* healthy.

1: Do good acts. When we do good things for others, our sense of spirit is invigorated. An act of kindness or thoughtfulness done without expectation of any benefit to oneself creates a climate in which one's spirit can blossom.

It is not sufficient to talk about good acts or to have good intentions. To fulfill the spirit, the act must actually be done.

2: Think good thoughts. When our thoughts are positive, we allow the good graces to soothe our mind. Bad thoughts like those stemming from *envidia* (envy) create a negativity that only hurts oneself.

3: Meditate. Give yourself quiet time to reflect and not act. Too often we act or do or say quickly, without giving enough time to thought.

4: Pray. Regardless of our religion, prayer is an important part of faith. Prayer can take many forms, from the reciting of the rosary to the work we do in our everyday lives. It is this prayer through our actions that is often seen as nourishing to our *espíritu*.

5: Listen. Leave your heart and ears open to hear private revelation.

Summary

More often than we Latinas admit publicly, our sense of *espíritu* is based on a devout relationship with God. Religion, faith, and spirituality are the basis for many of our concepts about ourselves and our health. Religion gives us the framework in which to demonstrate our faith and to take care of our health. Our faith and spirituality help us determine when and for what we seek help.

Latinas are the product of a cultural and religious history that sees health as a function of the complex *espíritu*-mind-body relationship. Latinas know that health is about the combined state of our body, with all of its organs and systems; our mind, which experiences the spectrum of feelings ranging from joy to sadness and the great in-between; and our *espíritu*, which is the underpinning for our total sense of well-being.

For Latinas, being healthy is the integration of our body, our mind, and our *espíritu*. That is what makes us *sanas*.

RESOURCES

General

Organizations

National Mental Health Association
1021 Prince Street

Alexandria, VA 22314-2971
(703) 684-7722 or (800) 969-6642
www.nmha.org

National Mental Health Consumers' Self-Help Clearinghouse
1211 Chestnut Street Suite 1207
Philadelphia, PA 19107
(800) 553-4539 or (215) 751-1810

National Institute of Mental Health
6001 Executive Blvd.
Rm 8184, MSC 9663
Bethesda, MD 20892-9663
(301) 443-4513
www.nimh.nih.gov

American Institute of Stress
124 Park Avenue
Yonkers, NY 10703
(914) 963-1200
www.stress.org

Books

Berkow, Robert, and Mark H. Beers, eds. *The Merck Manual of Diagnosis and Therapy*. 17th ed. Rahway, NJ: Merck Research Laboratories, 1999.

Boston Women's Health Book Collective. *Our Bodies, Ourselves for the New Century: A Book by and for Women*. New York: Simon & Schuster, May 1998. Also Nuestros Cuerpos, Nuestras Vidas, May 2000.

Braiker, Harriet B. *The Type E Woman: How to Overcome the Stress of Being Everything to Everybody*. New York: Signet, 1992.

Carlson, Karen J., Stephanie A. Eisenstat, and Terra Ziporyn. *The Harvard Guide to Women's Health*. Cambridge: Harvard University Press, 1996.

Catechism of the Catholic Church. New York: William H. Sadlier, 1994.

Epps, Roselyn P., and Susan C. Steward, eds. *The Women's Complete Healthbook*. New York: Delacorte Press/Bantam Doubleday Dell Publishing Group and the American Medical Women's Association, 1997.

Horton, Jacqueline A., ed. *The Women's Health Data Book: A Profile of Women's Health in the United States*. 2d ed. Washington, DC: Jacobs Institute of Women's Health, 1995.

Powell, J. Robin, and Holly George-Warren. *The Working Woman's Guide to Managing Stress*. Englewood Cliffs, NJ: Prentice Hall, 1994.

Publications and Pamphlets

"A Consumer's Guide to Mental Health Services." NIH Publication No. 94-3585. National Institute of Mental Health, National Institutes of Health, 5600 Fishers Lane, Rockville, MD 20857; (301) 443-4513.

"Coping with Stress." Information on how to identify the physical and mental health problems caused by stress. Structured Exercise in Stress. Mental Health Association, Duluth, MN.

"Social Ties and Susceptibility to the Common Cold." Cohen, Sheldon; William Doyle, David P. Skoner, Bruce S. Rabin, and Jack M. Gwaltney. *Journal of the American Medical Association*. June 25, 1997. Vol. 277, No. 24, pp. 1940–44.

"Women and Mental Health: Issues for Health Reform," March 1995. Background paper by Sharon Glied and Sharon Koffman of Columbia University describing overall rates of disorder among women. The Commonwealth Fund, Commission on Women's Health, New York; (212) 305-8118.

3

Where the Traditional Meets the Conventional

Lo Mejor . . . The Best

Rosa liked her doctor a lot, even though he did not know about the traditions passed from her mother and grandmother to her. Sometimes she was unsure of how to answer his questions. When he asked her what she had been taking for her sleeplessness, she simply replied, "Nothing." She wanted to tell him about the special teas she drank, which seemed to soothe her uneasiness, but felt that he would not understand about the benefits of té de manzanilla *(chamomile tea)* o el té de tilo *(linden flower tea).*

Rosa feared that if he knew about them he would think less of her. And yet she knew that the tea had been better for her than all the pills he had given her. The tea did not upset her stomach the way the pills did.

She did not want to offend him, and so she said nothing. Rosa smiled and thanked him for his care. When she got home, she took the medicine that he gave her and put it in the drawer with the other pills he had given her.

Our knowledge of the soothing effects of *té de manzanilla* is part of the tradition we have received with our Latina heritage. Many of us were drinking *té de manzanilla* to calm our nerves long before chamomile tea became a feature on restaurant menus. When we were growing up, *tés* and *cocimientos* (medicinal brews) were among the medicines we took to make us better.

Each one of us has a set of *remedios* (medicines) that were given to us by our mothers, and although we may be unable to identify the active ingredients that make them work, we *do* know that they make us feel better. Each of us also keeps the memory of the special attention and care involved in making our soothing preparations. And we cherish both, our traditional *remedios* and the memories that go with them.

We may even believe that our problems or ills are due to *mal de ojo* (evil eye) or the more contemporary "bad karma." If this is the case, we have our *remedios* too. Consistent with our beliefs, we may find the appropriate provider to help us with either the cleansing that is necessary, or we may wear little bags filled with special herbs or turn to prayer to free us. When we follow those steps that are based in our beliefs, we find that often times life does seem a little better.

As adults, we have in many cases kept some of these folk or traditional beliefs, and many of us still accept that there are alternative systems to healing. Yet some of us still feel uncomfortable sharing with our health care provider the fact that we are using traditional remedies. We may even feel reluctant to speak about them.

And we know why this is so. Early in our experience we learned that when we seek care from a conventional provider, there are things we say and things we do not say. It isn't that we do not want to be forthright. It is rather that we believe the provider would either not understand our methods or think less of us for believing that they can help us.

We receive dissonant messages about our traditional practices, but the good news is that science is changing its views about them.

> *Consejos*
>
> Home remedies can be risky.
>
> Ephedra (ma huang), in which the active ingredient is ephedrine, has been sold for a variety of health reasons. Since ephedra is classified as a food, it does not have to undergo any clearance by the FDA before it is sold to consumers. The supplements industry that produces ephedra and the public health community have been at odds over the safety of its use as the number of reports of adverse reactions to ephedra continue to mount.

Conventional and Alternative Therapies

Since the 1970s and the opening of relations with the People's Republic of China, there has been an increased interest in non-Western medical methods. In the beginning, Western researchers and providers rushed to either praise or curse not only acupuncture but an unfamiliar assortment of Chinese herbal treatments as well. At the same time, those desperate for treatment tried whatever new potion was available, while pharmaceutical companies tried to identify the key molecules in herbs that were claimed to produce a desired effect.

In the area of scientific research, a great divide markedly separated Western and non-Western medicine. In many ways this was an artificial division, however, because Western medicine did not present a unified front. The term *conventional medicine* became more popular to embrace those forms of medicine and health care that are based on "objective" science.

During the next twenty years, efforts to study alternative medicines, folk medicines, and similar practices expanded beyond the field of medical anthropology. In addition to looking to the East for alternative medicines, researchers began to examine all the practices existing in the West, including the southern hemisphere. As it began to be accepted that there were medical treatments that worked and were not explained by conventional medicine, it became necessary to look critically at alternative treatments.

In 1992 Congress established the Office of Alternative Medicine (OAM) within the National Institutes of Health. The office was created to "support research to investigate the effectiveness of alternative therapies and provide public information about alternative practices."

By 1997 the number of persons who used an alternative therapy had risen to 42 percent from 33 percent in 1990. The most commonly reported alternative therapies were herbal medicine, massage, megavitamins, self-help groups, folk, remedies, energy healing, and homeopathy. These therapies were used as an alternative to conventional therapies (alternative approach) or in combination with conventional therapies (complementary or integrative approach). The $27 billion in out-of-pocket costs in 1997 for these therapies represented an amount greater than the total out-of-pocket costs for all hospitalizations during the same time period. It is clear that these alternative therapies are widespread.

In 1998 Congress elevated the office by changing it into the National Center for Complementary and Alternative Medicine (NCCAM) and increased the budget to $68.6 million in 2000 (in 1993 the budget was $2 million.) Additionally, Congress established the White House Commission as Complementary and Alternative Medicine Policy.

Just as the marriage of alternative and conventional medicine is in its early stages, there is still much progress that needs to be made in trying to understand the underlying science, safety, and effectiveness of CAM therapies.

The uneasiness of this new alliance is best exemplified by the question posed in the title of the December 1994 OAM symposium, "Botanicals: A Role in U.S. Health Care?" As Latinas, we know the answer to that question—it is a resounding yes! The issue is how to facilitate the exchange between traditional and conventional medicine in a positive way.

Limits of Conventional Medicine

Esther was sure that the doctor would cure her tuberculosis. She wasn't even worried about her physical health. What did disturb her was her conviction that she had lost her sense of espíritu. *How could she ever explain that to her doctor? He would think she was talking about an emotional problem, and that wasn't it at all. She had followed the doctor's orders, but she wasn't getting better. Esther sighed as she closed her eyes and began to pray for the first time in a long while. She needed to make her spiritual connection.*

Technology and science can take us a long way with respect to our physical and mental health. But there are limits. Sometimes when we do not feel well, we reluctantly admit that our physical illness is closely related to nonphysical factors. Among ourselves we may say that someone is not really sick—that it is just in his or her head. Conventional medicine sometimes disparagingly refers to this type of unwellness as "somatization." Nevertheless, when our body is ill due to nonphysical factors, we need care too. The problem is determining who will provide this care.

> **Fact**
>
> Hispanics are just as likely as any other community to use alternative medicine.

The typical health care provider is trained to care for our body and sometimes for our mind. This requires extensive training, knowledge, and ongoing participation in continuing education courses. The care of the spirit, however, is usually beyond the scope of the training the health care provider receives.

Given the framework of medical training, the role of our health care provider should be to rule out organic problems and recognize when there is unrest in our mind or spirit. The care of the spirit is best left to other accredited providers (priests, ministers, and rabbis) and, most important of all, to ourselves. Many Latinas use a dual system of care—one for the body and one for the spirit.

Recognizing the limits of conventional medicine is a key step in defining our responsibilities as active participants in our own health care.

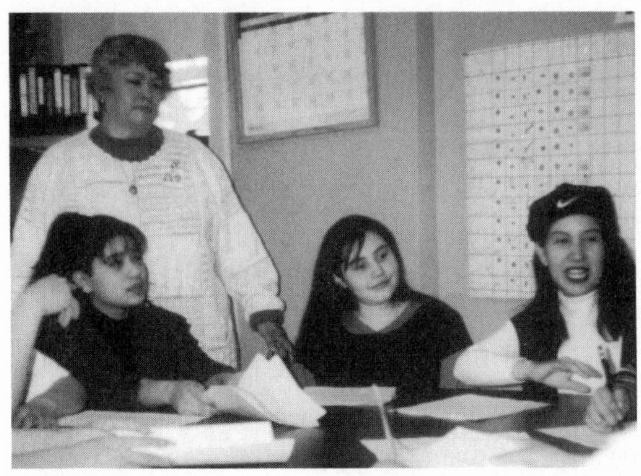

We learn much of what we know from talking to each other.

Empowering Patients

Health care used to be about the relationship, *confianza* (trust), and *respeto* (respect) between a Latina and her health care provider. We enjoyed the relationships we established with our doctors. We valued the time we spent talking to them and felt that these conversations were critical to their care for us. Some of us even remember when we were so ill that our physicians made house calls.

We trusted and believed whatever our health care providers told us because we knew they always had our best interests at heart. We even accepted knowing that sometimes they would not tell us everything, because they were "protecting" us.

Today the profound changes occurring throughout our health care system have changed all that. When we visit our health care provider, it is rarely in an office that feels warm and nurturing. The typical health care setting is increasingly large, cold, and sterile, with prompt "in and out" care. As we are rushed in to see our provider and quickly moved through the system, we often find ourselves at a loss for words. The reality is that we are functioning under new and changing models of health care delivery.

The biggest shift in the provision of health care is the one affecting the assumptions that define the role of the physician and the role of the patient. The fundamental nature of how we relate to our provider is evident in the sad fact that physicians no longer have much freedom in determining the amount of time they spend with each patient. In the name of efficiency, 2 out of 3 physicians estimate that they spend less than 15 minutes talking to a patient.

Just as problematic for Latinas is the increasing reality that one may not see the same provider on subsequent visits. The written record in your file (increasingly replaced by an electronic record), along with your statements, becomes the basis for making decisions about how to proceed with your health care. The management principle is that there is no need to have one health care provider talk to another about the patient, because the written record provides all the necessary information. While this may be sufficient for tracking objective measures—such as blood pressure, weight, or glucose level—what is lost is the valuable information the provider obtains by seeing the same patient over a series of visits.

We also hear that the role of the patient has changed from one of passive recipient of medical intervention to that of active consumer. The truth is different, though. While the health care system expects us to take more responsibility for our health, outside of the occasional suggestion box or consumer survey little has occurred to truly empower patients. Too often what we see is that patients are released from hospitals so quickly that they *must* manage their own care. The concept of "patient dumping" is taking a new twist as we see responsibility being pushed onto patients who haven't previously been provided with adequate training or support.

In the cost-cutting environment that many health care providers and patients alike are forced to endure, too often what is cut is human relationships, which provide the essential nuances by which health is assessed and treated. The amount of time that provider and patient spend talking to each other has decreased to unacceptable levels. And things are not going to go back to where they once were.

For the sake of our health and our lives, we have to learn new ways of interacting with our health care providers. We have to develop skills to make maximum use of the time we spend with them. The first step is for us to track our health on an ongoing basis.

Tracking Our Health

Probably the only thing that we Latinas usually track on a regular basis is when we menstruate. Too many of us have been taught to define our health status based on our menstrual cycle. But truly caring for our health requires that we monitor more than just our menstrual cycles on an ongoing basis. A health journal (see Appendix B) is a good starting place for all of us as we track the status of our body, mind, and spirit.

As frequently as is reasonable, preferably on a daily basis, we should rate how we feel and describe changes in our feelings. It will take less than 4 minutes to complete your journal entry. This record keeping will be very valuable as we begin to take control of our health.

> *Consejos*
>
> **For Your Health Care Visit—Just the Facts**
>
> 1. Symptoms—day, time, and nature of your symptoms
> 2. Changes—any major changes in work, home, or family
> 3. Medications—name and dose of all over-the-counter or prescription medicines you take
> 4. Extras—any special teas or natural products you have taken
> 5. Questions—be specific

Preparing for the Health Care Visit

Having so little time to talk to our health care provider, we need to make certain that we use the time wisely. We must be prepared to give details about our health so that a diagnosis is made with the maximum amount of information. By doing this we will be helping our provider decide how to make us better.

A review of recent entries in your health journal would be a good place to start, in writing down what you want to tell your health care provider. Although we may want to chat—and indeed, having more time to talk with our provider could be helpful—the reality is that the time we have with him or her needs to be spent answering questions in a timely and accurate manner. We need to stick to just the facts about our symptoms, major life changes, medications, and extras. We should also be prepared to ask questions.

1: Symptoms. Before you go to see your health care provider, make a record of when you started to feel ill. In as much detail as possible, keep a listing of when you felt ill and what was the nature of your symptoms. Make sure to note fluctuations in how you felt.

2: Changes. As painful or irrelevant as it may seem, make note of major changes in your work, family, or home life.

3: Medications. Make a list of all medicines (over-the-counter, home remedies, or prescription) you are taking. Be sure to include name and dose.

4: Extras. List any special teas, natural products, or medicines you have taken.

Consejos

How to Have a Good Visit with Your Health Care Provider

1. Tell your health care provider that you need to write down what they say because you want to be able to take better care of yourself.
2. Provide all the information that is requested.
3. Ask what your diagnosis is and write it down.
4. Ask how you should proceed and write it down.
5. Read what you have written to your health care provider.
6. Make changes that are recommended.
7. Ask any additional questions.
8. Ask if there is any other reading you can do.
9. Thank the provider and let them know that you appreciate the extra time they took with you (remember, current systems do not encourage a health care provider to take time to talk to you).

5: Questions. Try to limit yourself to the three most important questions you want answered. For some of us, this is the hardest part of preparing for the visit. Sometimes we are afraid to ask a question because of the answer we may get. In the groups of Latinas who talked to me during the writing of this book, a remarkable number related undergoing surgery for ovarian problems and waking up to find that they'd had hysterectomies. The major lesson that Latinas have to learn is to ask questions. We should be as thorough in our search for understanding our bodies as we are about any other aspect of our lives.

The Visit

Take a copy of the "Visit Summary" (see Appendix B) and something to write with. Write out the questions you have and take them with you. You may need to take someone with you when you are especially worried about your health to help you understand and remind you of what the health care provider actually said as opposed to what you heard when you were stressed out by your own fears. In order to get the most out of your visit, be sure to complete the "Visit Summary" by following the *Consejos* above.

Patients' Rights

The changes in our health care system have made it essential to be clear about the role of patients and health care providers. These relationships are increasingly complex as payers/insurers learn that there are severe consequences to cost-cutting decisions. For example, reducing costs by not giving the health care provider support so that care can be provided in the language of the patients served, is no longer acceptable.

In August 2000 the President signed a Presidential Executive Order for Improving Access to Services for Persons with Limited English Proficiency (LEP). To help carry out the intent of the Executive Order, the U.S. Department of Health and Human Services issued a policy guidance that states "in order to avoid discrimination against LEP persons, health and social service providers must take adequate steps to ensure that such persons receive the language assistance necessary to afford them meaningful access to their services, free of charge." This landmark guidance should help us in obtaining services that are more effective.

Another ongoing struggle has been the many attempts to develop a Patients' Bill of Rights. The National Health Council's 1995

"Patients' Bill of Rights and Responsibilities" is still the best.

This document was the result of meetings with every major voluntary health agency as well as with more than a hundred other organizations in the health field. In what follows, each of the bill's articles has been expanded to explain what it means for Latinas.

Patients' Bill of Rights and Responsibilities

All patients have the right to:

1. Informed consent in treatment decisions, timely access to specialty care, and confidentiality protections.
2. Concise and easily understood information about their coverage.
3. Know how coverage payment decisions are made and how they can be fairly and openly appealed.
4. Complete and easily understood information about the costs of their coverage and care.
5. A reasonable choice of providers and useful information about provider options.
6. Know what provider incentives or restrictions might influence practice patterns.

All patients, to the extent capable, have the responsibility to:

7. Pursue healthy lifestyles.
8. Become knowledgeable about their health plans.
9. Actively participate in decisions about their health care.
10. Cooperate fully on mutually accepted courses of treatment.

Source: National Health Council, 1995.

Rights

1: All patients have the right to informed consent in treatment decisions, timely access to specialty care, and confidentiality protections.

Respeto is the operating word to keep in mind. Respect is the underpinning for the interaction between a Latina and her provider. To maintain *respeto* means that there is private and confidential communication between you and your provider. It means that you and your provider speak the same language, in a way that goes beyond speaking in English or Spanish. It means that the language you are using is at the same technical level.

Your provider has to be able to tell you everything that is known about your health. This means that the provider will explain to you what is wrong with you and what your possible options are. This may mean that your provider describes what is going on during your physical examination.

You may find that your providers explain things but you do not understand what they are saying. This is very natural because usually when we see our provider we do not feel well or are under stress. Under these conditions, our ability to comprehend is diminished.

In providing information to you, your provider needs to do it in words that you understand. There are several things to remember:

- It is all right if you do not understand what your health care provider says.
- It is OK to ask for a simpler explanation when you do not understand what a word means or what is being said.
- Your provider may ask another member of the team taking care of you to answer some of your questions.
- Sometimes it will not be possible for the provider to know what is wrong with you.

Providing information is not supposed to be a dumping of medical jargon but rather an instructive exchange of ideas. Keep in mind that it is probable that your provider has had considerable training in the technical aspects of taking care of you but has not been taught how to treat you as an equal partner in maintaining your health.

The best patient is one who understands what is wrong with him or her and what the options are for getting better. As part of this principle, it is important for providers to feel comfortable saying that they do not know what is wrong. Latinas have to understand that health care providers do not have a diagnosis for every list of symptoms and that even when there is a diagnosis, sometimes there is no treatment. There is not a pill for every illness.

It is also important to recognize that you should be referred for qualified second opinions in a timely manner and that you should have access to needed specialty care and other services.

Respeto also applies to our requests as we state them in our legal advanced directives or living wills (see Chapter 23).

2: All patients have the right to concise and easily understood information about their coverage.

Given the changing health care system, we need to know what is covered under our health plans. Some of the better health plans have an ombudsman who serves as a helper to answer your questions and represent your needs to the health care organization. At the very least, we need information about medicines, hospitals, and nonhospital coverage.

Medicines

Some plans cover the cost of medicines, while others do not. In some plans, experimental or new medicines are not included as part of the benefit. Some over-the-counter medicines are available in higher doses as prescription medicines. Since over-the-counter medicines are not covered by most health plans, you may want to ask your provider if it is possible to prescribe the higher dose, which requires a prescription. We need to make sure that we know what medicines are covered.

Hospitals

Lucy had made arrangements for a private room so that her daughter, Anita, could stay with her in the hospital. The nurses were nice, but none of them spoke Spanish, and more than anything Lucy was scared. She was not looking forward to surgery the next day.

When visiting hours were over, the head nurse came into the room and told Anita that she had to leave. Lucy did not understand how this could be. The head nurse stated, "You have to remember that when you come into a hospital you give up your rights." Anita responded, "This is a hospital, not a prison. Most important, we are consumers paying for services."

It is important to know the extent of hospital care covered, the hospitals you can go to, and the procedures for getting admitted to a hospital. In some plans, all hospital stays have to be approved in advance. Other plans require that for certain procedures you obtain a second opinion. You also need to have detailed information about which hospital services you are likely to use and which ones are included in your plan.

> **Warning**
>
> More technology is not necessarily better. The best health care professionals use technology appropriately, which sometimes means using less.

Nonhospital Care

While the average length of stay in a hospital has been decreasing, there have been increases in the amount of care provided outside of the hospital in a variety of alternative care settings, such as nursing homes, intermediary care facilities, skilled nursing facilities, and patients' homes. You need to know the amount of coverage and out-of-pocket expenses related to the costs of specialized health care, supplies, and equipment. Do not assume that you can go to any clinic or emergency room. Sometimes you need advanced approval from your health plan.

3: All patients have the right to know how coverage payment decisions are made and how they can be fairly and openly appealed.

Sometimes we are told that our health care plan will not cover some aspect of our medical treatment. It is important to find out from the administrator of our health plan how these decisions are made. In plans with an ombudsman, that person will provide you with this information. We also need to know how to appeal decisions that are made, especially if we feel that those decisions may be damaging to our health.

4: All patients have the right to complete and easily understood information about the costs of their coverage and care.

When you go on a trip, you make sure that you know how much you are going to spend on food, transportation, and hotel. Yet when we are sick, many of us have no idea of what the things we need are going to cost. In order to prepare for a "rainy day," we need to have a better understanding of how much health care will actually cost.

We feel relieved when our health plans cover 80 percent of costs. But what if the costs amount to $100,000, an amount that could easily be reached if several operations and providers were involved in our treatment. That would leave us with a $20,000 bill, which we would have to pay ourselves. Many of us believe that our health plan will cover all our expenses, and it is not until we get the final bills that we realize our health plan covered only part of them. We are similarly taken by surprise when we have to pay deductibles. Some of us have catastrophic health insurance and think it will cover all expenses for any catastrophic illness. The reality is that most plans have limits on the total catastrophic costs they will cover.

Before you agree to any treatment, be sure to ask about the long-term and short-term costs of the different treatment options as well as what your quality of life is expected to be after the procedure. In some instances you may be able to take part in a clinical trial (see Chapter 22).

5: All patients have the right to a reasonable choice of providers and useful information about provider options.

For Latinas, the trust relationship with the provider is of the utmost importance. Thus it is essential that Latinas be able at least to select their own provider. Your plan should also explain how you can change providers if you become dissatisfied with the care you receive. On the other hand, if your provider leaves the plan, there should be some accommodation so that you can continue to see the same provider. Increasingly plans are allowing patients to go outside of their network.

Usually your health plan will give you a list of providers and facilities. Make sure you know how your plan selects these providers and facilities. An acceptable list of providers would include a variety of listings based on geographic proximity, hours of operation, areas of expertise, ability to speak in languages other than English, and other factors. Before choosing providers, you should know where they were trained, what special licenses and accreditations they have, and their areas of expertise. With respect to facilities, you need to know whether they are accredited, their hours of operation, and whether day care is available.

6: All patients have the right to know what provider incentives or restrictions might influence practice patterns.

Practice patterns, in this context, means the diagnostic services or treatment you receive. All patients should familiarize themselves with the parameters within which a provider has to frame decisions about care. Current systems focus on reducing immediate costs and therefore on reducing the options your health care provider has for providing you with quality care. In some health care plans, a provider receives a fixed amount for providing services to you. This is called *capitation*. Regardless of whether you go for one visit or one hundred, the provider receives the same amount of money. In these kinds of systems, perverse incentives sometimes operate so that providers are rewarded financially or in other ways for providing less care. In a capitation system, all the incentives are directed at having you use fewer services.

Another way systems try to reduce costs is by limiting the number of times a provider recommends a procedure. This results in a de facto rationing of services. Providers are told that they can only perform a procedure or order a test a fixed number of times. To exceed the target may mean that the provider is penalized, or the provider may receive an incentive for being below the target.

To counter this trend, health systems sometimes develop treatment protocols or practice guidelines. Unfortunately, since what we know about the health of Latinas as a group is relatively new, sometimes these guidelines may not be the best for determining the care we are to receive. A similar concern is raised by protocols for quality assurance procedures.

Responsibilities

Along with rights come corresponding responsibilities to help reduce the need for medical intervention and benefit our health.

7: All patients, to the extent capable, have the responsibility to pursue healthy lifestyles.

Latinas should make their lifestyles healthier by doing those things that insure a healthy body, mind, and spirit (see Chapter 2).

8: All patients, to the extent capable, have the responsibility to become knowledgeable about their health plans.

We need to become familiar with what is and is not included in our health plans. If there is something we are not sure about, we should seek additional information.

The National Patient Empowerment Council developed the checklist on the next page to suggest the right questions to ask about your health plan.

9: All patients, to the extent capable, have the responsibility to actively participate in decisions about their health care.

Although Latinas are reluctant to see a health care provider when they are well, it is something we need to do. We need to go for regular preventive checkups even if our plans do not cover them. It is a financial investment that we must make.

When we go to see our health care provider, we should take with us as much information as possible about our current health problem. We should also bring a paper and pencil so that we can take notes, have the provider review our notes, and ask additional questions. If we do not understand what is being explained, it is our responsibility to ask questions.

It is important to remain patient if the health care provider seems annoyed or impatient with our questions. Keep in mind that most providers were not trained to talk to patients, and moreover that most health care plans do not reimburse providers for taking lots of time to talk.

Whenever possible, Latinas need to find

Checklist for Reviewing Your Health Plan

COVERAGE

1. How will the plan cover preexisting conditions?
2. Will the plan cover preventive care or wellness visits?
3. Will the plan cover immunizations?
4. Is there a maximum amount the plan will pay per illness?
5. Is there a maximum lifetime amount the plan will pay for my family?
6. Will my child be covered while he or she is away at school?
7. What happens if we're out of town and need medical help—must I call for approval before seeing a doctor; must I get approval before going to the hospital or emergency room?
8. Does the plan limit the number of days of hospital stay for each illness?
9. Does the plan cover dental exams?
10. Does the plan cover dental expenses?
11. Does the plan cover eye exams?
12. Does the plan cover the cost of eyeglasses/lenses?
13. To what extent does the plan cover mental health treatment?

ACCESS

1. Can I choose my own obstetrician?
2. Can I choose my own pediatrician?
3. Can I choose my own family doctor?
4. Will I be allowed to change my doctor if I am not satisfied with the one I have?
5. Can I choose my hospital if I am sick or need treatment?
6. Must I get approval before going to the hospital or emergency room?
7. Must I get a second opinion before treatment?
8. Is the expense of a second opinion covered?
9. Will I be limited in the number of times I can visit the doctor?
10. Must I wait a specific amount of time after each visit before I can return to the doctor?
11. Will I have to pay an extra fee to see a specialist?
12. How long will I have to wait to get an appointment with a specialist?

RESTRICTIONS

1. Does the plan cover experimental treatments?
2. Will my doctor have access to all FDA-approved medications, or will my doctor have to choose from a limited list of drug options?
3. Are prescription medications covered?
4. Is there a lifetime maximum amount the plan will pay for prescriptions?
5. Are plan doctors provided financial incentives or disincentives in relation to their practice patterns?

EXPENSES

1. Is there a co-payment per doctor's visit?
2. Is there an extra charge for seeing a doctor outside the plan's provider network?
3. What is the monthly premium?
4. What is the deductible?
5. What is the lifetime maximum coverage per person?

HELP

1. Is there a toll-free (800) number I can call if I have a question?
2. Is a patient ombudsman available to assist plan members?
3. Is there an open-appeals process available if the plan refuses to pay for treatment or service?
4. Will the plan respect advance directives and living wills?

Source: National Patient Empowerment Council, 1995.

out the potential risks, benefits, and costs of treatment alternatives. Remember, the health care provider may not have all the answers, so you should look for information about your condition. The resource section at the end of each chapter in this book will help you find such information.

10: All patients, to the extent capable, have the responsibility to cooperate on mutually accepted courses of treatment.

When we go to health care providers and work with them to develop a treatment plan, it is our responsibility to make sure that we carry it out. Sometimes we make the mistake of assuming that because we did not get any better after the first day of treatment, the treatment is not working. As Latinas, very often we then consult with our *comadres* to find out what they did to get better and make a change from our treatment plan.

We have to remember that it is also our responsibility to keep the provider informed of how we are doing. If the treatment is going well, we should let the provider know. If the treatment is not going well, we should contact the provider and together decide on a new plan of action. It might very well be that once again the *comadre* was right but we must talk to our health care provider.

As Latinas, we may want to supplement our treatment with some traditional methods or medicines. Our providers need to be told of these remedies because sometimes the interactions among different treatments can produce negative side effects. While providers used to consider home remedies harmless, recent evidence from the Food and Drug Administration suggests that many over-the-counter substances are more potent than we think. If our providers make us feel uncomfortable talking about home remedies, then we need to find new providers.

Finally, we must make sure to tell our health care providers about all the nonprescribed substances we consume on a regular basis, e.g., teas, over-the-counter remedies, supplements, etc.

Where to Complain about Your Health Plan

There is no 800-number hotline for consumer complaints about health plans or health care organizations. Individuals should contact their health plan's patient representative or their state insurance commissioner.

Contact your state Insurance Commissioner; also let the Joint Commission on Accreditation of Healthcare Organizations (JCAHO) know about your concerns. The Joint Commission evaluates and accredits nearly 19,000 health care organizations and programs in the United States. Complaints filed by consumers can have a significant impact on a health care facility's ability to obtain the accreditation from JCAHO that it needs to operate and get reimbursed for services. If you have questions about how to file a complaint, you may contact the Joint Commission toll free at (800) 994-6610 from 8:30 am to 5 pm, Central Time, weekdays. Only English speaking operators are available. You can also visit the JCAHO on the web *(http://www.jcaho.org/compl_frm.html)* for information in English or Spanish on filing a complaint.

The JCAHO also has a "Quality Check" service on the web *(http://www.jcaho.org/qualitycheck/directry/directry.asp)*. You can enter a request for health care organizations by geographic area or the name of a specific health care organization and get links to the JCAHO accreditation and performance reports for those health care organizations.

Medicare patients can contact their State Health Insurance Counseling Program. To find out the number for your state program, call Medicare at 1-800-MEDICARE (633-4227). Phone counselors are available Monday through

Health Insurance Commissioners (Selected States)

AZ	Arizona Department of Insurance 2910 North 44th Street, Suite 210 Phoenix, Arizona 85018-7256	 Fax	602-912-8400 602-912-8452
CA	California Department of Insurance 300 Capitol Mall, Suite 1500 Sacramento, California 95814	 Fax	916-492-3500 916-445-5280
CO	Colorado Division of Insurance 1560 Broadway, Suite 850 Denver, Colorado 80202	 Fax	303-894-7499 303-894-7455
CT	Connecticut Department of Insurance PO Box 816 Hartford, Connecticut 06142-0816	 Fax	860-297-3800 860-566-7410
FL	Florida Department of Insurance State Capitol Plaza Level Eleven Tallahassee, Florida 32399-0300	 Fax	850-922-3101 850-488-3334
IL	Illinois Department of Insurance 320 West Washington St., 4th Floor Springfield, Illinois 62767-0001	 Fax	217-785-0116 217-524-6500
MA	Division of Insurance Commonwealth of Massachusetts One South Station, 4th Floor Boston, Massachusetts 02110	 Fax	617-521-7301 617-521-7758
MI	Michigan Insurance Bureau Office of Financial and Insurance Services 611 W. Ottawa St., 2nd Floor North Lansing, Michigan 48933-1020	 Fax	517-373-9273 517-335-4978
NJ	New Jersey Department of Insurance 20 West State Street CN325 Trenton, New Jersey 08625	 Fax	609-292-5360 609-984-5273
NM	New Mexico Department of Insurance PO Drawer 1269 Santa Fe, New Mexico 87504-1269	 Fax	505-827-4601 505-476-0326

NV	Nevada Division of Insurance 788 Fairview Drive, Suite 300 Carson City, Nevada 89701-5753	775-687-4270 Fax 775-687-3937
NY	Agency Building One Empire State Plaza Albany, New York 12257	518-474-6600 Fax 518-473-6814
PA	Pennsylvania Insurance Department 1326 Strawberry Square, 13th Floor Harrisburg, Pennsylvania 17120	717-783-0442 Fax 717-772-1969
TX	Texas Department of Insurance 333 Guadalupe Street Austin, Texas 78701	512-463-6464 Fax 512-475-2005
WA	Washington Office of the Insurance Commissioner 14th Avenue & Water Streets PO Box 40255 Olympia, Washington 98504-0255	360-753-7301 Fax 360-586-3535

Friday from 8:00 am to 4:30 pm, Eastern Standard Time. Spanish-speaking counselors are available.

If your health plan's patient representative or Medicare State Health Insurance Counseling Program does not resolve your complaint, you should contact your State Health Insurance Commissioner. Their office is responsible for overseeing all health plans operating in your state and resolving consumer complaints. When you contact the Commissioner's office, ask to speak to a consumer representative. To find out who your Commissioner is, contact the National Association of Insurance Commissioners; 2301 McGee, Suite 800; Kansas City, MO 64108-2604, or call (816) 842-3600. The addresses and phone numbers for the Health Insurance Commissioners in the fifteen most populous Hispanic states are listed in the resource section.

Finally, read your newspapers carefully for changes in health insurance coverage and patients rights. Every elected official wants to be the one who makes history by making it possible for everyone to have health insurance and have good health care. This may be the decade when it happens.

Summary

Today it is much more common for everyone to use some sort of alternative medicine. Latinas use both conventional medicines and different types of *remedios* (remedies) to make us feel better. In order to ensure that we have the best care we must be able to discuss with our health care provider all the *tratamientos* (treatments) that we use. We also need to learn to formally track our own health status and learn how to discuss our concerns with our health care provider. In the best of all situations we will develop a partnership with our health care provider. The Patient's Bill of Rights and

Responsibilities is an important starting point for laying out the details of the new health care environment. The checklist for reviewing health plans helps us to evaluate some of the critical elements of a health plan.

Just as health care has changed, we must also change.

RESOURCES

Organizations

American Association of Naturopathic Physicians
8201 Greensboro Dr., Ste 300
McLean, VA 22102
(703) 610-9037
www.aanp.net

American Osteopathic Association
142 East Ontario Street
Chicago, IL 60611
(800) 621-1773 or (312) 280-5800
www.aoa-net.org

National Center for Homeopathy
801 North Fairfax Street, Suite 306
Alexandria, VA 22314
(703) 548-7790 or (877) 624-0613
www.homeopathic.org

National College of Chiropractic
200 E. Roosevelt Road
Lombard, IL 60148-4583
(630) 629-2000 or (800) 826-6285
www.national.chiropractic.org

National College of Naturopathic Medicine
Clinic:
11231 SE Market Street
Portland, OR 97216
(503) 255-4860
www.ncnm.edu
College:
049 SW Porter Street
Portland, OR 97201
(503) 499-4343

National Health Council
1730 M Street, NW, Suite 500
Washington, DC 20036-4505
(202) 785-3910
www.nhcouncil.org

National Patient Empowerment Council
56 Maple Lane
Blairstown, NJ 07825
(908) 362-5498

National Center for Complementary and Alternative Medicine
National Institutes of Health
NCCAM Clearinghouse
PO Box 8218
Silver Spring, MD 20907-8218
(301) 589-5367
(888) 644-6226
www.nccam.nih.gov

Books

Isaacs, Stephen L., and Ava C. Swartz. *The Consumer's Legal Guide to Today's Health Care: Your Medical Rights and How to Assert Them.* Boston: Houghton Mifflin, 1992.

Kirchheimer, Sid, Debra Tkac, and the Editors of *Prevention* Magazine Health Books, eds. *The Doctors Book of Home Remedies; Over 1,200 New Doctor-Tested Tips and Techniques Anyone Can Use to Heal Everyday Health Problems.* New York: Bantam Books, 1993.

Guía Médica de remedios caseros: Mas de 1200 técnicas y nuevas surgérencias que cualquiera puede utilizar para resolver un sinnúmero de problemas cotidianas (June 1996).

Moyers, Bill. *Healing and the Mind.* New York: Doubleday, 1995.

Starr, Paul. *The Social Transformation of American Medicine.* New York: Basic Books, 1984.

PART II

Being Female

4

Controlling Our Own Fertility

Just the Facts

I wish I knew all I needed to know to understand what goes on down there with my ovaries and everything else. No one ever talked to me about it.

I know that I have had children and should know more. But what is there to know? The Church tells me one thing and my husband . . . well, he has his own mind.

I know it is my body, but to me this body is a stranger.

—LEONOR, 45

Some of us learned about our reproductive system the hard way—after we were pregnant. Many more of us just ignored our reproductive system. Sure we kept calendars, talked about cramps and how heavy our bleeding was, but we did not talk about how it all happened.

If you ask, most Latinas will tell you that they did not even speak to their mothers about their reproductive system. What little we did learn about our bodies occurred haphazardly or through a biology class, which tried to avoid discussions that might be too embarrassing. Even now some of us have some unusual ideas about how things work. For many of us, having children defined our reproductive system.

Indeed, childbearing is extremely important to the majority of Latinas, even more so than for the general population, according to data from the Alan Guttmacher Institute. Historically, it was essential to have many children for two reasons: (1) the high rate of child mortality before the age of five and (2) to meet the labor demands of the agrarian societies that were the norm until the twentieth century.

For Latinas, life is different today. Not only do a far larger majority of our children thrive into adulthood, but few of us live in agrarian societies. Moreover, good medical advice indicates that for the well-being of the child and for the physical health of the mother, it is a good idea to space children at least two years apart.

The issue remains of how are we to do this. Often the conflicts we experience make it very difficult for us to make good decisions. The results of our inability to make responsible choices about our bodies can be alarming.

Such indecision is understandable when one considers the varied messages we receive, as well as the existence of our own contradictory desires. For instance, while our bodies might be in prime childbearing mode, our minds may tell us that we are not ready to care for a child. On the other hand, we might be sensitive to taboos regarding some methods of birth control. Yet we know that as Latinas, our body, mind, and spirit need to be well balanced so that we can accept the choices we make.

Perhaps the most concrete proof of our confusion is that while Latinas are overwhelmingly Catholic, we are more likely than non-Hispanic white women to have abortions. How could this be?

Some attribute these data to our ignorance about birth control or our reluctance to go to family planning clinics. But it is more than that. Many of us have not been encouraged either to understand or to take control of our own fertility. Childbearing has been considered something that is God's will, when in fact, as the old saying goes, God gave us brains so we could think.

Mark wants to have a baby. I'm just not ready. But how can I have some say over what will happen? He won't use a condom, and I'm not sure what I should do. Take pills? The Church says I should have children, but I have to earn money to support the children I already have. My mother is sick, and I must take care of her. I don't know what to do. No, that's not true. I know what I have to do, but I do not know how I can do it.

—*Carmen, 29*

For too long, men selected women as partners based on their belief that a woman would be able to have lots of children—preferably male. In most instances, whether or not a woman became pregnant was left up to husbands and lovers, who controlled when and where women would have to make themselves sexually available. Yet, slowly, things have changed, and Latinas have looked for other ways to control our fertility although we remain reluctant to use effective methods of birth control and continue to be hesitant to ask our partners to use birth control.

We only complicate matters when we do not entirely understand our fertility. Out of ignorance comes a greater likelihood that there will be an unwanted pregnancy. In such situations some women, whether alone or with the support of their partner, decide to keep and love the child. In other cases a woman might be faced with the wrenching decision to have an abortion.

The first step in preventing unintended pregnancies is understanding your reproductive organs. The second step is taking control of your fertility and accepting it as your responsibility. With that in mind, let us begin at the beginning.

In this chapter we will focus on the internal sexual organs that make up our reproductive system and on how we can understand and control our reproduction. In the next chapter we will review what we know about sexuality. This separation of reproduction and sexuality has the purpose of emphasizing that although there is overlap between the topics, sexuality has many purposes, only one of which is reproduction.

It is essential to recognize that sexuality is separate from reproduction because, unlike our female ancestors, who had much shorter lives or died in childbirth, we live most of our adult lives beyond our reproductive years. And there is, of course, sexuality after we can no longer have children. But that is the subject of Chapter 5.

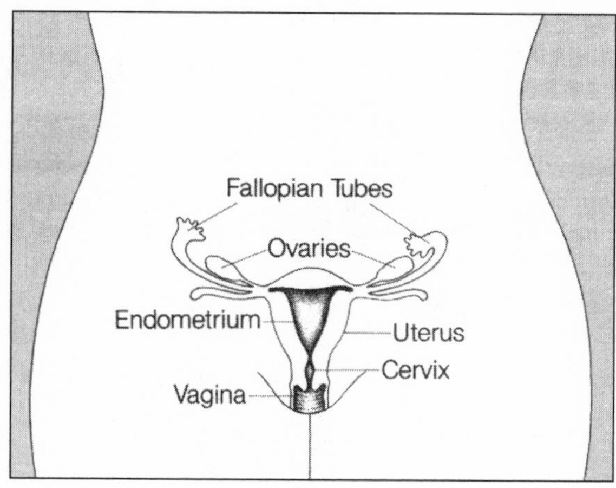

Reproductive System

The Mechanics

The female body is a complex system. Our internal sex organs are the ovaries, fallopian tubes, uterus, cervix, and vagina. Each of these organs undergoes dramatic changes during the menstrual cycle and changes in appearance as a result. Pregnancy changes the functioning and appearance of these organs even more radically.

Ovaries are small. They are roughly the shape and size of a small almond (1¼ inches long and ¾ inch wide). Ovaries are responsible for (1) the monthly release of eggs, (2) the production of estrogen throughout the menstrual cycle, and (3) the production of progesterone.

Each woman is born with all the eggs that she will ever carry. Most women are born with approximately two hundred thousand eggs per ovary. The exact number of eggs is determined while she is still in her mother's uterus. No more eggs are produced after birth.

Within the ovaries there are follicles, which surround the eggs. They also provide all the necessary nourishment and support for the eggs. It is the follicle cells that are responsible for the production of estrogen and progesterone.

During puberty, hormonal changes make the substances surrounding the egg follicles change, making it possible for three hundred to five hundred of the eggs to fully mature. After puberty, ten to twenty eggs begin to develop each month. Usually only one egg reaches full development.

The work of the ovaries is stimulated and directed by two hormones: luteinizing hormone (LH) and follicle-stimulating hormone (FSH). FSH helps ripen the egg, and LH prepares the uterus to receive the fertilized egg. Both of these hormones are produced by the pituitary gland, which is located in your brain.

The ovary releases an egg during what is called ovulation, which occurs only once in a menstrual cycle. When this occurs depends on the length of your cycle.

The **fallopian tubes** are the passages through which the developed egg travels and where the egg and the sperm (released from the penis into the vagina during penile-vaginal intercourse) first meet and fertilization takes place. These hollow tubes are only ⅓ inch in diameter and extend approximately 4 inches from the ovary to the uterus. Each month, one of the fallopian tubes carries one egg to the uterus.

One end of the tubes is near the ovary. That end looks like a trumpet, with edges that seem to be feathered or to have fingerlike projections (called fimbria). The feathered edges have hairlike projections (called cilia), which draw the egg that is produced toward the inner part of the fallopian tube.

The other end of the fallopian tube is attached to the uterus and is much more narrow.

The **uterus** is often described as having the shape of an upside-down pear. It is usually 3½ inches long and 2½ inches at its widest point. During pregnancy, this muscular organ

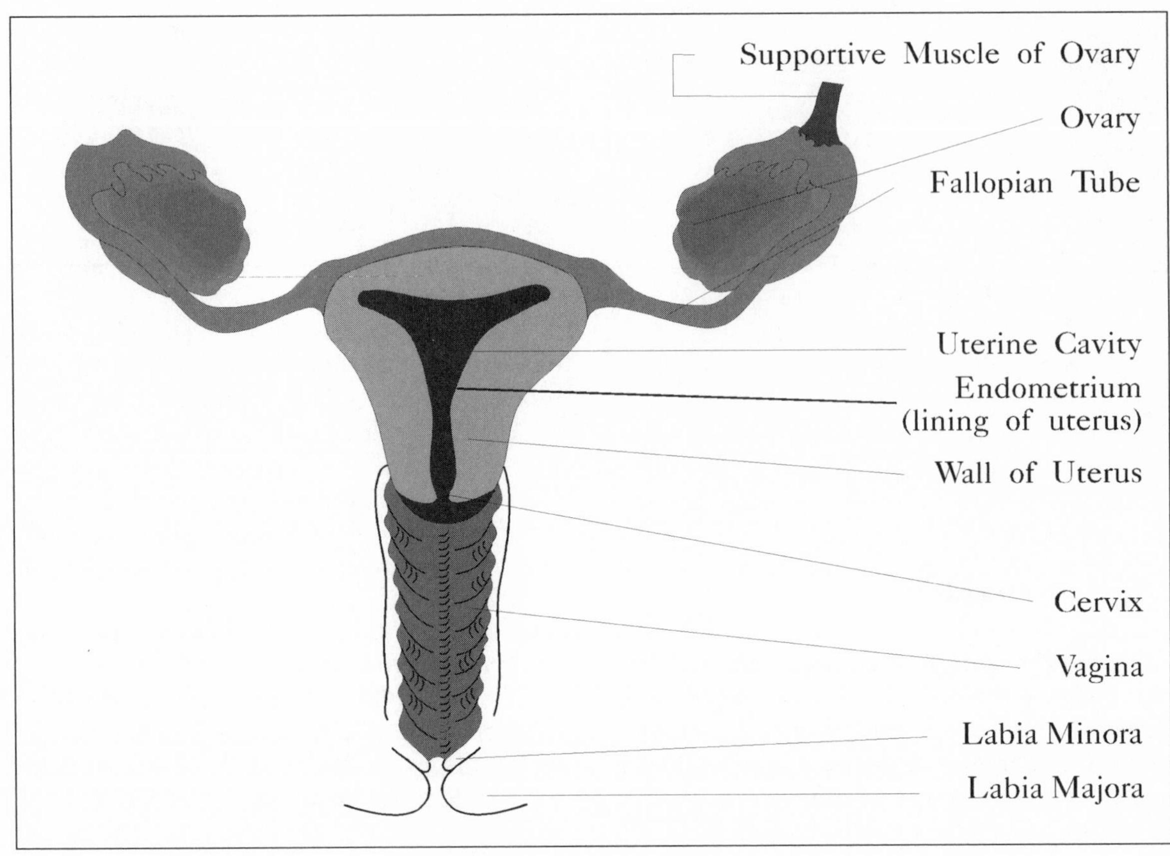

Reproductive System

expands to as much as thirty times its size. This expansion is possible because the walls of the uterus are made up of flexible muscle fibers.

The lining of the uterus is called the endometrium. The endometrium is a layer of cells, which thickens during the month in preparation for possible implantation of a fertilized egg along its surface. A fertilized egg will travel out of the fallopian tubes and attach itself to the walls of the uterus. If there is no fertilized egg, the lining that was built up during the cycle is released as menstruation.

The **cervix** is at the bottom of the uterus and leads into the vagina. It is the gateway between the uterus and the vagina. There is a small opening in the center of the cervix called the cervical os. This opening allows for the blood to flow out during menstruation and also expands to allow for childbirth. The cervical os is the opening through which the sperm has to travel in order to fertilize the egg.

The cervical os is lined by glands that release a mucuslike substance. The cervical mucus changes in color and consistency at different times of the month. These changes match the hormonal fluctuations of your menstrual cycle.

As the time of ovulation approaches, there is more mucus, and it is clear and watery in consistency. This increases the ability of sperm to swim through the cervical os to the uterus and arrive at the fallopian tube, where it can fertilize the egg. After ovulation the mucus changes again, but this time it becomes thick and semiopaque. When the mucus has this consistency, it is difficult for the sperm to get through.

The **vagina** is a hollow, muscular tube that is like the finger of a glove—flat when nothing is inside but increasing in size during intercourse and childbirth. The vagina extends from the cervix to the outside of the body. It is about 3 to 4 inches long when at rest. The vagina has three layers: the inside vaginal lining (mucosa), a muscular layer, and a layer of connective tissue.

There are changes in the vaginal lining as a function of estrogen levels. When there is more estrogen, there is an increase in glycogen (the way the body stores carbohydrates) in the vagina. The normally occurring bacteria in the vagina metabolize the glycogen and make the vagina slightly acidic, which is critical to a healthy vaginal environment.

Our vaginas are very sensitive to some of the medicines we take. For example, when we take antibiotics, not only do they kill the bad bacteria that are making us sick, they also often kill the healthy and necessary bacteria in the vagina. Without these bacteria to metabolize the glycogen, the vaginal environment may favor the growth of fungi or other bad bacteria.

Understanding Our Menstruation

I remember seeing a list of booklets you could get about a girl becoming a woman. You could get them for free by just sending away for them. Free sounded good to me. So I sent away for lots of information. I liked the idea of knowing what it would be like to grow up. For certain, it would mean that I could use lipstick and dark eye shadow too.

When the booklets arrived, they talked about menstruation and had diagrams of girls about my age with curly round things drawn by their bellies. It looked pretty strange to me.

Then, one day when I was in school, I went to the bathroom and found that there was blood on my panties. I did not know what had happened.

I guessed that somehow I must have cut myself down there. I could not imagine how I had done it, so I just put toilet paper in my panties to help stop the bleeding until I got home.

When I told my mother what had happened, she smiled and said that now I was a woman. I didn't understand.

I looked in the mirror and I still looked the same. All I knew was that this becoming a woman wasn't like in the pamphlets I had received. It was messy, and my mother still wouldn't let me use lipstick. And you can forget about eye shadow!

—Sara, 21

Each one of us has her own story about what we thought when we got our first period. Most of us faced that first messy day with a mixture of anguish and confusion.

Onset

There is great variability in the age when menstruation begins. Onset of menstruation can occur between the ages of ten and seventeen. In the United States today, the average age of onset is 12.8 years of age, while in 1840 the average age of onset was between sixteen and seventeen. When you begin to menstruate is a function of your genetics, overall health, physical activity (intense exercise, common in athletics, ballet, or gymnastics, can delay onset), nutrition, and other factors.

Cycle

The menstrual cycle lasts 21 to 35 days in most women. The cycle begins when the ovaries begin to produce estrogen. The length of the cycle can vary for many reasons, including changes in physical activity, stress, sleep, frequency of sexual activity, and general health. Sometimes a change in cycle may indicate an underlying physical problem.

The menstrual cycle is actually the process by which our bodies prepare for possible pregnancy. The first part of the cycle occurs when estrogen, which is produced by the ovary, accumulates and stimulates the pituitary gland to begin to produce FSH.

FSH helps the egg develop. As the days pass, the level of estrogen increases and there is an increase in LH. At this point, which is about midway through the cycle, an egg is released and moves down the fallopian tubes. Simultaneously, the inner lining of the uterus (endometrium) begins to build up in preparation for a fertilized egg to implant itself on the walls of the uterus.

If an egg is not fertilized, it is released as menstruation, together with all the material built up in the lining of the uterus. Then the cycle begins all over again. By recognizing where we are in this cycle, we are able to control our own fertility—and this is one of the most self-empowering things we can do.

Myths and Facts

Myth: You should avoid intercourse during menstruation.

Fact: There is no medical reason to avoid intercourse during menstruation.

Myth: The earlier you begin menstruating, the later you will reach menopause.

Fact: Age of onset of menstruation is not correlated with age at which menopause will begin.

Myth: People can tell when you are menstruating.

Fact: The only way other people can tell if you are menstruating is if you make a public announcement or are not practicing good hygiene.

Understanding Our Own Fertility

As women, we spend a lot of time and energy worrying about whether we are pregnant, whether we can be pregnant, and about whether our menstrual cycle is normal. We also practice birth control, even though we often feel uncomfortable talking about it.

Natural Methods/Fertility Awareness

For generations Catholic women were told that the only acceptable way to control fertility was the rhythm (calendar) method. This largely discredited method too often resulted in pregnancies.

Very few women realize that while the rhythm method has become synonymous with natural family planning (NFP), there are actually several other forms of NFP that are far more effective. In fact, while rhythm is the most well-known method of NFP, it is also the one with the highest failure rate.

Today the term *NFP* is meant to encompass all the natural methods of child spacing that are based on a couple's practicing abstinence during the time when the woman is most fertile. These methods are consistent with the teachings of the Catholic Church and various other religions.

If you are considering practicing this form of birth control, it is important to realize that *abstinence* is a misleading term. To practice successful NFP means that during certain times of the month a couple has to abstain from penile-vaginal contact. However, that leaves a lot of room for showing each other physical affection in other ways. Perhaps a more satisfying and accurate description of NFP methods would refer to the fertile days as creative loving days instead of periods of abstinence. Given what we know about sexuality and orgasm in women (see Chapter 5), these days may actually turn out to be most enjoyable for both partners.

Josefina was a practicing Catholic and admitted that throughout her years of marriage she had always practiced natural methods of birth control. For her the most difficult part was not the record keeping. She had realized somewhere along the way that those very moments when she felt great and her body was feeling most desirous were the very moments when she was supposed to abstain.

She knew, however, that she was one of the lucky ones. She had also learned that abstinence did not mean that you didn't have any sex. It meant that it was a time for discovery of other ways of giving and receiving pleasure from her partner.

But this pleasure part . . . well, it was just not something you talked about. It was easier to just say "abstinence."

Latinas' interest in NFP methods is on the upswing because there is increasing reluctance to use methods, such as birth control pills, that introduce hormones and other chemicals into the body. Unfortunately, natural methods do not offer protection against sexually transmitted diseases (STDs).

The major drawback to natural methods is that their success in preventing pregnancy is a function of three factors: (1) the regularity of a woman's cycle, (2) the accuracy of the schedule of days she keeps, and (3) her commitment (and that of her partner) to adhere to the rules.

Given the variability in each of these factors, it is not surprising that 1 out of 5 women who use NFP methods become pregnant each year. For women who strictly adhere to the calendar method, the rate is 1 out of 11, and for women who monitor all three variables described below (time of month, body temperature, and mucus), the rate of pregnancy is 3 out of 100 in a year.

Cervical Mucus Method (Billings Method)

Close monitoring of vaginal secretions (mucus) provides the most accurate single method for natural family planning.

Vaginal secretions are a normal part of our reproductive system. Vaginal secretions are what you find on your panties or on toilet paper after you wipe yourself. They should not be confused with the discharges that are found with vaginal infections.

Before using this method, you need to track your vaginal secretions for at least three months. On a daily basis, keep a record of (1) whether you have a vaginal secretion, (2) the consistency of the secretion (thick or slippery), and (3) the color of the secretion (clear or cloudy). You are most fertile when you have secretions that are slippery and clear.

The cycle of secretions is quite predictable. After you menstruate, there are a few days when you have no secretions. Your fertile time occurs when you begin to have secretions again. These first secretions are cloudy, pasty, and/or somewhat thick. Once the secretions become more slippery and clear, it is likely that you are ovulating. Next your secretions either go away or become pasty and thick again. This is the time when it is once again unlikely, assuming your calendar is accurate, that you will become pregnant.

Your fertile period will vary based on the length of your menstrual cycle, which may be from 21 to 40 days. Most women are considered fertile for about one-third of their menstrual cycle.

Temperature Method (Basal Body Temperature, or BBT)

This method is based on the changes in your body temperature at different points in your menstrual cycle. Body temperature rises at least 0.4 degrees Fahrenheit during ovulation. This rise in temperature usually lasts about three days.

With a thermometer that measures in tenths of a degree (that is why it is called a basal thermometer), you must take your temperature as soon as you wake up in the morning (i.e., before you get out of bed, drink, eat, or engage in any other activity). According to some Latinas who practice this method, this simply becomes part of your sleep/wake-up routine.

Before you go to sleep, you shake down the thermometer to below 96.5 degrees Fahrenheit. Then you place the thermometer conveniently by your bed. As soon as you wake up, you insert the thermometer in your mouth and lie quietly in your bed for 5 minutes—this may be a good time to plan your day. When 5 minutes have passed, remove the thermometer from your mouth and place it in a safe place. Later on, when you are more awake, you can look at the thermometer and record your morning temperature on your chart (see Appendix B).

The BBT method only tells you when ovulation has occurred. It does not provide information about when your fertile period begins. If you use this method, you will have to abstain from vaginal-penile contact from the first day of your menstruation (period) until three days after your temperature rises. To avoid pregnancy, vaginal-penile contact is limited to the end part of your menstrual cycle (i.e, the days before you menstruate).

Calendar Method (Rhythm)

This is the least reliable of the methods for natural birth control because it relies heavily on having menstrual cycles that are always 28 days long. As we know, however, various factors can change even the most regular of menstrual cycles—stress, change in weight, change in activity level, childbirth, and natural hormonal changes occurring during the late thirties and early forties. Additional variability is due to the fact that sperm can live up to seven days within a woman's body and that your egg can survive for more than 24 hours.

It will be at least six months before you can begin to use this system because first you have to know the length of your menstrual cycle. To do this, you must keep track of the day when you get your period for at least six months.

After you have this information, you need to count the days in each of your cycles; that is, the number of days from day 1 of the first menstruation you record to day 1 of your next menstruation, and so on. Write down the number of days in your longest cycle and the number of days in your shortest cycle.

If your cycle is every 28 days, you must abstain during days 9 through 18 from the beginning of your cycle. If, like most women, your cycle varies between 21 and 38 days, you need to abstain from day 7 to day 21.

Combination Method (Symptothermal Method)

The success of this method is due to tracking vaginal secretions and body temperature. Although some health care professionals will also add the rhythm method, the relatively high failure rate of the rhythm method makes it ineffective for predicting fertility. When used consistently, the combined monitoring of vaginal secretions and body temperature results in pregnancy in only 3 out of 100 women per year.

Using this combination method, vaginal-penile contact should be avoided for approximately 10 days during the middle of your menstrual cycle.

Postovulation Method

In this method, a couple agrees to abstain from vaginal-penile contact from day 1 of a woman's period until the morning of day 4 after her ovulation. Ovulation is monitored using either the Billings Method or BBT or both. Using this method requires that a couple refrain from vaginal-penile contact for most of the woman's cycle.

Barrier Methods

These methods are used by women to prevent sperm from reaching the egg. They are considered simple to use by some. Their effectiveness is based on proper placement of the device.

Female Condom/Vaginal Pouch

This device looks like a small plastic bag with a ring around the edge. It serves as a good barrier against the transmission of sexually transmitted diseases (STDs) and HIV. On the average, 13 out of 100 women who use it become pregnant. Although initially awkward, it has the advantage that it can be inserted several hours before vaginal-penile contact.

Diaphragm

Until the advent of the pill, this was the preferred birth control method for women. Most recently, there has once again been increased interest in using the diaphragm because it reduces the amount of chemicals that women have to absorb into their bodies. If used properly, only 6 out of 100 women will become pregnant; the average failure rate, however, is 18 out of 100. Failures of the diaphragm to work are usually due to movement of the diaphragm during vaginal-penile contact.

Diaphragms are not recommended for women who have a tendency to have urinary tract infections.

A diaphragm is used with a spermicidal jelly. In order for the spermicidal jelly to be effective, the diaphragm with the spermicidal jelly cannot be inserted more than 6 hours before ejaculation and must remain in place for at least 6 but less than 24 hours after ejaculation. Sometimes a woman or her partner may have a reaction to the spermicidal jelly. Usually a change in brands will resolve this problem.

Once you have decided to get a diaphragm, you will have to see your health care provider. The diaphragm will be fitted to meet the contours of the uppermost part of your vagina. You should be instructed on how to insert it and allowed to feel what it is like when it is in its proper place. When you get your diaphragm, make sure that you practice putting it in a few times before you leave your provider's office.

You also need to practice taking your diaphragm out. If you feel uncomfortable doing this with your health care provider present, you should ask another health care provider to assist you.

Correct use of this medical device is essential for it to be effective. If you wear contact lenses, you know how much care was taken showing you how to put them in. You should receive at least as much attention with repect to your diaphragm. Given the difficulty usually experienced when first using a diaphragm, it seems reasonable to have your health care provider provide the necessary guidance. Don't be embarrassed to ask for more instructions.

Your diaphragm should be washed (mild soap and water), dried (powdered with cornstarch), and properly stored between uses (in its case and away from light).

Intrauterine Devices (IUDs)

In 1974 the U.S. banned the use of the Dalkon Shield. Also banned were the Majzlin Spring and Birnberg Bow. Today the only IUDs available in the United States are Progestasert and Copper T 380A (Para Gard).

Insertion of the IUD must be done by your

health care provider and checked one month after insertion and then on an annual basis. There is a greater risk of pelvic inflammatory disease (PID) in women who use IUDs. Additionally, the IUD provides no protection from STDs. IUDs are rarely recommended in the United States.

Hormonal Methods

These methods work by suppressing production of a mature egg and changing the lining of the uterus so that it cannot support a fertilized egg. If you use any of the hormonal methods available and monitor your cervical mucus, it will always be thick and sticky. Part of the effectiveness of this method depends on changing the consistency of the cervical mucus and making it less conducive for sperm to travel through.

Side Effects

Many women have no side effects, due to the newer low-dose pills. In the early years of birth control pills, the doses of hormones were much higher than in the low-dose pills available today. Nevertheless, some women do have side effects. Side effects vary from woman to woman and may include bloating, breast tenderness, weight gain, nausea, excessive hair loss, increase in hair growth, and skin problems. In conjunction with your health care provider, you have to decide whether the side effects are bothersome changes you can cope with or sufficiently significant for you to discontinue use of hormones.

Studies indicate that it is safe for women who are nonsmokers in their forties to take birth control pills. Women who are over thirty-five and smoke should not use birth control pills. Keep in mind that hormonal methods of contraception are relatively new, and long-term studies of their effects on women have not been completed.

Pills

Oral contraceptives were first widely used in the 1960s. Since then they have become the method of choice for most women. More than half of the women who use a reversible method use birth control pills.

The reason most women take birth control pills is their ease of use and their low rate of failure. Only 3 out of 100 women taking birth control pills become pregnant, and this is usually because the woman forgets to take a pill. Moreover, some Latinas report that they enjoy the spontaneity that comes with not having to think about and plan when they are going to have penile-vaginal contact.

Recent research indicates that taking the pill may protect women against ovarian and endometrial cancer. At the same time, for women who are smokers, there appears to be a possibility that taking the pill may increase their chances of getting stroke, breast cancer, and cervical cancer. Also, women who have diabetes, heart disease, stroke, or circulatory problems are just some of the women who are not encouraged to take the pill. Finally, the pill does not protect against STDs.

The pill usually comes in packages containing a 21- or 28-day supply. The 28-day package includes 7 days of placebo pills. It is believed that a 28-day package helps women acquire the habit of taking a pill every day.

With respect to the chemistry of the pills, there are four major kinds:

1. Monophasic: gives a steady amount of hormones throughout the month
2. Triphasic: varies the hormones to more closely follow a woman's pattern
3. Combination: gives estrogen and progesterone
4. Mini: gives only progesterone. For this pill to be effective, it is essential that the woman not deviate from her pill-taking schedule.

Injections

In 1992 Depo-Provera Contraceptive Injections became available in the United States. The birth-control effectiveness of these injections lasts 90 days. Although there is a 30-day period after the 90 days when the likelihood of pregnancy is decreased, women are reminded that during this period the likelihood of pregnancy is higher than during the first 90 days after the injection. Only 1 out of 300 to 400 women get pregnant with this method. One of the concerns raised about Depo-Provera is that once you stop taking the shots, it can take you up to two years to regain your fertility.

The injection is made up of a synthetic hormone that is similar to progesterone. From day 14 to day 90 after an injection, a woman has protection from pregnancy. Since there is no estrogen in the injection, those side effects related to estrogen are eliminated. Nevertheless, other side effects occur, including irregular bleeding, weight gain, headaches, and depression, and should be reported to your health care provider. You are the one who must decide whether the side effects are acceptable or not. Your health care provider will help you decide whether the side effects are sufficiently severe for you to discontinue injections in the future.

Implants (Norplant)

In 1990 the FDA approved the Norplant system, which requires the implantation in a woman's arm of six capsules made of flexible tubing. The system provides birth control for up to five years through the slow release of progestin. During the first year, only 1 out of 500 women become pregnant.

To place the implant, your health care provider will anesthetize the area (the underside of the upper arm), make the necessary incision, and insert the capsules. Implantation results in at least some tenderness the first few days in the area of insertion. Women who have thin arms will be able to see the capsules under the skin.

The implant usually causes difficulties (scarring, pain) when it has to be removed. Removal involves minor surgery, which is more difficult than when the implant was first inserted because skin tissue forms around the capsules. Some women have had to return for two visits to have the implant completely removed.

If you take other medication and are thinking of using the Norplant system, you need to discuss this with your health care provider because some anticonvulsants and some antibiotics may reduce the effectiveness of the Norplant system.

Surgical Methods

Throughout the world, surgical sterilization is the most commonly used contraceptive method. In this ostensibly nonreversible procedure, eggs are prevented from traveling through the fallopian tubes from the ovaries. Specifically, your surgeon will cut the fallopian tubes and clip or cauterize them. At most the procedure may involve an incision that is less than 2 inches long and poses minimal surgical risk. There are no known long-term complications from this procedure.

A hysterectomy (i.e., removal of your ovaries or uterus) is not necessary for contraception.

Male Methods

Male Condom

Condoms were originally developed as a protection against STDs. They are a somewhat effective barrier method of birth control when they are used from the outset of any penile-vaginal contact. On the average, only 12 out of 100 women become pregnant when their partners use condoms.

Some men complain that they do not enjoy penile-vaginal contact when using a condom. For this and other reasons, it is recommended that couples incorporate placing the condom on the penis into their foreplay.

When placing the condom on the penis, be sure to leave a little pouch about ½ inch long at the tip to hold the semen. As soon as the man ejaculates, his penis decreases in size and it is important to hold the base of the condom firmly, to prevent any release of fluid into the vaginal area. It is also important to withdraw the penis and the condom from the vagina at the same time. This also offers protection from STDs. Often a condom is used to supplement other female methods of contraception to increase the effectiveness of both and offer protection from STDs.

It is helpful if both partners know how to use a condom.

Vasectomy

This surgical procedure prevents sperm from traveling to the ejaculatory area from the testicles. It has minimal risks and has no effect on physical performance or hormonal levels. Although the amount of fluid a man ejaculates is reduced by 5 percent, this is not easily detected. The sperm the man continues to produce is absorbed by the body as part of its natural processes. While men may experience some discomfort from the operation, they usually do not have to take time off from work to recover.

Although the success in reversing vasectomies is much higher than in reversing the surgical sterilization of women, both of these procedures are considered permanent.

Withdrawal

Withdrawal is not an effective method of birth control. At some undetermined time prior to ejaculation, the Cowper's gland releases thousands of sperm. While this amount is less than the hundred thousand sperm that are released during ejaculation, it only takes one sperm cell to fertilize an egg.

Myths and Facts

Myth: When you are breast-feeding, you cannot get pregnant.

Fact: If you are breast-feeding, you can still get pregnant.

Myth: The Catholic Church does not allow the use of birth control.

Fact: The Catholic Catechism states in section 2370: "Periodic continence, that is, the methods of birth regulation based on self-observation and the use of fertile methods [NFP], is in conformity with the objective criteria of morality. These methods respect the bodies of the spouses, encourage tenderness between them, and favor the education of an authentic freedom."

Mind and Spirit

The choice of how to control fertility is now ours. As Latinas, we can use this as an opportunity to define who we will be or let our partners make that determination for us. Science has provided us with knowledge and technology to control our fertility, but we are the ones who ultimately decide what we will do. The choice has to be consistent with our realities and our beliefs.

Summary

So, how are you going to control your fertility? The information is here, and the decision is yours. Whatever you choose to do will have consequences, which will have a long-term impact on your life.

Understanding your reproductive system should help you decide what method is consistent with your body, mind, and spirit.

RESOURCES

Organizations

American Society for Reproductive Medicine
Patient Information Dept.
1209 Montgomery Highway
Birmingham, AL 35216-2809
(205) 978-5000
www.asrm.com

Association of Reproductive Health Professionals
2401 Pennsylvania Avenue NW, Suite 350
Washington, DC 20037-1718
(202) 466-3825
www.arhp.org

National Family Planning and Reproductive Health Association
1627 K Street NW, 12th floor
Washington, DC 20006
(202) 293-3114
www.nfprha.org

National Women's Health Network and Women's Health Network Clearinghouse
514 10th Street NW, Suite 400
Washington, DC 20004
(202) 347-1140
www.womenshealthnetwork.org

National Women's Health Resource Center
120 Albany Street, Suite 820
New Brunswick, NJ 08901
(877) 986-9472
www.healthywomen.org

Planned Parenthood Federation of America
810 Seventh Avenue
New York, NY 10019
(212) 541-7800
www.plannedparenthood.org

Publications and Pamphlets

"Birth Control: Choosing the Method That's Right For You," 2000. Pamphlet No. 1524. AAFP Family Health Facts series. Information on various birth control alternatives. American Academy of Family Physicians 11400 Tomahawk Creek Pkwy, Leawood, KS 66211-2672; (800) 944-0000. Other titles include "Vasectomy: What to Expect from a Vasectomy," 2000. Pamphlet No. 1561.

"Choosing a Birth Control Method," July 1994. Information on various birth control alternatives (also available in Spanish). Association of Reproductive Health Professionals, 2401 Pennsylvania Avenue NW, Suite 350, Washington, DC 20037-1718; (202) 466-3825. Other titles include:

"Questions and Answers about Birth Control Shots," July 1994. Information about obtaining shots when using contraceptives (also available in Spanish).

"La Selección de un Método Para el Control de la Natalidad," February 1994. Spanish language information on contraception.

"Birth Control" Pamphlet No. AP005. Information on various birth control alternatives. American College of Obstetricians and Gynecologists, 409 12th Street SW (P.O. Box 96920), Washington, DC 20090-6920; (800) 762-2264 www.acog.com.

"¿Cuál es Mejor Para Usted? Cómo Escoger un Método Anticonceptivo." Pamphlet No. OF2531/PB2535. Education Programs Associates, 1 West Campbell, Suite 40, Campbell, CA 95008-1039; (408) 374-3720.

5

Sexuality and Pleasure

I never really enjoyed sex. But I knew I was a good lover. I allowed Estevan to make love to me whenever he wanted to. Sometimes I was too tired and other times I did not feel very sexy, but we did it anyway. He always came, no matter how I really felt. I could fake an orgasm and knew the noises that I could make to excite him.

I knew I was a good lover because Estevan always had an orgasm real fast. I liked that because once he had an orgasm, then I could just relax and do whatever I really wanted to do—sleep, clean, or just be by myself. It really was good for me when he came, because then it was over.

All that business you hear about orgasm and pleasure is just talk to me. Those things are for women who do not know that their obligation is to please their mate. Oh yes, I know all there is to know about sexuality. I am a very good lover.

—CLARA, 43

In the United States, sex is about release of pressure and tension.

—ANITA, 31

When my husband and I got married, we were both virgins. We were very young, and both our families were pleased with the match. There was much celebration about the life that we would share. I did not know very much. I didn't even know what we would share.

I knew he would work and I would work. Each of us had our responsibilities to the new family we had created. Although I did not know very much, the one thing that was certain was that I was for him.

It was hard to tell what that meant completely. At the very least it meant that in the house, as well as away from the house, we were to do whatever he said should be done. When it came to what we did in our bedroom at night, I thought that meant that the only thing that mattered was his pleasure. But I was wrong.

I do not know how, but somehow in the bedroom things changed.

I guess it sounds silly, but we truly did love each other, and with time I changed too. Yo aprendí *(I learned). And because he loved me and cared about my pleasure, he changed too.* Aprendimos *(we learned).*

—JULIA, 68

Most of us learn about sex the hard way. There is so much painful experience associated with sex . . . the pleasure aspects got lost in the experience.

—Sandra, 27

We see lots of sex everywhere in society—television, movies, advertisements. Whenever manufacturers want to convince us of the goodness of their product, they show us how it will make us sexier. Leading magazines know they will sell more copies if they have feature articles that detail how to look sexy, have good sex, have great sex, and even why some of us do not want anything to do with sex. We buy magazines to fill out the checklists of how we should dress and what we should say in order to appear sexy.

Sometimes when we read the suggestions we may think, "I am a Latina—I do not do that!" But descriptions of sex intrigue us, with their range of possibilities from the clinical to the tawdry. One Latina told me she was certain that the experts who wrote about sex probably never even went on a date, and if they did, she added, they were probably never asked to go on a second one.

Too often society adds sex to everything around us in the same way that some of us sprinkle salt on food. Sex is added indiscriminately to whatever is put before us, regardless of how much is already there. The assumption is that more is better. But just as excess salt is not good for us, too much sex may leave us numb. On the other hand, too little sex may leave us feeling wanting and incomplete.

What is the right amount of sex to have in our lives? What makes us sexy? Are men really different? The answer to all those questions and more is the same—it all depends on the individual. A brief overview of historical and scientific trends is necessary to help us define our own response to these questions.

History

For generations the sexuality of women in Western cultures was defined as either dangerous or nonexistent, and women struggled between the two extremes. In the dangerous interpretation, there was Eve in Eden with Adam. Then along came the snake, who convinced Eve to taste the forbidden fruit, and the rest we all know too well. In the nonexistent view, the female role model was the Virgin Mary, who conceived and gave birth while still remaining pure. She also dedicated her life to her son.

Consequently, throughout history, women's sexuality was treated as something best left unexpressed because when expressed it only led to unfortunate events. Women were depicted both as sexual temptresses and as creatures who were easily fooled and consequently needed protection from bad influences. Ironically, men, who were always depicted as all-knowing and all-powerful, were not held responsible for acting on the temptations. Whatever temptations men felt were ultimately the woman's fault. And women had to be protected from themselves.

The need to protect women deteriorated into the necessity to subdue and shackle them. In order to save women from their poor judgment and impulsivity, it became necessary to make them subservient to men. To avoid the devastation to which unleashed female sexuality would lead, and to help women remain pure and obedient, female sexuality needed to be controlled. Humanity would be saved again.

Historically, most societies found mechanisms to protect girls from themselves. As soon as their bodies began to show that they were maturing sexually (usually between the ages of nine and thirteen), young girls were kept under constant supervision by their families or were betrothed. Ideally, the lucky girls were the ones who were betrothed. Control of their sexuality was then transferred to the men they married. The unfortunate ones were those for whom the family could not find a mate; these girls often became servants within their own families.

Science

Regardless of the unflattering historical treatment of women's sexuality, science makes it clear that sexual activity is part of normal human development. Unfortunately, too often the only aspects of female sexuality that have been studied are those related to reproduction—even though we know that sexuality does not exhaust itself in reproduction. Reproduction is only one of the outcomes that sexuality achieves.

Although sex may be all around us, most of what we see is not based on science. Factual data about sexuality are not that easy to find. Although the physiology of sexual arousal has been studied in animals, cultural taboos have limited the amount of research focused on the human sexual response. Somehow, people associate any scientific investigation of sexuality with an implicit support for promiscuity.

If there is limited research into the mechanics of the human sexual response, still less is known about how women respond sexually. Taboos imposed by culture and religion, and the mythology—or is it wishful thinking?—propagated by men about what is desirable female sexuality, serve to bury or obscure the facts. Thus our knowledge of women's sexuality tends to be of a purely technical nature or colored by a male point of view.

The technical perspective focuses on sex as a purely physical aspect of life. Books written from such a point of view discuss, for example, the biology and psychobiology of sex. In their attempt to be clinical, their authors typically include diagrams, which are often line drawings of organs and parts of bodies that have little to do with what we know to be our own bodies or sources of pleasure. Moreover, the breasts they show tend to be upright, and bellies do not hang, revealing the natural passage of time. Often these are drawings based on the male point of view of female sex and sexuality.

The male point of view that has dominated much of research and erotica gives little importance to the role of women in sex. Women are seen as receptacles designed to passively accept the lust and pleasure of men. As one Latina summarized it, "I was for him." Thus, for many researchers, female sexuality has remained undefined: it is nothing in and of itself, but rather a consequence of the biological needs of humanity.

Needless to say, the technical descriptions of sex are woefully inadequate. Further, views of sexuality based solely on the views and culture of men are not meaningful for women, particularly for Latinas.

Today there is growing evidence that for women, sex and sexuality are more than a physiological need. And most important of all, women, including an increasing number of Latinas, are no longer allowing their sexuality to be defined in terms of what others want.

Sex is more than mechanics and more than reproduction. The problem is that the "more" consists of thoughts, and thoughts are not easily measured. The little research that exists indicates that for most women, thoughts mediate feelings about sex and sexuality to a larger extent than for men. As women, when we think about sex or want to express our sexuality, we are more likely to be inspired by the nonphysical aspects of our partners than by their physical attributes. What women think and feel about sexual activity and their own sexuality is difficult to measure.

Latinas and Sex

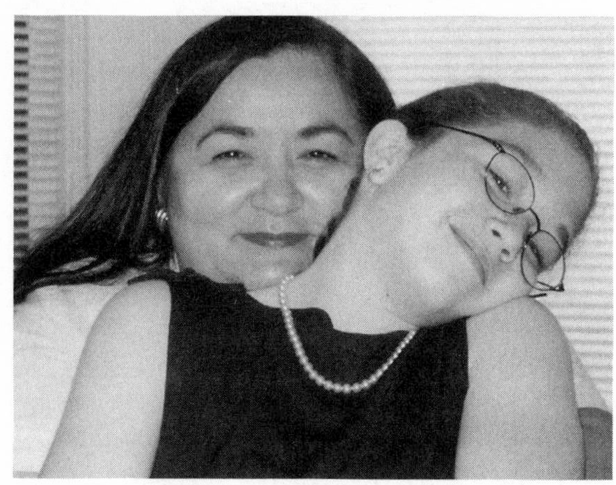

Mothers and daughters should talk to each other about sexuality.

Sex is about many things: intimacy, pleasure, power, strength, and love. We see sex as anything from the sublime to the superficial to the downright repulsive. Some try to exalt sex as the closest thing to communion with God, and others devalue it to the point where it becomes a cheap thrill.

Although sex refers to a broad array of topics, sexuality is best defined as each individual's expression of sex. How we express our feelings about sex is determined by our knowledge, attitudes, needs, and desires. For Latinas to have a healthy sense of sexuality requires honest introspection as we come to grips with our individual and collective histories.

For many of us, our familia *(families) treated sex as a never-ending mystery novel. This experience in itself has had a profound impact on slowing our sexual developmental growth. Thank goodness I am going to live to be a hundred years old, so I can make up for lost time!*

—*Cassandra, 51*

Perhaps the best way to illustrate the meaning of sex for Latinas is to relate what a Latina mother of two children told me. She said she never learned about sex. Her comment held a core truth that Latinas understand: sex is not synonymous with having children. Latinas with children as well as Latinas who have had more than one sexual encounter will often admit that they do not know very much about sex, despite having had sex on at least several occasions. Just as we may cook without understanding the basics of health and nutrition, some of us have had children without understanding sex or even thinking about our own sexuality.

That should not be surprising, given the lack of research on either the physiological or cognitive aspects of female sexuality. Moreover, for Latinas there is an added dimension to our sexual behavior that current research does not capture. This dimension is made up of the cultural, religious, and spiritual traditions that permeate who we are. It is rooted in the Catholicism that is part of our background regardless of whether we define ourselves as Catholics.

It is unreasonable and unhealthy for us to view ourselves as either Eve or the Virgin Mary. Although we may learn lessons from the mistakes and lives of these women, our sexuality must be defined somewhere between these two extremes. How we define it is often a mystery even to ourselves. Whether we are seventy-five years old or twenty-five, when asked about sex, as Latinas, we simply smile. The smile conveys the whole gamut of experiences from "Yes, I know what sex and pleasure are about" to "Sex was never about pleasure, and I am glad that I no longer have to do it." A smile can say so very much . . . and at the same time it can say nothing at all.

I remember one time you said that since you were a little girl your mother always told you how beau-

tiful you were. That is a rare experience. For most of us, our mothers had such closeted sexual hang-ups they couldn't transfer any positive sexual meanings to their daughters. It took me a long time to deal with my mother's self-image.

—*TERESA, 25*

Do we have good role models of healthy sexuality? Are we free enough from our own issues of self-esteem or early life traumas to fully appreciate our own sexuality? What are the beliefs we have about sexuality? What were the messages we were receiving at the same time that men were getting messages that they should be sexually experienced and knowledgeable?

Sexuality, as an expression of ourselves, occurs at three levels: body, mind, and spirit. Our fulfillment at each of these levels is important to understand, and the fulfillment of all three at the same time can only be described as pure ecstasy. But there is much to discover about ourselves before we experience ecstasy. At a fundamental level, we have to understand the mechanics of sex.

Body

A man looks at and holds his penis several times a day. Since his infancy, his penis has been treated as some sort of magic wand with which he could conquer the world. As a boy, he played with it, gathered in circles with other little boys to pee in unison, and hopefully learned to put the toilet seat down.

Many men even have a nickname for the organ that is between their legs: One-Eyed Giant Squid, Baldheaded Champ, José, Herman, and even The Lizard. The names tend to imply size and strength.

As Latinas, our experience is the total opposite. As young girls, we were always taught to keep ourselves clean and covered. We were told to wipe and flush but never to look at ourselves. And we were *never* supposed to touch ourselves.

Ask a Latina what name she has given to the area between her legs, and she will become uncomfortable. During most of our lives, we have successfully avoided referring to our vulva; we refer instead to "that" part of our body and in most cases have no name for "it" beyond vague references to *ahí abajo* (down there). With a *tú sabes* . . . (you know . . .), we brush off the question of how we refer to our vulva.

In the name of healthy sexuality, we need to feel more comfortable with our bodies. Whatever name we choose for our vulva, the time has come to become familiar with this important part of ourselves.

It is OK to look. There are Latinas who have been sexually active, have had children, and yet have never looked at their bodies. That is something that has to change. The exercise below is a first step in getting better acquainted with your body.

Good health practices require that we know what our vulva looks like when it is healthy so that we can recognize the early signs of any problem. You must become familiar with how your body looks in order to know when something does not seem right.

Exercise: Looking at Our Genitals

You may not be able to do this exercise in one day. So do as much as you are comfortable doing.

In order to look at ourselves carefully, all we need is a room where we can comfortably be nude and a hand-held mirror so that we can see our bodies, our breasts, and what is between our legs.

Follow these simple steps to identify each of the parts of your body that appear in the diagram of the vulva.

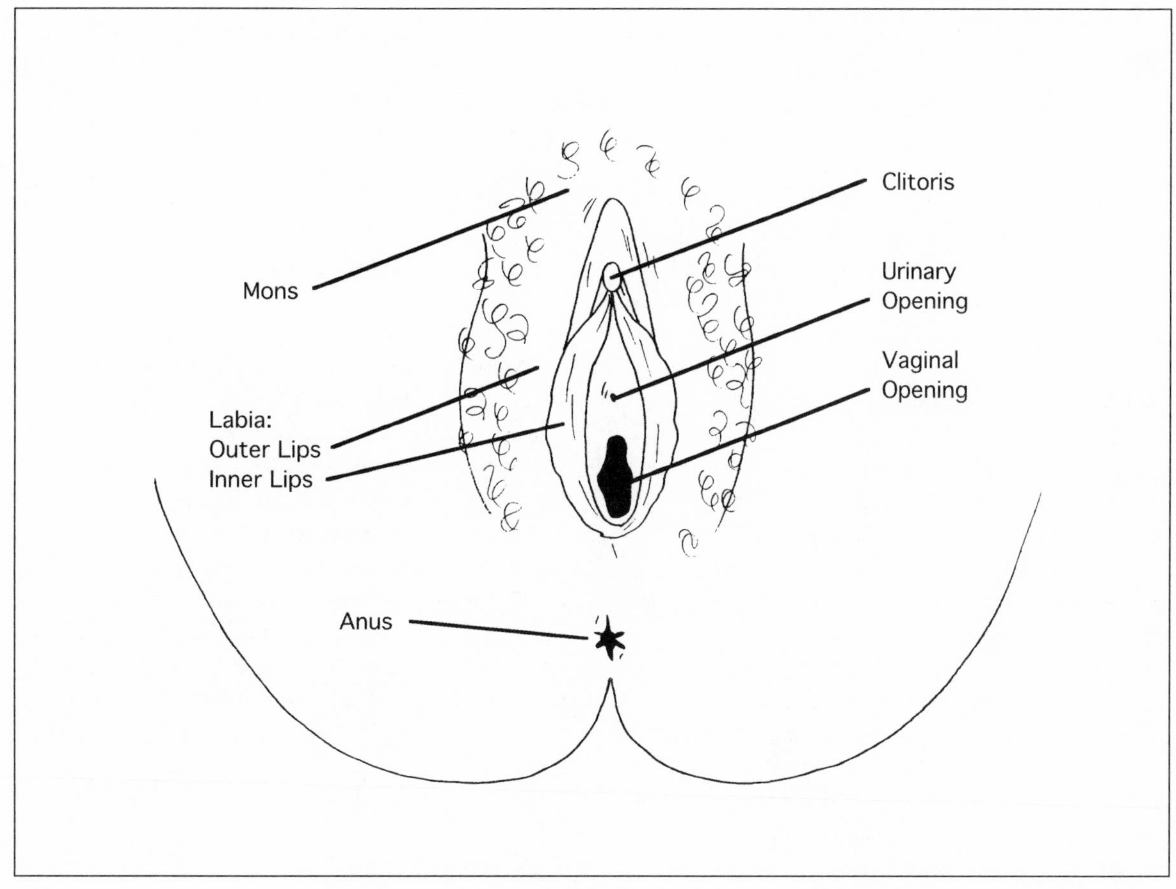

Vulva

1. Take a shower, and do not put your clothes on after you finish. If you feel more comfortable, wrap yourself in a towel, or put a towel around your shoulders to keep yourself warm.
2. Sit at the edge of your bed and spread your legs 2 feet apart.
3. Look down between your legs. Notice how much hair you have. Notice if your hair is straight, curly, or both. This area is called the mons pubis.
4. With one hand, hold the mirror between your legs about 8 inches from your vulva. The word *vulva* comes from the Latin word meaning "covering." This area is highly sensitive to touch. The vulva includes the outer lips (labia majora), inner lips (labia minora), vaginal opening, urinary opening (urethra), and clitoris.
5. With your other hand, spread your labia majora so that you can see what they protect.
6. Try to identify your labia minora, vaginal opening, urethra, and clitoris.
7. Notice how close to each other are the vaginal opening, urethra, and clitoris.
8. Now look at your breasts.
9. Notice the color and texture of your nipples.
10. Now look at your face and smile. Behind

> that face is the most important component of your sexuality and your sexual response—your mind.

Now that we are comfortable looking at ourselves, the next step is to feel comfortable touching ourselves. The best way to understand what arouses each one of us is by talking about one of the major taboos for Latinas—masturbation.

Touching Our Bodies

I can remember the first time I masturbated. I was eleven years old and already was menstruating. I was bathing myself and started to wash "real good" between my legs because I had heard that if you weren't clean, the boys in your class would be able to smell when you had your period. As I pressed the washcloth hard against myself, it began to feel good! The more I rubbed, the more I liked it. So I kept rubbing and rubbing, and in a while I erupted into something so pleasurable that it made me tremble and quiver. I did not know what I had done, but it felt so good that I just knew it had to be a sin. I did not masturbate again until I was thirty-two.

—*Sara, 34*

I still have scars on my back from the beating my mother gave me whenever she found me masturbating.

—*Magda, 54*

When I got married, I didn't know anything and neither did my husband, . . . but we learned [laughter].

–*Jasmin, 63*

As hard as it may be for some of us to accept, Latinas masturbate, just as other women do. It is not something we talk about comfortably, but it is something we do. Ironically, some of the women who masturbate have never looked at their vulva.

Masturbation provides relief for our bodies by reducing the tension that sometimes builds up when we do not have a partner with whom to fully share all aspects of sexuality. Masturbation can also be part of sexual intimacy with a partner.

Satisfying Ourselves

I just use my pillow.

When I check into my hotel, I go to my room and order a hamburger. I then review the selection of adult videos available and decide whether or not I am going to watch one. I then take a shower. By the time room service has arrived, I am feeling more relaxed. I eat my hamburger slowly, and I may watch an adult video too. And once my belly is full, I know it is time to give myself pleasure. I lie back on the bed and begin to caress my body with one hand while the other becomes reacquainted with the pleasure bumps and folds of my vulva.

Now I find myself beginning to get aroused as soon as I order the hamburger [giggles].

—*Esther, 39*

Although some Latinas learned how to masturbate surreptitiously, others have more elaborate scenes that they create to satisfy themselves. For most women, masturbation involves getting into a mind-set that leads to truly focusing on themselves. That, of course, is difficult for some of us. But we can do it.

Masturbation is also a way of learning about your own sexual response—what gives you pleasure. In healthy relationships, your partner will value learning what you enjoy from you.

You can think of masturbation as a process that takes you through the following six levels: Level 1, establish the setting; Level 2, make yourself focus on your body; Level 3, let your hands explore your body; Level 4, focus on what is arousing to you; Level 5, continue to arouse yourself to the point of maximum pleasure; and Level 6, relax.

Depending on your own past experiences, you may be able to go only as far as Level 1, while other Latinas will go through all the levels and repeat them again.

- Level 1: Establish the setting. Think of the settings that make you feel aroused. Perhaps you can escape mentally when you are in your bedroom or taking a bath. For some women it helps to create a routine for masturbating, so that all the elements associated with your pleasure become pleasurable too.
- Level 2: Make yourself focus on your body. You have to clear your mind of all of your thoughts and focus on your body. This may mean that you have to schedule some private time to please yourself.
- Level 3: Let your hands explore your body. You already know where your genitals are, so close your eyes and let your hands touch your body. You may want to use a vibrator (not in the bathtub or shower) or other object to stimulate yourself. All you have to do is allow yourself to touch your body in a variety of ways.
- Level 4: Focus on what is arousing to you. Fantasizing may be helpful. Once you begin to feel aroused, you may want to explore other ways of stimulating yourself. Try to just think about your body and how it feels when you touch it.
- Level 5: Once you have identified your arousal points, continue to arouse yourself to the point of maximum pleasure. You may want to continue until you have an orgasm.
- Level 6: Relax. When you have experienced the degree of arousal you desire, you will find that you can relax.

By going through these levels, you can learn what to tell your partner about what pleases you. You may prefer direct stimulation of the clitoris or just a light pressure in the surrounding areas. Each one of us can learn what makes us feel good.

Although masturbation is part of healthy sexual development, for many of us it is not a permanent substitute for the expression of sexuality that can be enjoyed in a committed monogamous relationship.

Orgasm

I knew I had orgasms. The pleasure was just too intense to miss. I imagined that all women had orgasms in the same way. But then I watched the famous faked orgasm scene in When Harry Meets Sally*. I wondered what that was all about. Why did she bang on the table and make all that noise? Maybe non-Latinas have orgasms in a different way. Mine certainly did not involve all that noise. My orgasms felt like waves of pleasure that reverberated throughout my body until I could not even take the slightest touch as I exploded into feelings of joy and fulfillment.*

—Tensia, 31

I am so embarrassed to have an orgasm. I can't help the sounds I make. It is as if I have to scream out with the overwhelming feelings for which there are no words.

–Amelia, 43

I have had sex with my husband for many years. We have a good sex life, but I do not think I have ever had an orgasm.

–Alina, 46

I can't help the sounds I make, the passion that pumps through my body. I know the children must wonder what are all the muffled sounds they hear in our room. But that is as quiet as I can be.

–Carmen, 34

Orgasm is probably the most frequently discussed aspect of sexuality.

At a physiological level, orgasm occurs as a

result of direct stimulation of the clitoris. Some women have indicated that they prefer vaginal orgasms, yet the limited research that exists indicates that all orgasms are clitoral. For some women, however, the clitoris is stimulated during vaginal penetration in a unique way that increases pleasure.

Physiological Phases of Sex

Often orgasm is seen as the end point of sex, when in fact it is only one of the four major stages in the continuum that makes up sexual activity: initial arousal, plateau, orgasm, and resolution.

Initial Arousal. This phase, which includes foreplay, can last from a few minutes to several hours. Foreplay includes all sorts of activities, from a romantic meal to actual touching. Our bodies signal arousal in a number of ways: our nipples harden, our pupils enlarge, and there is an increase in our heart rate and blood pressure. And it all feels good. We feel happy and wonderful.

Plateau. This phase is actually an intensifying of our initial arousal. Our heart rate increases even more, our breathing is heavier, and we may feel that our bodies begin to tense as we come closer to having an orgasm.

Orgasm. With continued and appropriate stimulation, most women will experience an orgasm. Clinically speaking, an orgasm is described as a series of contractions, but the orgasmic experience can cover the gamut from an explosive release of tension to waves of warmth to involuntary spasmodic movements. Each of these expressions of orgasm is equally valid and pleasurable. An orgasm is pleasure for each one of us in the way we feel most comfortable and satisfied expressing it.

When I was younger and had sex, I thought that it was bad that I could have more than one orgasm and that the man only had one. So I learned to enjoy my orgasms quietly and to myself.

—Eliana, 48

For women, there is often an additional stage, which occurs between orgasm and resolution—further orgasm. It is this capacity to have more than one orgasm that distinguishes the pattern of sexual arousal and response of females from that of males.

There are some women who have never had an orgasm. As many as 95 percent of these women can be helped to achieve orgasm through (1) therapy to understand their feelings about sex and their own self-esteem and (2) training so that they can become comfortable with their own sexuality and communicate their needs more easily. It is important to recognize that physical conditions account for only 5 percent of women who have not had an orgasm.

Resolution. This is when our heart rate slows down and we go back to an unaroused state. Some individuals experience a sense of oneness with their partner; others want to get up and take a shower.

Afterplay. Latinas asked about the phases of sex felt it was important to add a fifth major stage—afterplay. Afterplay is the continued stroking and cuddling that occur after orgasm and resolution. It is the hugging and intimate conversation that emphasize that sexuality involves the mind and the spirit.

What we know is that those who are generous participants in afterplay are rewarded with partners who are more likely to be desirous and responsive in the future.

Orgasms are delightful, but they are part of a continuum of intimacy, which for most of us includes the mind and the spirit.

Body: Myths and Facts

Myth: If you love a man, you can cure his impotence.
Fact: Love alone cannot cure impotence.

If a man is impotent, then he should discuss it with his health care provider to develop a treatment strategy. In many cases, treatment will alleviate the problem.

Myth: Penis size does not count.
Fact: Penis size does count.

The "one size fits all" view of the vagina is a myth. The more Latinas shared with me their experiences, the more obvious it became that a penis can be too big or too small. Each woman has her own range of "just right" sizes. For some women, appropriate size has to do with the ability of the man to stimulate her clitoris during penetration. For other women, it is the angle of penetration as a function of penis size that allows for the most pleasurable clitoral stimulation during penetration. Most important of all, in a loving relationship, couples learn to give each other pleasure in many ways.

Myth: Women with large breasts are more sensitive.
Fact: Breast size is not correlated with sensitivity to sexual stimulation.

The only thing with which breast size is correlated is bra size. Too often we have been made to feel that our breasts or nipples were too small, too large, drooped too much, or had some other quality that made us feel we were lacking, that we were less than complete. In fact, there is no evidence that size of breasts has anything to do with pleasure. What is important is to make sure that your partner handles your breasts in a way that you find pleasurable. Remember that your breasts are meant for mutual pleasure.

To have a healthy, pleasurable sex life:

Consejos

For a Healthy, Pleasurable Sex Life—

1. Talk to your partner about what you like.
2. If something hurts, don't do it.
3. If something feels uncomfortable, don't do it.
4. Be monogamous.
5. If either you or your partner is not monogamous, use a condom.

1: Talk to your partner about what you like. Sex and sexuality require that you share your body, mind, and spirit with your partner. If one of these aspects is missing, you should be honest with yourself about why you are involved in the relationship. If you cannot talk to your partner, it is difficult to have a healthy or happy relationship.

2: If something hurts, don't do it. Sex is supposed to be about pleasure. Let your partner know if it hurts you to engage in certain activities.

3: If something feels uncomfortable, don't do it. You should feel comfortable during sex. If you are uncomfortable, let your partner know. This should make your partner reconsider whatever the two of you are doing. For example, although much is written about mutual oral-genital pleasure (commonly referred to as position 69), the reality is that most couples find this an awkward and thus an unsatisfying activity. Much more satisfying is alternating giving each other oral-genital pleasure.

4: Be monogamous. Persons who are monogamous tend to have better and more frequent sex. The reasons are fairly self-evident in that monogamy is a means of establishing commitment, and commitment is the key to fully enjoying the cognitive and spiritual aspects of sex.

5: If either you or your partner is not monogamous, use a condom. Given the severe danger posed by sexually transmitted diseases, it is important to use a condom. If your partner cannot make the commitment to being monogamous, at the very least he should care enough about you to use a condom. If your partner is not monogamous and refuses to wear a condom, you should consider whether you are willing to lose your life or risk your health by having unprotected sex. Even if both partners are now monogamous, they must remember that they are going to bed with a history, i.e., all the previous partners.

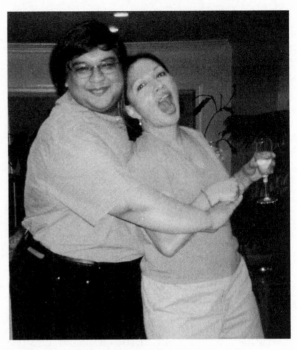

Pleasure and fun do not mean that you must be involved sexually.

Mind

The largest sex organ is the brain, and the most potent aphrodisiac is your mind. It is in the cognitive area that there is the greatest difference between men and women. For women, arousal is much more cognitive than we are led to believe. This difference is exemplified in the relatively new field of female-oriented erotic movies, which tend to have romance and story lines, as compared to male-oriented movies, which focus more on nudity.

What you think about yourself and your partner determines how much pleasure you will have. If you like and love your partner, sexuality is a way of expressing that intimacy in a nonverbal way. How well your partner treats you, whether your partner focuses on your pleasure, and all the other aspects of intimacy determine whether you will be able to enjoy sex with your partner.

There is a myth that if we love somebody, they will instinctively know how to give us sexual pleasure. The reality is that no one is a mind reader in such circumstances, and it is very natural, even desirable, to teach your partner what you enjoy.

This is particularly important for women because the ability to experience orgasm is more complex in females than in males. This does not mean that you should just give up or that you should come prepared with a flip chart of your preferences and a diagram of the vulva. It means that you have to talk to your partner. This may seem difficult or embarrassing, but if you are comfortable enough to have sex with someone, you should be able to talk to them about what you enjoy and do not enjoy.

If you feel more comfortable with less direct means of communicating your desires, you can try guiding your partner's hand to those parts of your body that are more sensitive. You can also shift your body to improve the angle of penetration. Your responses and the sounds you make will be your partner's best indicator of what you prefer.

MIND: MYTHS AND FACTS

Myth: All women should want to give oral-genital pleasure (fellatio).

Fact: Giving oral-genital pleasure is a matter of choice.

Some women do not feel comfortable giving their partner oral-genital pleasure. As in most aspects of sexuality, although you may want to try new things, if you do not like to do something, you should not do it. Sexuality is supposed to be a mutually satisfying activity.

Myth: All men want to receive oral-genital pleasure.

Fact: Most men enjoy receiving oral-genital pleasure and are typically quite enthusiastic in their praise and appreciation of their partner's efforts.

Some men do not enjoy receiving oral sex, however—they also tend to be the ones who do not like giving their partners oral-genital pleasure.

Myth: If you truly love someone, semen will taste good.

Fact: There is great variability in the taste of semen.

Although love may suppress our visual sense, as in "love is blind," it does not change our sense of taste. Latinas have stated that although they may love their partners, semen is not always on their list of the most appetizing or flavorful substances.

Myth: Men do not enjoy giving oral-genital pleasure (cunnilingus).

Fact: Most men enjoy giving oral-genital pleasure.

As Latinas, we are so used to giving that receiving oral-genital pleasure is difficult for some of us to accept. Some of us, however, have learned to appreciate oral-genital pleasure and to take it for what it is—a wonderful way to show love and trust. Your partner should be concerned about your enjoyment and attentive to your response in order to improve his technique.

Myth: You can tell when your partner has been unfaithful.

Fact: Partners who cheat know how to lie.

By their very nature, unfaithful partners lead triple, not just double, lives. They lie to us, they lie to their other partners, and they lie to themselves. When you lie that much, you get good at it. No matter how much you love someone, if they have been with someone else and want to hide it from you, they will. That is a lesson many of us have learned only too painfully. To avoid this pain, some of us may have ended up lying to ourselves instead, as we try to pretend that we do not see that there is a *casa grande* and a *casa pequeña* (a big house for the family and a small house for the "other" partner), regardless of which *casa* may be ours.

Myth: As you get older, you get less interested in sex.

Fact: Age is not a predictor of one's interest in sex.

Studies showing that with increased age there is less sexual activity have often failed to take some intervening factors into account. One such factor is the impact of menopause: women going through menopause may experience a period of time when there is less sexual activity, but they typically resume an active sex life after going through the changes. Another factor is that there may be fewer available older partners. The availability of partners may limit options for older women who are looking for mates their age or older. The solution to the smaller pool is simple: women should consider younger partners. Or women should reevaluate what they need to do for themselves in order that they may feel sexual *and* sensual.

When I speak about being sensual rather than sexual, I am talking about another aspect of the mind component. I have had women correct me by saying "You mean sensual,*" and they were right. The physical act of sex has nothing to do with what I am talking about, and Latinas should feel comfortable with themselves (body and all) without thinking about sex per se.*

—*Sofia, 55*

Spirit

I thought that when I had sex with someone I would see angels, but I didn't.

—*Alexandra, 28*

Of the many Latinas who shared their experiences, some felt that sex with their partners had gone beyond the physical and mental aspects and into a realm of intimacy that was beyond words. This makes it difficult to fully describe the experience. Nevertheless, there were some similarities in what was described.

Contrary to what the media portray, this type of intimacy did not necessarily require any special sexual gymnastics. That is, sex did not involve hanging from the chandeliers or rolling in the sand on the beach (which in reality ends up getting sand in the most uncomfortable places). What was involved was a deep sense of commitment, which transcended the day-to-day lives of the couple. The bonds that were reinforced through the mutual expression of sexuality generated the type of ecstasy that is only achieved in the total freedom of a committed monogamous relationship.

Spirit: Myths and Facts

Myth: The Catholic Church says you should not enjoy sex.
Fact: The Catholic Church says you should enjoy sex.

Too often Latinas feel that sexuality is their obligation and duty as wives. It is something they do because it is expected of them and is part of their childbearing responsibility. But sexuality is more than childbearing. It is also a means of expressing deep love and devotion. At its most powerful, it is a union of the mind and the spirit. That is why it should not be surprising that the new 1994 Catechism of the Catholic Church states, "Sexuality is a source of joy and pleasure" (The Love of Husband and Wife section, part 2362).

Myth: Foreplay is not important.
Fact: Foreplay and afterplay are extremely important.

A recent survey of men indicated that the average male spent 10 minutes having sex. I do not know with whom these men were having these 10-minute encounters, but in all likelihood 10 minutes was not enough for their female partners to fulfill their physical needs. To fulfill the spirit's needs, we need the time and affection involved in foreplay and afterplay.

Women enjoy not only overt sexual foreplay, but also all the romance and courtship that surrounds lovemaking. Even after decades with the same partner, an act of tenderness can make our hearts dance again.

We often have to remind our partners of how much we value afterplay and foreplay. Foreplay and afterplay encompass all the affection, hugging, kissing, stroking, laughing, and massaging that demonstrate our affection. Touching each other with our hands, bodies, and tongues is what ignites the fire within us. The chemistry between two totally committed partners can produce a sensation to the skin that is electrifying.

Summary

Latinas must recognize the historical factors and lack of scientific inquiry that have limited what we know about women and sexuality. The role of sex and our own sexuality must be clearly defined. These are not things we can hide from, but aspects of being human that we must celebrate.

As uncomfortable as it is for many of us to admit, masturbation is an important part of normal human sexual development. It is how we learn about our own sexual response so that we can share our knowledge about ourselves with our partner.

We also need to understand sexuality in terms of body, mind, and spirit. To do this requires recognizing that there is a continuum, from knowing our own arousal to afterplay. Finally, when there is complete commitment between partners, the experience of sexuality is about our body, mind, and spirit working together to produce a state of ecstasy.

RESOURCES

Organizations

American Association of Sex Educators, Counselors and Therapists
P.O. Box 238
Mount Vernon, IA 52314-0238
www.aasect.org

American College of Obstetricians and Gynecologists
409 12th Street SW
Washington, DC 20090-6920
(202) 638-5577 or (800) 762-2264
www.acog.org

National Latino/a Lesbian, Gay, Bisexual, and Transgender Organization
1612 K Street NW, Suite 500
Washington, DC 20006
(202) 466-8240
www.llego.org

Sexuality Information and Education Council of the United States
130 W. 42nd Street, Suite 350
New York, NY 10036-7802
(212) 819-9770
www.siecus.org

Books

Comfort, Alex. *The New Joy of Sex* and *More Joy of Sex*. New York: Pocket Books/Simon & Schuster, 1998.

Fischman, Yael. *El Lenguaje de la Sexualidad Para la Mujer y la Pareja*. San Francisco: Volcano Press, 1992.

Kitzinger, Sheila. *Women's Experience of Sex: A New Approach. The Facts and Feelings of Female Sexuality at Every Stage of Life*. New York: Penguin Books, 1985.

Westheimer, Ruth. *Dr. Ruth's Encyclopedia of Sex*. New York: Continuum, 2000.

6

Common Problems

Elena did not like having to go for her annual pelvic exam. She knew exactly what it would be like. It was always the same.

She'd be asked to undress from her waist down. Usually someone would give her a "modesty cover" so that she could cover her naked belly. That always amazed Elena. "How could anyone ever be modest in this situation?" she wondered.

Then Elena would undress as directed and lie on the table. She hated the way it felt to be so exposed—her legs would be spread apart, and there would be more bright lights on than she would ever let shine on her nakedness.

Elena closed her eyes, thinking of how humiliating it still felt to have her most private parts seemingly on display on the table. It didn't matter that she did this every year or that she knew that her health care provider saw upwards of thirty women a day from this unique angle.

As she placed her feet in the stirrups, she could feel how they directed the angle of her legs even further apart. The health care provider would soon come in and poke around and press down on her belly. Then he would use the cold ducklike thing to expose her insides even more. Then he would stick some long cotton swabs inside of her. She didn't actually feel when he did that, but he always described what he was doing.

Elena sighed when it was over. She did not like going for either her pelvic exam or her Pap test. But she did. Elena didn't have cancer in her family and intended to keep it that way. She knew that an annual Pap test was something she had to do.

Vaginitis, fibroids, ovarian cysts, endometriosis, premenstrual syndrome (PMS), hysterectomy—when you talk to Latinas, it is obvious that we seem to have more gynecological problems than other women. At the same time, we have to understand that our health care providers will not always have the answers to our problems or may not be able to give us the answer we want. There is much to share with each other and with our health care provider so that together we can take better care of our bodies. Things do go wrong with our reproductive system, and we must learn to be alert to early signs so that we can work with our health care provider to make things right.

Too often we take better care of our nails, hair, and teeth than we do of our reproductive system. Preventive and ongoing maintenance of all parts of our bodies is essential, yet research shows that Latinas are not taking even the most basic measures to protect their reproductive health. Latinas have the highest rates of infertility, the highest rates of cervical cancer, increasing rates of untreated sexually transmitted diseases, and we are less likely than non-Latinas to get a Pap test.

The low rates of Pap tests and our lower rates of prenatal care suggest that we do not visit our health care providers for the most routine of procedures. Latinas say that they only see a health care provider if they are sick. Yet the concept of wellness visits in the form of well baby clinics is something we readily accept for children. We must also acknowledge that we too need wellness visits. That is what taking care of ourselves is all about. If the concept of taking care of yourself seems selfish to you, consider that if you don't keep yourself well, you can't take care of anyone else who might need you. There is a lot for us to learn so that we can take care of ourselves.

At a minimum, to maintain our overall health, we Latinas need to see our primary health care provider once a year. This is true whether or not you still have sexual relations. You also need to see your health care provider regularly if you have stopped having your period. Remember that cervical, ovarian, and uterine cancer are most common in women over sixty years of age.

If you have had a hysterectomy, depending on the kind it was, you may or may not need a Pap test. Whether or not you need a Pap test will be determined by your health care provider. Nevertheless, at the very least, all women over eighteen, as well as those under eighteen who are sexually active, need a pelvic and Pap exam on an annual basis.

Scheduling Your Annual Pelvic Exam and Pap Test

When trying to decide on a good time to schedule our Pap test, we normally focus on when it is convenient for us and when there is an appointment available in our health care provider's practice. That is the wrong way to go about it.

We need to schedule our visit in order to get the best sample of cervical cells. To obtain an accurate sampling of cells from your cervix, you should not schedule your Pap test during your menstrual cycle. The ideal time is 10 to 20 days after the first day of your menstrual cycle.

If you have an infection, remember that the infection must be cured before you have your Pap test. If it is not cured, you will have to redo the test. Also keep in mind that you should not use creams, douches, or birth control foams during the two days prior to your exam. The use of these substances makes it harder to find abnormal cells.

The Pelvic Exam

The actual pelvic exam including Pap exam takes only a few minutes and should not be painful. There are seven key steps to a pelvic exam and Pap test.

1: Making you feel comfortable. At the outset, your health care providers should do whatever they can to make you feel comfortable. Some may dim the lights in the room and use a more focused and brighter light on the areas being examined.

2: Looking at the outside. The health care provider will first look at the outside (vulva) to see if there are any growths or abnormalities.

3: Inserting the speculum to widen the opening of the vagina. Some health care providers place the speculum in warm water so that it is not cold. The placing of the speculum and the widening of the opening of the vagina are usually done in a gentle manner.

4: Getting a sample of cells from the cervix. Once the opening of the vagina is widened, the health care provider may use a tiny brush and tiny spatula to obtain cells from the cervix.

If a colposcopy examination is also performed, the following additional steps occur:

- Your health care provider will use a large cotton swab to liberally coat the vagina and cervix with 5% acetic acid (common table vinegar).
- The lights in the room will be dimmed.
- Your health care provider will wait at least 60 seconds after coating the vagina and cervix and then look at the coated areas using a low-powered magnification source to identify any signs of abnormal cell growth.
- The lights in the room will be adjusted to their normal position and the speculum removed.

5: Examining the vaginal area with a gloved hand. Your health care provider will then insert two gloved fingers into your vagina and with the other hand feel through your abdomen from the outside to feel if there are any lumps or if you experience pain. Some tenderness is usually expected.

6: Performing a rectal exam. Using one gloved finger, your health care provider will examine your rectum for any obvious abnormalities.

7: Then it is over. You will be given a tissue to wipe yourself and remove any lubricants that may have been used to make the examination more comfortable for you. Then you will be asked to get dressed. At the very least, you should congratulate yourself for having taken a giant step toward maintaining your wellness.

Results of Your Pap Test

When was the last time you called your health care provider and asked for the results of your Pap test? Too many of us assume that no news is good news. If we are to take control of our own health, we have to learn to ask questions and listen to the responses.

Remember that it is best to write the answers down. Do not feel that you have to listen and respond at the same time. Writing the answer down will give you an opportunity to think about what you were told. You can always call back if you later realize there is something you do not understand.

Key Questions

1. What did you find?
2. What does that mean?
3. What do you recommend I do next?

Always end by saying, "Thank you!"

1: What did you find? In most cases, you will be told that your test results were normal and that you should come back in a year for your next Pap test. You may be told, however, that the test results were not normal. In this case you can proceed with questions 2 and 3, as appropriate.

2: What does that mean? A Pap test identifies changes in cells and helps detect when these changes indicate a precancerous or cancerous condition. In 10 to 15 percent of Pap tests, the results indicate atypical squamous cells of unknown significance (ASCUS). This means that the Pap test needs to be repeated because what was found was not usual (atypical), and the meaning of this is unclear (unknown significance).

3: What do you recommend I do next? If your Pap test results are not normal, your health care provider will probably want to obtain more information to further understand what is going on.

Common Problems

Marlene had always had strange menstrual cycles. Her periods were very irregular and so light that all she ever had to use was a panty liner.

The surgery was supposed to help her have easier periods, but it didn't help very much. Her surgeon also told her that her uterus was tipped and that he had sewn it so that it would now point in the right direction. Marlene didn't know what it all meant. She was twenty-one and had full confidence in the surgeon because he was a friend of the family.

Now, at twenty-seven, Marlene was reconsidering her surgery and her surgeon. She was having more severe cramps, and whenever her period decided to show up it was still very light. She decided it was time to find her own gynecologist and talk to that person directly.

The first doctor she saw told her to take birth control pills to regulate her period and that would take care of the pain. She decided to be a good consumer and get a second opinion.

The second doctor said that since the pain was so severe, there was a nerve he could sever so that she would no longer experience pain. That made her nervous, so she decided to get another opinion. She had obviously picked the wrong health care provider to give her a second opinion.

A third doctor told her that surgery was her only choice because he could feel that she had tumors and that she probably had adhesions from her earlier surgery. The idea of surgery again was unappealing, so she went to a fourth doctor. His recommendation was that she should learn to live with the pain and be happy that her periods were light.

Marlene had gone to four doctors, and no two of them had given the same recommendation. Marlene was more confused than when she started. So she just did nothing.

Much of what we know about the reproductive systems of healthy women is limited because until recently we did not have the diagnostic procedures to look inside the body without making an incision. Surgery was performed on women who were having symptoms, often without clear proof that such an intrusive procedure was necessary. As ultrasound and other less invasive procedures have advanced our knowledge, we have learned more about the natural changes in our reproductive system.

We have also made progress in understanding the role of hormones in controlling our very sophisticated internal reproductive organs, although we still have much to learn. For example, estrogen is crucial for stimulating changes in the lining of the uterus to produce a surface on which a fertilized egg can implant itself. Estrogen also maintains the right conditions for the uterus throughout pregnancy.

While we know that emotions and stress may change the regular menstrual cycle (i.e., the way our hormones work), we have not documented the mechanism that connects our mind, hormones, and body.

Unfortunately, most of us became adults believing and expecting that the only thing that was supposed to grow in our reproductive system was a baby and that if anything else was growing in there it was cancer and we would die. It is not surprising that when we are told that something is growing in our uterus or on any of our reproductive organs, we are paralyzed with fear.

As a result, sometimes when there are

Consejos

What to Expect with Ultrasound

Ultrasound is a relatively safe way to look at your reproductive system. The most difficult part of this test is that you will be given lots of water to drink until your bladder is full, and you will not be allowed to go to the bathroom until the procedure is over. Although this is uncomfortable, it is bearable and not painful.

You will be asked to take off your clothes from the waist down and to put on a gown. After you drink the water, you will be asked to wait a few minutes. You will then be brought into a room and asked to lie down. A lotion will be applied to your belly, and then the technician will move a wand on your belly. As the sound waves bounce off the belly, a picture appears on the screen. If the bladder is not sufficiently full, you will be given more water to drink.

Another method of ultrasound involves inserting another kind of wand (a transducer) through the vagina. Both of these procedures are painless and produce minimal discomfort.

symptoms we try to minimize their significance. Too often we just leave things alone, hoping they will get better on their own, and in the process pass by all the advances in science that have benefited other women. We cannot do that anymore.

Ignorance and denial only make any problem we might be having worse; often the problem is less serious than we feared, and the knowledge that our condition is treatable can be a tremendous load off our minds. By being well informed about the most common problems with our reproductive system and understanding the possible solutions, we *can* make things right.

Vaginitis

Teresa did not normally look at herself down there—after all, what was the point of that? She knew what was there. She had had three children.

But she had become so very itchy, and today she had some sort of discharge on her panties. In a moment of desperation, Teresa took a mirror in her hand and spread her legs to see what was happening.

What she saw in the mirror was not what she expected. Her cosita *(little thing) was red and raw. She was so embarrassed. "Yes," Teresa thought to herself, "I have something there . . . but how could I?"*

Teresa had no idea how she had gotten whatever she had, but she knew that she had something.

The vagina is more than just an opening. It is a home to healthy and naturally occurring fungi, bacteria, and other substances that a well-functioning body keeps in balance. When these substances are in balance, they work together to make sure that the vagina is clean and free of infection. The balance may be easily disrupted by a variety of factors, however, such as stress, medication, and douches. If we women were born with an instruction manual for our bodies, one of its first statements would be "It is extremely likely that we will experience vaginitis at least several times in our life."

There are no exact numbers on how many women have vaginitis, but look in any pharmacy and you will see an abundance of over-the-counter medicines that claim to prevent, treat, and manage all types of vaginitis. You can be certain that at some point you will have the major symptoms of vaginitis, itchiness or

> *Consejos*
>
> **Know Your Healthy Scent**
>
> It is a natural part of being a woman that our vagina emits a mild scent. You should be able to recognize your healthy scent. To maintain it, it is important to keep your vulva clean and dry. Trying to cover or mask your healthy scent may actually cause a problem because some of the chemicals in soaps, douches, or deodorized products can upset the delicate balance that exists in your vagina.
>
> You should be aware of when your scent changes or becomes unpleasant. That may be a signal that the balance in your vagina is upset.
>
> Remember that your healthy scent is a natural and appealing part of your sexuality.

irritation around your vulva, and sometimes it will be accompanied by a discharge.

Vaginitis is a symptom, not a disease. There are many reasons why we may have vaginitis. To get better, we need to be able to identify the source of the irritation.

Vaginitis may be caused by infections or be a side effect of some medications. Chemical irritants, certain health problems (such as diabetes), or some natural changes in your hormonal balance can also cause vaginitis. The most common reason for vaginitis, however, is infection. Excluding sexually transmitted diseases (Chapter 18), there are three major types of infection: yeast infections, bacterial infections, and trichomoniasis.

Yeast Infections

Yeast infections, also known as candidiasis, are one of the most common vaginal infections. They occur when the environment in your vagina changes and encourages the few yeast that are naturally there to reproduce in greater numbers than usual. The change may be due to diabetes, pregnancy, or an immune system that is not working properly. The most common cause, however, is being given antibiotics to take care of a problem in some other part of your body. The antibiotics that attack the bad bacteria that cause an infection in one part of your body can kill the good bacteria in your vagina and allow yeast to flourish.

A yeast infection typically results in itchiness, redness, and a burning sensation. If there is a discharge, it usually has no odor and is white. Although there are many yeast treatments that can be bought without a prescription, you should see your health care provider if you:

- Have never had these symptoms before
- Are worried that you may have been exposed to a sexually transmitted disease
- Used an over-the-counter treatment, but the symptoms have not gone away
- Have a discharge that has an odor and is yellow or green

The treatment of yeast infections is usually successful, but some yeast infections seem to resist treatment. Your health care provider may need to treat you with different types of medications and for an extended period of time.

Bacterial Infections

Bacterial vaginitis (i.e., bacterial vaginosis, nonspecific vaginitis, or Gardnerella vaginilis) occurs when there is an overproduction of bacteria that are naturally found in the vagina.

A bacterial infection is recognized by a thin, watery, grayish-white or yellow discharge, which often has a fishy odor that is more noticeable after vaginal intercourse. Other symptoms include mild burning or irritation. You do not usually have redness or itchiness.

Like most bacterial infections, bacterial vaginitis is treated with antibiotics. It is most likely that you will be prescribed either metronidazole or clindamycin in pill form. Alternatively, both of these antibiotics may be prescribed in a gel form that is placed directly in the vagina.

Very often there will be a need for repeat treatments. While under treatment, you should either not have vaginal intercourse or use a condom.

Trichomoniasis

Trichomoniasis, or trich, is caused by a tiny one-celled organism. Most women get trich from having unprotected vaginal intercourse with men who carry the organism. In most instances, men have no symptoms.

Your symptoms include a yellowish-gray discharge that has an unpleasant odor; burning, redness, swelling, and a tendency for symptoms to become severe before and after you menstruate. There may also be some burning during urination.

Both you and your partner should be treated with metronidazole. If the symptoms do not go away, you may have to take larger doses of the medication.

Other Causes

Sometimes the nice-smelling things that are sold to make us feel clean are the very things that may give us vaginitis. Each one of us is different, so one of us may find a particular soap or sanitary napkin to be wonderful while for someone else it upsets the natural environment of the vagina and leads to vaginitis.

The changes that we go through during menopause, pregnancy, and even as a result of stress may all change the balance in our vagina. And of course in some instances, the symptoms of vaginitis may also be due to sexually transmitted diseases (see Chapter 18). It is important to consult your health care provider about any recurring vaginal irritations.

Consejos

How to Reduce the Chances of Getting Vaginitis

1. Keep your vulva clean and dry by washing with water and mild soap.
2. Try not to trap moisture near your vaginal opening. Wear cotton panties or pantyhose with a cotton crotch. Avoid pants so tight that air cannot circulate (i.e., your vagina cannot get air).
3. When you use toilet paper, wipe yourself from the front (vaginal opening) to the back (rectum) to prevent infecting your vagina with bacteria from your rectum or feces.
4. When antibiotics are prescribed for you, ask your health care provider how you can decrease the likelihood that you will get a yeast infection. In some instances your health care provider may recommend that you use an over-the-counter yeast medicine as a preventive measure.
5. Do not use scented or deodorized tampons, sanitary napkins, douches, toilet paper, or hygienic sprays.
6. Make sure that whatever objects you insert into your vagina (e.g., diaphragms, applicators, sex toys) are cleaned after use and stored in a sanitary place.
7. If you are not in a long-term, mutually monogamous relationship, you should use condoms and consult your health care provider about any recurring irritations.

Uterine Fibroids

Fibroids (fibromyomas, leiomyomas, myomas, or myofibromas) sound a lot worse than they actually are. Uterine fibroids are noncancerous tumors that grow on the inside, outside, or within the walls of the uterus. Although they may grow and get bigger, they do not change into cancer. The one exception is that 3 out of 1,000 women with fibroids will also have a rare uterine cancer, which on an ultrasound examination looks like a fibroid.

While the vast majority of fibroids are not dangerous, in some cases they can cause a change in the shape of the uterus. This is a problem only when the change is so great that the uterus presses on other nearby organs, causing pain. At least half of all women have fibroids, and the majority of women who have them never know that they are there. Most fibroids shrink or disappear after menopause.

There is no specific information about Latinas and fibroids. We do know that African-American women are much more likely to get them than non–African-American women.

Diagnosis

Some women with fibroids complain of heavy and irregular periods or of pain around their internal organs. In doing your pelvic exam, your health care provider may find that you have fibroids. At that point it may be suggested that you have an ultrasound to make sure that it in fact is a fibroid. The ultrasound picture of what was felt during the pelvic exam will show whether it is a fibroid, cyst, or some other type of growth. The presence of fibroids is not a major cause of infertility, although sometimes fibroids may grow within the uterus and create problems during pregnancy.

Treatment

For most women with fibroids, no treatment is necessary. When treatment is called for, it is typically geared to reducing the heavy menstrual bleeding that is found with fibroids. Only twenty years ago, women with fibroids were routinely recommended for hysterectomy, even when the fibroid was not causing any symptoms.

Medication

New research shows that the growth of fibroids may have something to do with the production of estrogen and/or progesterone. The use of medication to temporarily suppress the production of estrogen induces a pseudo-menopause (see Chapter 9) that makes the fibroids shrink in size. There has been some success in reducing pain and bleeding with the use of synthetic versions of gonadotropin-releasing hormone (a hormone released by the hypothalamus, which stimulates the pituitary gland) agonists (brand names Lupron, Synarel).

Surgery

In severe cases of pain or bleeding, surgery may be recommended. The size and location of the fibroids will determine the surgical procedure that is recommended.

For women who may still want to have children, surgery may be limited to removing tumors. A hysterectomy may be recommended for women who do not want to have children. This surgery may be done in a variety of ways—conventional abdominal surgery, hysteroscopy (entering through the vagina into the uterus), or laparoscopy (see pages 86–87).

Ovarian Cysts

Ovarian cysts are common and found in most women. Cysts are saclike structures filled with fluid. As part of ovulation, your body naturally produces some cystlike structures. If these structures do not disintegrate during the menstrual cycle, they are called functional cysts.

Functional cysts are a normal part of your system. They usually do not cause pain and consequently do not require treatment. Most functional cysts disappear within three menstrual cycles. While commonly found in women who menstruate, they are rare among women who have reached menopause or who use oral contraceptives.

Abnormal cysts may cause pain, discomfort, or irregular periods. Even though they are usually noncancerous (benign), they require some sort of treatment to reduce the discomfort and careful examination to make sure that they are not cancerous (malignant).

There are four kinds of abnormal cysts: dermoid, cystadenoma, endometrioma, and polycystic ovarian disease.

Dermoid cysts are filled with different kinds of tissues, including hair, teeth, and bone. These tissues are not a by-product of a missed pregnancy but result from the woman's body giving cells in the cyst the wrong message as to what they should become, so they develop into hair, teeth, and bone.

Cystadenoma cysts are produced by cells that are on the surface of the ovary.

An endometrioma (sometimes called an endometrial cyst or chocolate cyst) is a cyst formed by endometrial tissue (i.e., the tissue that forms the inside lining of the uterus). These are found in women who are diagnosed with endometriosis (more on this on page 81). These cysts are filled with blood, which darkens over time and imparts a deep reddish-brown (chocolate color). An endometrioma may range from the size of a pea to larger than a grapefruit.

In polycystic ovarian disease, the single cystlike follicle that is released during healthy ovulation is not released. They accumulate, covering the outside of the ovary.

Consejos

When the Words Are Not as Bad as They Sound

Dysmenorrhea: You have cramps when you menstruate.
Primary dysmenorrhea: When you first menstruated you had bad cramps, but as you got older, and especially after you had children, the cramps went away.
Secondary dysmenorrhea: When you were in your twenties or later you began to get menstrual cramps.

Diagnosis

Latinas who have symptoms usually describe a constant pain that feels like soreness on the inside. In a few cases ovarian cysts may also cause pain during intercourse. Some Latinas say that their stomachs get distended, while others indicate that they have severe cramps during their periods. Periods are usually irregular.

There are three ways to diagnose ovarian cysts: a pelvic exam, ultrasound, or laparoscopy. In some instances your health care provider may feel a cyst as part of your pelvic exam. If there is reason to believe that you have a cyst, you will be sent for an ultrasound exam. Ultrasound may provide details on the type, size, and location of cysts.

Laparoscopy is usually done as both a diagnostic procedure and as an intervention. You should discuss with your health care provider the two major options you have:

1. Diagnostic only: Your surgeon looks inside at your reproductive system and makes a definitive diagnosis. After surgery, you and your health care provider make a decision about the best way to proceed.

2. Diagnostic and intervention: After diagnosis, your surgeon treats the condition by removal of your ovary(ies), cysts, or other damaged structures. Before you have your laparoscopy, you need to have a discussion with your health care provider about what you would agree to have removed after a diagnosis is made (in other words, what may be removed during the laparoscopy).

Treatment

There is great variability in treatment, depending on you (your age, health, choices about fertility, and the size, type, and location of the cyst) and your health care provider (training and expertise). Here are some of the options.

1. No treatment: Since functional cysts disappear within three menstrual cycles, your health care provider may decide to wait and see what happens.

> *Consejos*
>
> **Take Time to Heal Fully—Laparoscopic Surgery Is Hard on the Body**
>
> Too often women believe that the invasiveness of surgery is mainly a function of how large an incision is made. This common sense would imply that laparoscopic surgery, with its little incisions, requires no recovery time. Although the recovery period is shorter for most procedures, it still requires time to heal. Don't be fooled by looking at the surface of your body—your skin—the fact is that most of the work was done under your skin and requires a lot more healing time than is apparent.
>
> So be sure that if you have laparoscopic surgery, you give your insides time to heal, no matter how good your outside may look.

2. Hormonal treatment: Oral contraceptives are sometimes successful in shrinking cysts. Some research suggests that they also reduce the likelihood of cysts that are cancerous.
3. Surgery: Surgery is recommended when the cyst is large or is twisted (referred to as "torsion"). Surgery may also be recommended for women who experience severe pain or have completed menopause.

   The extent of the surgery may involve removing the cyst, part or all of an ovary, or the uterus. Make sure you talk to your doctor and give written instructions about what you prefer not to have removed.

Endometriosis

The pain felt like a knife twisting in my ovaries up into my stomach. I would be unable to move—scared that something inside would burst. Sometimes days would go by between attacks, sometimes weeks or months, but the pain always came back.

The first doctor I saw diagnosed an infection and gave me antibiotics. They didn't help. The next doctor offered the same pills. He, too, thought I had a sexually transmitted disease. Because I'm Hispanic, he probably assumed I had many sex partners. "Only one," I insisted, but no one ever seemed to believe me.

I saw a third doctor and a fourth. When the fifth man handed me yet another prescription for antibiotics, I had had enough. Like most Latinas, I was raised to defer to authority, but by then I was sure I didn't have an infection. I knew that there was something very wrong with me.

I insisted on a laparoscopy to find out what was wrong. When I woke up from surgery, my surgeon said in a light manner, "No wonder you were in such pain. You have a tumor the size of a small grapefruit and endometriosis."

—Lisa, 26

If you talk to your Latina friends and family, you may be surprised to find how many of them have been diagnosed with endometriosis. There are no national or state data that tell us how many Latinas have endometriosis. What we know about endometriosis we know from how the disease acts in the general population.

Endometriosis is when the endometrium, the tissue that forms the inner lining of the uterus, spreads and grows (implants itself) in other nearby structures—the lining of the pelvic cavity, the outer surface of the uterus, the internal area between the vagina and rectum, the ovaries, and the fallopian tubes. In rare cases, the tissue may grow on the intestines, rectum, bladder, vagina, cervix, or vulva or in scars from abdominal surgery.

Regardless of where it grows, the implant acts like the endometrial tissue that is in the uterus: it responds to the hormonal cycle. As part of the hormonal cycle, the endometrium grows and thickens (from roughly day 5 through day 14) and prepares itself for implantation by a fertilized egg (days 14 through 17). If there is no fertilized egg, hormones induce the endometrium to break apart, bleed, and be released by the 28th day. The endometrial cells are also responsible for production of prostaglandins. Prostaglandins are the chemicals that make the uterus contract, resulting in menstrual cramps.

I was a young woman when I was first diagnosed with endometriosis. I had no idea what it was then, and I really do not know everything I probably should know about it now. After all the treatment and all the surgery, it is still with me.

I even have a nickname for when I can feel it. At those times I grimace and tell myself that the pain in me is only "Endo" acting up again.

I know it is not going to kill me, and hopefully when I go through menopause it will just go away.

—*Priscilla, 42*

Consejos

Use a Sanitary Napkin Instead of a Tampon

Given the backup theory of endometriosis, it is recommended that women use sanitary napkins rather than tampons whenever possible. This allows for the natural flowing out of the endometrial tissue.

Changes in the endometrium occur every month, wherever there is endometrial tissue. While the endometrium in the uterus is released as menstruation, the blood from the endometrium that grows in other parts of the body has no place to go. The misplaced endometrial tissue also produces prostaglandins. As a result, nearby tissues become swollen and inflamed, which over time creates scar tissue.

Some scar tissue (adhesions) tends to be weblike and may connect or cover some of the pelvic structures. Other scar tissues develop and may take several forms: small superficial patches (lesions or implants), thicker patches that penetrate the area where they are growing (nodules), or cysts or growths (endometriomas).

There are three major theories about the cause of endometriosis: genetic predisposition, backup of menstrual tissue, and delayed childbearing.

- The genetic predisposition theory states that endometriosis is a condition that is passed on within a family.
- The backup theory states that some of the endometrial tissue flows back into the body instead of being released as menstruation. The reason for this is not certain, although it is suspected that it may be due to changes in the immune system.

- The delayed childbearing theory suggests that as part of pregnancy, hormones are released that protect women from getting endometriosis. Women who do not have children or who delay childbearing may not have the benefits of this protection.

Even though there are many theories, the actual cause of endometriosis is still not known. What we do know suggests that it is a major problem: approximately 10 to 20 percent of women of childbearing age have endometriosis. We also know that 30 to 40 percent of women with endometriosis are infertile.

The good news is that less than 1 percent of women with endometriosis get endometrial cancer. The prognosis for women who get endometrial cancer is better than expected, with five-year survival rates of 85 percent for women who are diagnosed in stage I and 60 percent for women who are in stage II (see Chapter 12).

The one consistent finding in all research with respect to endometriosis is that there is no single answer to diagnosis or treatment for all women. The individual's experience with the condition varies, and the choice of intervention is tailored to each situation. Nothing is clear-cut. Here is the best of what is known; keep in mind that most of it applies only to some of us, some of the time.

Diagnosis

Women with endometriosis usually complain of pain. While some women have painful menstrual cramps, other women have pain during or after sexual activity. The degree of pain, however, is not an indicator of the size or extensiveness of the implants. Some women with severe endometriosis experience less pain than women with mild or minimal cases. Nevertheless, most women with endometriosis tend to have painful periods.

The severity of endometriosis is described as stages:

- Minimal or mild when the implants are small and localized
- Moderate when there are larger implants or more extensive scar tissue
- Severe when the implants are large and there is extensive scarring

A diagnosis may be suggested based on your history, physical exam, and pelvic exam. A definitive diagnosis is possible only by laparoscopy. Laparoscopy will allow your gynecologist to determine the stage of the disease.

Treatment

There is no cure for endometriosis. The treatments that are available offer varying degrees of relief.

1: Hormonal. One of the facts about endometriosis is that after menopause the symptoms of endometriosis seem to go away. Hormonal treatment creates a chemical menopause (see Chapter 9). Although this is considered a pseudomenopause or a reversible menopause, the fact is that you may have all the symptoms of menopause, such as hot flashes, vaginal dryness, and acne. Also, during this time you will not be able to get pregnant.

Danazol, a weak synthetic male hormone, is given as a temporary treatment and is successful 80 to 90 percent of the time when given in the minimal or mild stages. Other drugs that are given to control endometriosis are gonadotropin-releasing hormone analogs. These drugs are the synthetic equivalent of the naturally occurring gonadotropin-releasing hormone found in your body, which is essential to the production of estrogen and progesterone. Neither of these drugs, however, seems to have an impact on large endometriomas.

During pregnancy the signs of endometriosis also improve. Another form of treatment involves taking birth control pills every day to create a pseudopregnancy.

Some health care providers prescribe progestins, the synthetic form of progesterone, for endometriosis. Research continues to establish the full benefits of each of these treatments.

2: Surgery. You should consider surgery if you want to become pregnant at some point or if the pain is severe. You are most likely to get pregnant within the first year after surgery. The goal of surgery is to save as much healthy tissue as possible and remove the diseased tissue.

The surgery may be performed in a conventional manner (full abdominal surgery) or by using a laparoscope. In most hospitals, a laser is used during laparoscopy to vaporize abnormal tissue. It is important that you discuss these options with your health care provider.

Consejos

Talk to Your Surgeon

It is always a good idea to get to know your surgeon before you have surgery. This is especially true in the case of surgery to treat endometriosis because it is often impossible to know the extensiveness of the endometriosis until you have surgery. Be sure you make clear what things you do not want done and under what circumstances.

The importance of clarity with your surgeon cannot be stressed enough; some Latinas have been surprised to find out upon awakening from surgery that they had a full hysterectomy.

Hysterectomy (total removal of ovaries and uterus) is becoming increasingly rare for the treatment of endometriosis.

The different interventions for endometriosis are undergoing further comparative research to fully understand their long-term impact.

Premenstrual Syndrome (PMS)

Eliana couldn't help but be furious at John. Once again he was late. Once again he had kept her waiting. It was so like him. He was just so inconsiderate. When he finally called her, she was fuming.

John apologized for being late but said his computer had crashed and he had been trying to retrieve all his files. Eliana listened and responded with a hurt "Just come home." All she could think was that as usual he just did not have her on his mind. He always seemed to be putting her last on the list of his priorities.

By the time John finally arrived, Eliana was even more upset with him. As soon as he walked in the door, she let loose with a tirade, saying a lot of things that would have been better left unsaid. He looked at her quietly.

John realized that Eliana was not herself and gently asked if her period was due. Eliana became furious and stormed out of the room. When a few days later she got her period, his words echoed in her head.

Was her behavior the other night so extreme because her period was due? Did she have PMS? "No," thought Eliana, "not me. That's what happens to other kinds of women."

In our office, the majority of the staff are Latinas. And we laugh about PMS. Those of us who get it know enough to warn everyone else the first few times. After a while, we know when someone is PMSing, as we have grown to call it. If someone seems particularly edgy, we just ride it out, understanding that it happens.

I really don't know what the big deal is about PMS. So we get it? At least it is predictable—once a month.

—JENNY, 44

There is more myth about PMS than fact. The facts are few because science is unable to explain why it occurs or how to control it. In the absence of science, the media have provided a steady stream of testimonials that "prove" how out of control women can get because of their hormones. The raging hormone theories of why women need not bother to apply for some jobs has been fueled by lack of knowledge about PMS. As a result, there are people who still believe that women are not suited for work that requires careful judgment or consistency (i.e., management jobs). Similarly, because women, and especially Latinas, are thought to be so emotional, we are often not considered good candidates for decision-making roles.

What is most damaging is when we ourselves accept as fact the myth that somehow our emotions or hormones or even PMS makes us all dangerously unstable and unproductive. Hormones and their natural fluctuations are part of being female and male. We all know too well that men's hormones make them violent and aggressive—over 90 percent of prison inmates are male. Nevertheless, those male hormonal tendencies have not stopped them from reaching decision-making positions. For our own sake, we have to learn to accept that fluctuations in our moods are normal.

Diagnosis

It is estimated that 1 to 5 percent of women have the most serious cases of PMS. PMS is defined by some as a consistent physical or emotional change that occurs before a woman's menstrual cycle and interferes with at least one aspect of her life. Your health care provider may ask you to keep a chart of your physical and emotional symptoms as well as your menstrual cycle for several months to determine your pattern. You may find that your health journal is a rich source of information (see Appendix B).

Physical changes include acne, bloating, breast pain, fatigue, headaches, joint swelling, pelvic pain, and weight gain. These physical changes may make you uncomfortable as you try to pursue your usual activity.

For some of us PMS may mean that all of a sudden we seem to become sad, and the sadness stays with us for a while. One Latina was reluctant to admit that for her, PMS was different. As part of her monthly cycle, PMS meant "Please More Sex"—she found that during these times she felt very desirous.

Emotional changes due to PMS cover the full spectrum—anger, anxiety, depression, difficulty concentrating, mood swings, nervousness, and sleep disorders. Such changes should be expected, given the hormonal fluctuations that a woman's body undergoes leading up to menstruation.

That hormones influence our emotions and our bodies is nothing new. Men and women both have hormones that determine their behavior. Unlike men, in whom there is no known pattern to hormone fluctuation, a woman's monthly menstrual cycle provides a relatively consistent predictor of how hormones and perhaps mood will fluctuate.

Research that has monitored the hormonal levels of women has produced some perplexing findings. Specifically, women who have the same hormonal levels may not have the same experiences with PMS. An interesting finding is that some women who have PMS and undergo hysterectomy still have symptoms of PMS after surgery.

Treatment

Since there is no single set of symptoms that defines PMS, treatment is highly individualized and focuses on healthy eating, regular exercise, stress management, and symptom relief. The treatments are based on the experiences of health care providers with women having similar problems rather than being scientifically based.

In terms of healthy eating, women with PMS may be told that in order to keep their hormone level stable they should eat several small meals a day. It is also recommended that they assess the effect of taking some things out of their diets, such as alcohol, caffeine, chocolate, and sugary foods. For some women the addition of calcium (1,000 mg each day), magnesium (during the second half of their cycle—200 mg daily), vitamin B6 (50 to 200 mg daily), and vitamin E (150 to 400 IU daily) may be helpful.

Aerobic exercise on a regular basis (at a minimum, three times a week, with each session lasting at least 20 minutes) benefits women who experience PMS. In some instances a support group has been recommended.

Medication

Given the variety of symptoms women with PMS have, a number of specific medications may be suggested to offer some relief. For example, women who experience joint and muscle pain may have an anti-inflammatory medication added to their treatment program, while women who become depressed may be given an antidepressant. The medications focus on symptom relief.

The expectation that safe treatment with hormones might resolve PMS is still to be realized. Current research challenges the use of hormones in controlling PMS.

Hysterectomy

By the time I was thirty-one I had been to the gynecologist more times than I could remember. There always seemed to be something wrong. My periods were irregular, I had severe cramps, and I also seemed to have growths.

So when my gynecologist saw me again, she suggested that perhaps I should just have everything cleaned out. In that way I would not have any more problems—no more periods, no pain, no growths.

"Cleaned out?" I thought to myself. I was not ready for that. I knew that the likelihood of my having children was small, but . . . well, I still wanted the possibility of a miracle. And more than that, I didn't think that my insides were "dirty" and needed to be cleaned out.

I decided against a hysterectomy.

At forty-four I know I made the right choice. Doctors do not know everything.

–Cristina, 44

For me a hysterectomy was the best thing that ever happened. My life became simpler. I didn't have to worry about birth control anymore or ovarian cancer. I had worried about both of those for so long.

–Alba, 53

Whether or not a hysterectomy is the best treatment for the problems a woman has in her reproductive system has been a subject of much debate. The scientific, ethical, and political issues of hysterectomies have brought us to a new view. Where once hysterectomies were the preferred procedure for health care providers, there is now a concerted effort by providers and patients alike to find alternatives.

Nevertheless, a hysterectomy is the second most common surgical procedure that women undergo (cesarean sections are number one). The extent of a hysterectomy may vary greatly: simple (uterus and cervix are removed), partial (cervix is not removed), radical (uterus, cervix, upper part of vagina, supporting ligaments, and lymph nodes are removed). The latest science suggests that for women under forty-five

> *Consejos*
>
> **Get a Second Opinion**
>
> Whenever surgery is recommended, you should get a second opinion. This is especially true if you are considering a hysterectomy. Remember that when it comes to surgery, many health care plans pay for and welcome a second opinion.

with healthy ovaries, it is more prudent to leave the ovaries intact.

If your health care provider is recommending a hysterectomy, you need to understand the reason for the procedure and how extensive it will be. You should be made aware of what are the nonsurgical options. Most important, no matter how much you trust your health care provider, it is important that, as always, you obtain a second opinion.

How It Is Done

Removal of the uterus is major surgery and will be done in a hospital. The operation will involve either abdominal surgery or laparoscopic surgery. Abdominal surgery is when either a "bikini cut" or midline cut (beneath the belly button to pubic bone) is made and the uterus is removed. In laparoscopic surgery the laparoscope is inserted through the belly button to view the organs. Two other incisions are made on your abdomen for inserting the slender instruments that will be used for cutting and cauterizing. The uterus is removed by entering through the vagina.

The recuperation period for abdominal surgery is three to five days in the hospital followed by four to eight weeks at home; for laparoscopy it is one to two days in the hospital and four weeks at home.

The decision about which procedure to use should be based on your condition and not just on your schedule or what your health care provider does best. Although you may want the laparoscopy, it might not allow for as thorough a procedure as may be required.

After the Surgery

How you feel after the surgery has a lot to do with your understanding about what the surgery will and will not do. If you needed a hysterectomy, then you should feel physically better with respect to whatever it treated. Unfortunately, there is no research that states how each one of us will respond psychologically to having a hysterectomy.

> **What Type of Surgery Am I Having?**
>
> A total or simple hysterectomy may mean different things. Be sure to ask specifically what will be removed: ovaries (one or both), fallopian tubes (one or both), uterus, cervix? Here are some key words.

Hysterectomy	Removal of uterus
Oophorectomy	Removal of ovaries
Ovariectomy	Removal of ovaries
Salpingo-oophorectomy	Removal of ovaries and fallopian tubes
Bilateral oophorectomy	Removal of both ovaries
Unilateral oophorectomy	Removal of one ovary

There are some facts about a hysterectomy that we need to remember. Specifically, a hysterectomy will:

- Make menstruation cease
- Make it impossible to become pregnant
- Reduce the symptoms that made the surgery necessary
- Not make us less feminine
- Not make sex less pleasurable (even when the cervix is removed)
- Increase the risk of urinary incontinence

It is best to assume that each Latina's experience will be different. A few Latinas will be devastated and will need to seek the support of loved ones through this difficult time. Some Latinas may find that they have to reorient their self-image and develop new attitudes about who they are. This is an important time to reach out to others for support. If the pain becomes too great, it may be beneficial to talk to a mental health professional.

Other Latinas will celebrate their newfound health. Since each Latina defines who she is in a different way, the feelings we have after the surgery will reflect the views we had about ourselves before the surgery. To complicate matters further, we will also undergo hormonal changes as a result of the surgical menopause that is produced in hysterectomies where the ovaries are removed (see Chapter 9).

Myth and Fact

Myth: Ovarian cysts are very dangerous for women.

Fact: Most ovarian cysts are harmless.

Myth: Most women who have endometriosis are infertile.

Fact: At least 60 percent of women with endometriosis are fertile.

Myth: Only sexually active women get vaginitis.

Fact: Vaginitis occurs in women regardless of whether they are sexually active.

Myth: Vaginitis can be treated without a prescription medication.

Fact: Over-the-counter treatment is available only for yeast infections.

Myth: A clean woman gives herself a douche on a regular basis.

Fact: Regular douching may upset the natural environment of the vagina. It is also not recommended because it may force bacteria and other organisms up through the cervix and into the uterus and fallopian tubes.

Myth: A vaginal discharge means that you have an infection.

Fact: Every day glands inside your vagina and cervix produce fluids that carry out a natural cleansing of the body. The discharge that is produced is the way the body keeps the vagina clean and healthy. A healthy discharge is clear or milky, and the odor is not unpleasant.

Myth: Fibroids are dangerous because they turn into cancer.

Fact: Fibroids may get larger, but they are not known to turn into cancer.

Myth: If I have a hysterectomy, I will be unable to have orgasms.

Fact: There is no physiological reason for a hysterectomy to have an effect on orgasms. Some Latinas report that they were able to enjoy vaginal intercourse more because they no longer had to worry about becoming pregnant.

Mind and Spirit

When Ricardo told Alina that he was leaving her, she was devastated. She could not believe they would no longer be together. But Alina knew that if she focused on how she felt, her life would fall apart. And she could not let that happen—too many people depended on her.

Alina had to keep working and doing all the

things that signaled to her family and friends that she was OK. So she decided to eat healthier and to exercise. She was going to focus on all the things in her life that were right.

The first month that Alina missed her period, she chalked it up to stress. She knew there was no way she could be pregnant. And more important, she knew that when she had been upset in the past, it had thrown off her menstrual cycle. When the second and third months passed and still there was no period, she became concerned.

Alina went to see her health care provider to discuss what had happened. Perhaps she had been exercising too much. That was met with, "Olympic athletes have that happen to them. Your walking three times a week would not be the same."

"Well," Alina responded, "maybe for me that was like being an Olympic athlete." Her health care provider said, "Alina, I don't think so."

Getting increasingly annoyed, Alina said, "Well, if everything is so right with my body, then what's going on that I haven't had my period in three months?" The health care provider looked her in the eye and said, "You have to calm down."

Alina responded, "But I am calm." And then she thought to herself, . . . well, maybe putting the Ricardo issue in the back of my mind was not OK. It was obvious then that it had been overflowing into all parts of her life.

That so much of what we do affects our hormones is not new. But how can we make that work for us? As Latinas, we know that our wellness is the totality of our experiences. And while we can do well by using all the information we have about how to maintain our bodies, we must be equally attentive to our mind and spirit. They all work together.

Balance is hard to maintain as we rush through our lives. Our reproductive systems, which are so sensitive to hormonal changes, must be the beneficiaries of what we feel and think. It is not that doing good things and keeping our spirit in synch will insure a life free of physical problems. But we make a lifetime of good health much more likely if we actively maintain it rather than try to deny any problem we might be having.

Staying at peace with one's inner self and keeping one's mind and emotions on a positive and stable plane are essential (see Chapter 2). This means that at the very least we must eat healthy meals, exercise, practice our faith, and have a healthy self-esteem. We know that when we do not keep ourselves balanced, our feelings and thoughts disrupt our menstrual cycle and impact every part of our body.

Science talks about how the body produces hormones and a variety of other substances that determine how the body functions. Often when our body signals problems to us, it is a way our mind and spirit communicate to us. When we block off the inner paths from our mind and our spirit, the only outlet left for turmoil is our bodies.

Our constant challenge in the absence of fully understanding the science of what is going on is to listen to our minds and spirits.

Summary

We understand relatively little about the healthy functioning of women's reproductive systems. It is only with the technology of the last forty years—diagnostic ultrasound and laparoscopes—that we have begun to document what is going on when a woman complains about pain or an irregular period.

Women need to know the facts about vaginitis, fibroid tumors, ovarian cysts, endometriosis, PMS, and hysterectomy. To help us manage these health conditions, we must understand what is being said to us, what our symptoms mean, what the best interventions are, and what we should expect from them.

To keep ourselves healthy, we must learn to recognize things that we thought we could or should ignore—from recognizing our own healthy scent to knowing when a vaginal discharge is a sign that something is wrong. We must also know that sometimes there is no definitive treatment.

Most important of all is the role our mind and spirit play. We are only now beginning to understand the intricacies of the relationship between hormones and our reproductive system. And we must learn to trust our instincts and feelings—if we think something is wrong, it may be necessary to seek a professional opinion. We also need to learn to chart our own physical, emotional, and hormonal changes to see if there are any patterns that emerge. All this will help to further our understanding of the critical role our mind and spirit play in controlling our hormones.

RESOURCES

Organizations

American College of Obstetricians and Gynecologists
P.O. Box 96920
409 12th Street SW
Washington, DC 20090-6920
(202) 638-5577 or (800) 762-2264
www.acog.org

American Society for Reproductive Medicine
Patient Information Dept.
1209 Montgomery Highway
Birmingham, AL 35216-2809
(205) 978-5000
www.asrm.com

Association of Reproductive Health Professionals
2401 Pennsylvania Avenue NW, Suite 350
Washington, DC 20037-1718
(202) 466-3825
www.arhp.org

Endometriosis Association
8585 North 76th Place
Milwaukee, WI 53223
(800) 992-3636 or (414) 355-2200
www.endometriosisassn.org

National Women's Health Network and Women's Health Network Clearinghouse
514 10th Street NW, Suite 400
Washington, DC 20004
(202) 347-1140
www.womenshealthnetwork.org

Publications and Pamphlets

"Dysmenorrhea and Premenstrual Syndrome." National Institute of Child Health and Human Development, National Institutes of Health, P.O. Box 29111, Washington, DC 20040. Other titles include "Endometriosis." Publication No. 91-2413; (800) 370-2943.

"Endometriosis: A Guide for Patients." American Society for Reproductive Medicine, 1209 Montgomery Highway, Birmingham, AL 35216-2809; (205) 978-5000. Available in Spanish

"Important Facts about Endometriosis," Jan. 2000. American College of Obstetricians and Gynecologists, P.O. Box 92920, 409 12th Street SW, Washington, DC 20090; (800) 762-2264. www.acog.org Other titles include:

"Ovarian Cysts," Sept. 2000.

"Vaginitis: Causes and Treatments," Jan. 2000.

"PMS: What You Can Do to Ease Your Symptoms," 1999. Pamphlet No. 1546. AAFP Family Health Facts. American Academy of Family Physicians, 11400 Tomahawk Creek Pkwy, Leawood, KS 66211-2672; (800) 944-0000.

"Your Colposcopy Exam." Education Program Associates, 1 West Campbell, Suite 40, Campbell, CA 95008-1039; (408) 374-3720. Other titles include "Your Pelvic Exam." Available in Spanish.

7

When Having a Biological Child Is Difficult

Sara's memories were filled with images of lots of children. At any family function, there always seemed to be someone with either a new baby or one on the way. And she truly enjoyed being with all the children—she even volunteered to babysit when the adults wanted time for themselves.

As Sara got older, she began a scrapbook of her life, so she could share it with the children she would have. She cut out pictures from magazines and added them to her scrapbook, so that one day she would be able to show her children what things were like when their mother was a little girl.

Throughout high school, her plans for the future were more or less the same. She knew that she would have to work and earn money, but she also knew that she was going to have a large family. She figured that it would be nice to have four children—two girls and two boys. Family and work—that sounded right.

As time passed, she realized that sometimes in life things take a little while to sort themselves out. Later than she had planned, Sara married Manuel, a loving and caring man. They were both eager to start their family, but after a year of trying to have children, there was nothing. Sara did not understand this inability of hers to become pregnant.

All the women in her family seemed to have as many children as they wanted, and sometimes even more than they wanted. How could this be happening to her? In her most private moments, Sara would ask herself why God was punishing her in this way. What had she done that was so wrong?

She could not believe that this was happening to her.

Beginning when we are very young, especially if we are Latinas, we are taught that girls grow up and have children. The shows on television, the pictures in magazines, the voices on the radio, all define us with a perception of ourselves with an abundance of children. We are taught to value our lives and ourselves through our children. And when we have none, it is hard to value ourselves for who we are with or without children. We are unprepared for what happens to us if we find out that we cannot have children.

There is the pain of seeing other women with their kids—your sisters or cousins with many more children than they can handle, while you are "barren." And then there are the constant questions, "When are you going to get pregnant?"

Our initial response to the possibility that we may not be able to have children is disbelief. After a while, when we know it is true, we are devastated. Moreover, our feelings are magnified by thinking that there is no one to talk to about this problem. Those of us who live with the knowledge of our own infertility know how hard it is to talk about our experiences. We believe that infertility just doesn't happen to Latinas. Unfortunately, infertility is much more common among us than most of us imagine.

The facts tell us some disturbing news. Although Latinas have the highest rate of becoming pregnant (fertility), we also have the highest rate of not being able to become pregnant (infertility). So those of us who have children are more likely to have more than the general population, while at the same time a high percentage of us cannot have children. It is hard to explain why Latinas seem to have such high rates of both fertility and infertility, even though these are at opposite ends of the spectrum. Our experience with these divergent findings is that we accept the information on our high rate of fertility and are kept unaware of the infertility that exists among us.

There is practically no information available to Latinas on the subject of infertility within our community. The bulk of the information available is provided by fertility clinics who make money by trying to make you pregnant. The lack of information results in uninformed people, who define infertility as a woman's problem. The word *infertility* itself implies that the woman is deficient in some way. Another term used to describe reduced ability to bear children is fecundity. The complete inability to produce offspring is sterility.

Infertility occurs when there is a diminished or absent capacity to produce offspring. Primary infertility occurs in couples who have never conceived. Secondary infertility occurs in couples who have previously conceived.

Infertility is not defined by the inability of an individual but rather by the inability of a couple to produce a child after having unprotected penile-vaginal intercourse for one year. The data on infertility also include situations where a woman is unable to carry a pregnancy to term and has a miscarriage.

The infertility may be due to the man (40 percent), the woman (40 percent), or both (10 percent). For an additional 10 percent of couples, the reason for the infertility is never identified. Nevertheless, all the numbers and all the definitions and redefinitions still leave us feeling incomplete. As Latinas, we often feel that we are responsible for any fertility problem, even when it is due to the man's low sperm count or other medical problem.

When we have to face infertility in our own lives, it is not surprising that we are left without any points of reference. Infertility seems as alien to us as a creature from another planet. At the same time that we lack knowledge, the effect of infertility reaches deep into our body, mind, and spirit.

The best way to overcome infertility is to understand what it is. The hope is that with knowledge and prudent action, most of us will be able to overcome our infertility, regardless of whether we are eventually able to have a biological child.

What Is Infertility?

The use of the term *infertility* is broader than we think for the following reasons.

1. It refers to a couple and not just to a woman.
2. It includes women who may have had at least one biological child, but were unable to have more children.

3. Infertility includes women who have been unable to carry a pregnancy to viability. Unfortunately, miscarriages occur much more often than they are discussed; 17 percent of all pregnancies end in miscarriages.

It made me proud that Angela had decided to have the baby and raise the child by herself. Too many other women would have rushed and had an abortion.

I naturally agreed to be the madrina *(godmother) and help Angela with raising the baby. Surely we both had lives filled with commitments and obligations, but as a friend I understood that I needed to be there for her. After all, a child is a gift from God.*

Angela was very nervous about her pregnancy because when she was younger she had had a miscarriage. To ease her mind, I also agreed to be her coach.

I can still remember how I felt when Angela told me that she was spotting. I suggested that she go to see her obstetrician. She asked me to go with her, and so I left work to be able to meet her at the doctor's office.

I breathed a sigh of relief when she came out of the office and sighed, "Everything is OK, but I need to get a sonogram to be sure." We drove over to the radiology center. Angela asked me to go into the examining room with her. I felt awkward being there. I mean, I was looking at her private parts in ways I never intended to see another woman.

The radiologist came in and began to do the ultrasound. He matter-of-factly said, "Yes, I can see that there was a baby there, but it looks like you lost it." And then he just left the room.

Angela looked at me in disbelief, and I fumbled trying to find the words to explain what had just happened. She had lost the baby.

—*Rosa, 31*

Stigma of Infertility

One of the major stumbling blocks in overcoming infertility is its stigmatization. Think of the very words we use to describe an inability to bear children—*infertile*, *barren*. They seem to suggest that a woman is somehow less womanly because of her inability to give birth. When the problem is due to the man, we use less value-laden language, speaking of low sperm count or motility. We do not refer to a man as infertile. And since men do not give birth to children, the stigma of the inability to bear a child is disproportionately suffered by women.

Underlying the misconceptions about infertility is a belief that any woman can become pregnant and can do so easily. Contrary to this popular perception, the data indicate that unprotected penile-vaginal intercourse does not always lead to immediate pregnancy. When no means of contraception is used, 25 percent of women become pregnant during the first month, 63 percent within six months, 80 percent within nine months, and 85 percent within one year. This means that infertility occurs in about 15 percent (1 out of 7) of all married couples.

Given the high rate of infertility, we should know a lot more about it than we do. But we do not. We know that with proper medical or surgical treatment, half of all infertile couples will have a child. Additionally, for reasons that are unknown, every month 3 percent of couples who have been identified as infertile conceive on their own. What we know about these couples is very limited. For example, the research does not describe the circumstances of the couple who are eventually able to have a biological child—whether, for instance, they are young or have given birth successfully in the past.

There is one thing that we do know with certainty, however—that whatever course of action a couple selects will require the support and collaboration of both of them. As soon as a couple begins to understand that infertility is occurring in their relationship, they should seek a mental health professional and, depending on the couple's faith, a religious counselor to guide them through what will be a very emotional and spiritually challenging aspect of their relationship. This type of professional should be approached at the very beginning. It is unreasonable to believe that one can or should address these issues by oneself.

The next step toward addressing infertility is understanding what it takes physiologically to become pregnant and carry a baby to term.

Body

Pregnancy involves four things: (1) an egg has to be released from the ovary; (2) fertilization must occur; (3) the fertilized egg must be able to attach itself to the walls of the uterus; and (4) the woman must be able to carry the child to term. To determine whether it is possible for steps one, two, and three to occur, a couple will have to be monitored by their health care provider for several months. This requires assessment of the couple, the man, and the woman.

Assessment of the Couple

As a first step, your health care provider will interview each of you about your general health. It will also be important to bring in whatever records or charts you may have been maintaining with respect to your menstrual cycle.

As part of the interview, specific information will be requested about frequency of penile-vaginal intercourse and the positions used. It is important that this information be accurate. You must learn to feel comfortable about talking in this descriptive manner. You will probably be referred to a reproductive endocrinologist for a careful assessment of both members of the couple.

Assessment of the Man

Medications, environmental and chemical factors, certain illnesses after puberty (e.g., mumps), work, smoking, drugs (over-the-counter, prescription, and illegal), sexually transmitted diseases (STDs), and other factors may all affect the ability of sperm to reach and fertilize the egg.

The man will be asked to provide a sample of sperm. The sperm sample will be analyzed to determine its volume, number, motion (motility), and shape. For the sperm to be able to fertilize an egg, each of these characteristics must fall within a specific range. Blood tests for hormonal levels may also be conducted.

Assessment of the Woman

There are some women for whom infertility is a temporary condition. For example, some women may become temporarily infertile due to excessive exercising or dieting. This is most likely to occur when the level of body fat has been excessively reduced. Women who are too overweight may also have fertility problems.

There are a variety of conditions that may make a woman unable to have a child: too much or too little thyroid hormone, too much of a hormone called prolactin, too many androgens, exposure to environmental toxins, endometriosis, uterine fibroids, cysts, congenital abnormalities, pelvic inflammatory disease, and STDs among them.

Yet just the fact that a woman has one or more of these conditions does not necessarily mean that she will be unable to bear children. Some of these same conditions exist in women who are able to bear children. As in most things, the unique combination of factors in each individual will determine her ability to become pregnant and carry a pregnancy to term.

Given the variety of conditions that may affect a woman's reproductive system, there is a spectrum of tests and procedures that are usually considered, from noninvasive to invasive. Your clinician will consider your history and may suggest that you not undergo some of the more invasive procedures. Other clinicians may feel that invasive procedures provide the quickest source of information.

Regardless of the approach suggested, you need to know the reasons for the recommendation and the consequences of the procedure. The decision about which diagnostic procedure to pursue must be made jointly by you and your clinician. If you do not understand something or are unsure, ask questions. That is not only your right, but your responsibility as a patient.

Generally the goal of diagnostic tests and procedures is to answer the following questions.

1. Is your overall health good?
2. Are you ovulating?
3. Are your fallopian tubes clear?
4. Does your cervical mucus facilitate movement of sperm?
5. Is there a problem with your uterus?

The answer to each of these questions helps to determine the possible treatment.

1: Is your overall health good? Sometimes the difficulty we experience is due to an underlying health problem. Your health care provider will do some routine tests to make sure that you are in good health, e.g., diabetes is under control, thyroid is working properly, and your weight is good.

2: Are you ovulating? When you ovulate, you release an egg. If lack of ovulation is the problem, the question is whether an underlying hormonal deficit exists that stops you from ovulating. Blood tests will be taken to determine blood levels of follicle-stimulating hormone (FSH), luteinizing hormone (LH), progesterone, and prolactin. Over-the-counter ovulation kits are the main source of information.

Some of the preliminary assessment in this area is similar to that monitored in fertility awareness as part of natural family planning (see Chapter 4). Specifically, for a few months you will be asked to monitor your basal body temperature (BBT) and the cervical mucus that you produce.

BBT is measured using a basal body thermometer. A basal thermometer measures your body temperature from 96 to 100 degrees Fahrenheit in increments of one-tenth of a degree. In most cases you will have to use a glass and mercury thermometer because current digital thermometers are unable to provide this level of detail. Moreover, the accuracy of the digital thermometers does not make them completely useful for fertility purposes. The basal thermometer is relatively inexpensive (under $10). It is a good idea to call your local pharmacy and make sure that they stock basal thermometers.

The information included with the basal thermometer makes the monitoring seem more complex than it is. The steps for using the basal thermometer may be simplified as follows: before going to bed, shake the thermometer down to 96.5 degrees Fahrenheit; place the thermometer near your bed; as soon as you wake up, before you do anything else, insert the thermometer in your mouth; wait 5 minutes; take out the thermometer and set it aside; continue your morning routine; when you are more awake, record your BBT for the day. Monitoring your BBT gives you valuable information to determine whether or not you are ovulating. You will know you are ovulating when you see your temperature spike up (see Chapter 4 and Appendix B).

Your clinician may also ask you to monitor the consistency of your cervical mucus. You will be able to record this on the same chart where you record your BBT. Once a pattern of ovulation is determined, you may choose to use a home-test kit to confirm that ovulation has taken place.

3: Are your fallopian tubes clear? The fallopian tubes are where fertilization takes place. These narrow tubes must be unobstructed to allow the sperm to enter and fertilize the egg. They must also allow for the fertilized egg to travel out into the uterus. About 30 percent of women who cannot get pregnant have problems with their fallopian tubes.

A hysterosalpingogram is one method for determining whether the fallopian tubes are open. This involves placing a contrast dye into your uterus and fallopian tubes and then taking an x-ray. The best time to have this procedure done is after menstruation but before ovulation.

In this procedure, a clinician uses a thin tube to allow some contrast dye to pass through the cervix into the uterus. The dye is a harmless substance that is absorbed by the body after the procedure.

X-rays are taken of the dye as it travels through your uterus and fallopian tubes while the radiologist observes the flow of the dye. These x-rays are a concrete record that your clinician will have available to review.

The information you get from your health care provider in preparation for the hysterosalpingogram will probably say that you may experience some discomfort or cramping. To better prepare yourself, you should know that women who have undergone the procedure state that it is painful and that the cramps are severe. In some clinics, women are given local anesthesia or other medication to help them get through the process, which usually takes less than 15 minutes.

When the procedure is over, you should use a sanitary napkin to absorb the dye that is not absorbed by the body. You will probably have a bluish discharge, and it may last a few days.

Another way for your clinician to obtain information about your fallopian tubes is through a laparoscopy. This is an outpatient procedure that requires general anesthesia. A small incision is made by the belly button, and the gynecologist inserts a laparoscope through it. The laparoscope is a long, narrow, rigid tube with a fiber-optic light and a wide-angle lens at the end. The image from the laparoscope is projected on a viewing monitor so that the gynecologist can look at the uterus and the fallopian tubes. If there are adhesions or obstructions, they may be removed through the laparoscope using specially designed instruments.

4: Does your cervical mucus facilitate movement of sperm? Among fertility specialists there is debate about the usefulness of examining the interaction between sperm and cervical mucus. Only in rare instances will a woman's cervical mucus repel her partner's sperm.

The Sims-Huhner test is done after you and your partner have sex. This is referred to as a postcoital procedure. Specifically, a couple will be asked to have penile-vaginal intercourse right before the woman is expected to ovulate and 2 to 8 hours before the test is performed. The clinician will then obtain some of the woman's cervical mucus and view it under a microscope to observe the number of sperm and their motility and direction of movement. This test is not always reliable.

5: Is there a problem with your uterus? These problems are very rare. Some women are concerned when they are told that they have fibroids in their the uterus, but these do not usually cause infertility. For a fibroid to cause infertility it has to obstruct implantation of the fertilized egg in the uterus.

A hysterosalpingogram provides information on the shape of the uterus. Another procedure, hysteroscopy, provides information about the shape and walls of the uterus. This is an outpatient procedure. In hysteroscopy, an instrument resembling a small telescope is inserted through the cervix to view the uterus. Besides being a diagnostic tool, the procedure allows for treatment by removal of scar tissue or other small obstructions. A hysteroscopy is sometimes done at the same time as a laparoscopy.

MYTHS AND FACTS

Myth: Infertility is a woman's problem.

Fact: Infertility is a couple's problem. Men and women share equally as the causal factor in infertility.

Myth: To increase the chances of becoming pregnant, you should have intercourse every day.

Fact: It is best to have intercourse every other day during your fertile week. This makes for healthier and greater quantities of sperm.

Myth: As soon as you ovulate, you should have intercourse.

Fact: It is best to have intercourse the day or evening before ovulation, based on data from self-observation of mucus and BBT and ovulation detection kits.

Myth: It is easier to get pregnant if you are thin.

Fact: Women who are underweight may have temporary infertility.

Myth: If you adopt a baby, you will become pregnant.

Fact: Many women who adopt do not become pregnant.

> *Consejos*
>
> **All Providers Must Communicate with Each Other**
>
> When there are problems with both the man and the woman, it is essential that their respective health care providers, as well as the specialists who care for them, communicate with each other on a regular basis.

Treatment

At last I was a stockbroker. Everything was going so well. And now Mario and I were ready to have a family. We tried for a year. Nothing. After a while even lovemaking became a chore. We started to see doctors, who were surprised that I was having trouble getting pregnant—everybody knows Hispanics are supposed to reproduce like rabbits. We got tested and tested and tried all the new treatments, but there is no happy ending to this story. Only $14,000 down the drain for infertility treatment that didn't work.

—*MARÍA, 28*

The results of the diagnostic tests described above will determine the type of treatment that will be recommended. The treatment may involve surgery, taking strong hormones, or both. Regardless of the treatment recommended, it is important that the couple make the decision together about how to proceed. It is strongly recommended that the couple seek the services of a psychotherapist who is not affiliated with the infertility specialist to discuss these issues.

NO TREATMENT

Sometimes we begin to go down a path and find out that we don't want to go any further. After a series of diagnostic procedures, a couple may find that they do not want to take hormones or undergo surgery. Some couples may choose to adopt, while others may refocus their feelings and energies on other aspects of their lives.

The no-treatment decision is therefore the first option for a couple to consider. In arriving at this decision, the guidance and support of a mental health professional is crucial because sometimes a diagnosis of infertility can unravel a couple's relationship.

Treatment Options for the Man

The options for men are very limited because there are very little data on successful methods or the success rate of treating men. The findings from the sperm analysis will suggest a probable cause of the problem in the man and direct the kind of treatment.

If there is a low sperm count, treatment may focus on creating the ideal conditions for sperm. Since sperm are most efficient at 93.2 degrees Fahrenheit, prolonged fever or excessive heat is avoided. Some men may choose to undergo surgery if it is determined that they have an enlarged vein in their scrotum (varicocele) that theoretically increases the temperature in the scrotum. In uncontrolled studies, however, the pregnancy rate after this procedure is only 30 to 50 percent. The wearing of boxer shorts has also been recommended to reduce the temperature around the scrotum, but again there are no controlled studies to support this suggestion.

If endocrine or hormonal problems are found, the man might be treated with medications such as testosterone by injection, Clomid, or Pergonal. Very often the best alternative may be to collect and prepare the man's sperm for artificial insemination.

Unfortunately, treatment is not successful for men with low sperm counts who do not have a hormonal problem. There is no successful treatment for men with sperm that are defective in shape or movement.

Treatment Options for the Woman

Problems with ovulation. For women who do not ovulate or have a luteal phase defect (i.e., the walls of the uterus are not prepared for implantation or maintenance of a fertilized egg), a careful review of possible causal factors will be established. Some women who are obese will be told to lose weight, and some women who are too thin will be told to gain weight. If the infertility is due to excessive physical exercise, a woman will be told to exercise less.

In most instances, however, medication will be given to stimulate ovulation. The most common drug given is Clomid (clomiphene citrate). This is an estrogen-like substance that increases the release of FSH and LH. Most women (80 percent) who take Clomid will ovulate. If after three months on Clomid there is no pregnancy, the couple will be referred to an infertility specialist.

In all likelihood, the infertility specialist will prescribe stronger doses of Clomid and perhaps Pergonal (human menopausal gonadotropin, or HMG). With both of these medications you will have to be closely monitored because there is a potential for significant side effects. It seems that the medications that increase ovulation also tend to increase the growth of fibroids in the uterus and encourage the spread of endometriosis. There is also a risk of multiple births.

In the few cases of infertile women who have too much prolactin, they will probably be given bromocriptine to bring the prolactin level down to a normal range.

Problems with the fallopian tubes. If your tubes are blocked because of adhesions, laparoscopic surgery may be possible to clear the area. There has also been some success with laser surgery.

Problems with the uterus. Very few women have these problems. Depending on the problem, surgery may resolve structural problems of the uterus. Women who have had miscarriages may be given medications such as natural progesterone to make the walls of the uterus more suitable for implantation of the fertilized egg.

Problems with cervical mucus. The major treatment is to prescribe estrogen to improve the quality of the mucus.

Other Interventions

Adoption is a way to have a family. There are many children who are waiting to be adopted. The resource list at the end of this chapter provides suggestions about where you may find guidance in this area.

Assisted reproduction is an option for a couple if the woman is ovulating and the man has viable sperm or if the couple agree to have some third person donate an egg or sperm. These procedures place a heavy emotional, physical, and financial burden on a couple. Before pursuing this option, it is important that the couple seek psychological counseling from a therapist unaffiliated with the institution providing the assisted reproduction.

The success rates for these procedures is very low. In those instances where the assisted reproduction is successful (for in vitro fertilization, this is 14 to 16 percent of couples), there are usually several attempts. Each attempt takes ten days and costs between $10,000 and $15,000, which is generally not covered by most insurance carriers.

In these procedures, the woman is first given hormones and monitored. When she is ovulating, she undergoes surgery to remove some of her eggs. At this point, one of three options is then available.

1. In vitro fertilization (IVF) is the only option if the woman's fallopian tubes are damaged. This procedure involves extracting an egg from the woman, fertilizing the egg with sperm in the laboratory, and then placing the resulting embryo(s) into the woman's uterus through the cervix.
2. Gamete intrafallopian transfer (GIFT) requires that a woman's fallopian tubes be clear. In GIFT, the woman's unfertilized eggs and the man's sperm are injected surgically into her fallopian tubes to facilitate fertilization.
3. Zygote intrafallopian transfer (ZIFT) is a procedure in which the woman's egg and the man's sperm are fertilized in the laboratory, and the fertilized egg is then surgically placed in the woman's fallopian tube.

The option you choose is up to the two of you. There is a small chance of multiple births with these procedures. Be thoughtful, understanding that some of these options are riskier than one may think and the success rate is not very high. To make a good decision, you need to be sure you understand that both the mind and the spirit are an important part of infertility.

Mind: The Importance of Being a Biological Parent

Couple's View

Given that many of the treatments and even some of the diagnostic tests for infertility require a major commitment of time and resources on the part of the couple, it is critical to understand the reasons that motivate a couple to seek treatment for problems of infertility.

The healthiest mental attitude is to try what is reasonable and to stop before the interventions begin to change the dynamics of the couple. That is why both members of the couple need to feel that trying to overcome infertility is an important component of their relationship. That is also why therapy and counseling should be an ongoing part of the process of addressing infertility.

Becoming biological parents, however, should not be the defining factor in the couple's relationship. It takes more than having a biological child to bind two people to each other. Couples who state that having a biological child will bring them closer together are not being realistic.

Commitment to the process of trying to overcome infertility, and support for one another regardless of the outcome, are critical parts of the mental attitude needed to work through infertility. A couple must agree that the ability to bear children is not the sole indicator of their affection for each other.

Most important of all, couples must remember that raising a child and having a family do not require that one be the biological parent.

Man's View

There are an increasing number of men who view adoption as an alternative to having a biological child. These men genuinely enjoy children and welcome the opportunity to raise them.

Unfortunately, there are also men who feel that having children is one of their marital rights and who, regardless of the situation, will view the inability to have a child as failure on the part of the woman. Men with this point of view are usually not good long-term partners, because their resentment builds and is demonstrated in actions that attack the woman's self-esteem.

Other men will actually be relieved at knowing that there will be no children. These men may have gone along with the process of trying to have a biological child because they felt they had to but may secretly treasure knowing that they will continue to be the sole focus of the woman's attention.

Woman's View

As a Latina, what makes you a woman is how you see yourself. How you view yourself as a Latina is more than your ability to bear children. The ability to reproduce is only one way we can be a *madre* (mother).

We know that we care for and nurture others most of our lives. Perhaps because of this, Latinas are more accepting of their infertility than are other women. If we cannot have biological children, we know we can still care for other children and adults. That is part of who we are as Latinas.

Spirit: A Child Is a Gift from God

Since we were very small, we have been taught that children are a gift from God, so religious beliefs may temper how we proceed with the treatment for infertility. Regardless of how we proceed, when we are infertile it is hard to understand what is happening. Some of us feel guilty about things we did in our lives and may feel that infertility is our punishment and retribution. However, thinking that way would be contrary to what we know about forgiveness and redemption. For those of us who are infertile, our faith can provide an answer.

If we are unable to have children, it is certain that God has other plans for us. We may not know what these plans are, and they may not be the plans we had for ourselves, but still they are there. Our faith can help us to accept that our mission in life may not include biological children but we may still have *hijos de crianza* (children we raise).

Summary

Infertility is a problem that affects 1 out of 7 couples and has physical, psychological, and spiritual undertones. From the very beginning, couples need to seek professional psychological assistance to help them understand the complex feelings that arise from the diagnosis and treatment of infertility.

Diagnosis involves a thorough physical

workup of both the man and the woman. The treatment options for men are few and not very successful. For women there are more treatments, but the success rate with even the artificial methods is less than 25 percent.

Each couple has to carefully consider the psychological reasons for desiring a biological child. It may be that the healthiest alternative physically, spiritually, and psychologically may be not to undergo infertility treatment.

RESOURCES

Organizations

Adoption Network
PO Box 44047
Washington, D.C. 20026-4047
www.adoption.org

American College of Obstetrics and Gynecology
P.O. Box 96920
409 12th Street SW
Washington, DC 20090-6920
(202) 638-5577
www.acog.org

American Society for Reproductive Medicine
Patient Information Dept.
1209 Montgomery Highway
Birmingham, AL 35216-2809
(205) 978-5000
www.asrm.com

Compassionate Friends
P.O. Box 3696
Oak Brook, IL 60522-3696
(Offers support after pregnancy loss)
(877) 969-0010
www.compassionatefriends.org

Council on Adoptable Children
666 Broadway, Suite 820
New York, NY 10012
(212) 475-0222
www.coac.org

National Adoption Center
1500 Walnut Street, Suite 701
Philadelphia, PA 19102
(215) 735-9988 or (800) TO-ADOPT (862-3678)
www.adopt.org

National Women's Health Network and Women's Health Network Clearinghouse
514 10th Street NW, Suite 400
Washington, DC 20004
(202) 347-1140
www.womenshealthnetwork.org

RESOLVE
1310 Broadway
Somerville, MA 02144-1731
(617) 623-1156 or (617) 623-0744 (National Helpline)
(Helps people resolve their infertility)
www.resolve.org

Books

Gilman, Lois. *The Adoption Resource Book.* New York: Harper & Row, 1998.

Panuthos, Claudia, and Catherine Romeo. *Ended Beginnings: Healing Childbearing Losses.* New York: Bergin & Garvey/Greenwood Press, 1984.

8

Pregnancy

Tanya had arrived just in time to celebrate her boss's birthday. It was nice to work in a business run by a Latina because so much of what happened was like this—sort of family but not really family. It made for a supportive working environment. Tanya was greeted with hugs and laughter from her coworkers.

As Tanya spoke to her friends, she couldn't help but think about her own body and begin to smile at the changes that would be coming. Just as she was smiling to herself, her boss walked over and offered her a glass of champagne to celebrate.

Tanya fumbled with her words as she averted her eyes and said, "No, thank you." As she gazed down at her belly, she wondered if her boss knew the real reason she had said no to the champagne. Much to her joy, Tanya had just found out that she was pregnant.

Data from the National Center for Health Statistics indicates that Latinas have much healthier pregnancies than health researchers expected. The good news is that we usually have babies that are as healthy as those of non-Hispanic whites. Although there is little research to explain the reasons for these good outcomes, we can readily point to some of our habits and some characteristics of our culture that serve as protective factors.

On an objective level, we eat more fruits and vegetables and have more fiber in our diets than do non-Latinas. Our lower rates of alcohol and tobacco use are major contributors to our good birth outcomes. Our mental attitude is positive about birth and is strengthened by the belief at the spiritual level that having a child is a gift from God.

When a Latina is pregnant, she takes very seriously the responsibility of caring for herself, feeling that she is nurturing her child more than herself. In addition, throughout our pregnancies, most of us know that we are not alone. The expectation of our friends and family is that they are part of the network that will support us during our pregnancy. And those who find themselves physically alone often turn to the sense of God within them to guide and protect them.

Yet life in the twenty-first century is changing much of what we think about pregnancy and even how we view having children. To counterbalance the often conflicting messages we get, we need to reestablish what it means to have a healthy pregnancy. It should mean that we combine the best parts of our *cultura* (culture) with the best that science has to offer. How do we strike a balance? Well, that's what being a healthy Latina is all about.

Most Latinas describe being pregnant as one of the most important points in their lives. Since pregnancy is something we look forward to as a natural part of a healthy life, we do not see pregnancy as an illness or a medical condition. Therefore it is not surprising that we Latinas are reluctant to visit a health care provider once we have confirmed that we are pregnant.

Some Latinas report that acceptance of pregnancy as part of life made it unnecessary to see a health care provider until they were ready to give birth. Yet seeing a health care provider is a good way to become familiar with the health care system for both mother and baby. It is also essential to monitor the health of the baby as well as the mother's blood pressure, diabetes, and other health indicators.

This chapter assumes that you want to be in the best physical shape possible to give birth; that you want to have the healthiest mental attitude to support you during the many changes that will occur in your life; and that you wish to feel the most positive spiritually to fill you with thoughts of peace and love for your baby.

Preparing Ourselves for Pregnancy

Some of us like to plan everything. For those of us who do plan, it is good to know that *before* we are pregnant is the right time to schedule "preconception" care, our first prenatal visit. Preconception counseling is strongly recommended. During this visit your health care provider will ask you about your medical, reproductive and family history; what you eat; your exposure to drugs and environmental threats; and, social issues. The answers you give will be used to identify risks and provide educational counseling specifically for you. The more prepared you are for pregnancy the greater the chance for reduced complications for you and the baby. At the very least, your health care provider will tell you:

- To be careful about the medications you take (both prescription and nonprescription)
- Not to smoke
- To avoid being in smoke-filled rooms or around smokers
- To eliminate your alcohol intake
- To begin a program of moderate exercise
- To focus on healthy eating
- To have happy thoughts

Your provider should recommend that you take vitamins with folic acid, which is known to lower some birth defects if taken before pregnancy. These same practices will be helpful for you once you become pregnant and should continue throughout your pregnancy.

Camila and Mario had been married for a while now. And yes, even though they were Catholic, they always used birth control. But something had gone wrong . . . or right . . . or at the very least differently than she and Mario had planned. Camila wasn't sure how she felt.

One thing was certain, for the first time in fourteen years, she had missed her period. She bought one of those home-test pregnancy kits just to make sure that she wasn't pregnant. The test came out negative.

She scheduled a doctor's visit. He examined her and confirmed that she wasn't pregnant. She was to try to relax and go home. Then in one week, if she still had not had her period, she would undergo a menstrual extraction.

One week later, she still did not have her period, so she scheduled her menstrual extraction. Her health care provider decided to give her another pregnancy test and left the room to take care of another patient. As she sat there, Camila wondered what was going on with her body.

From down the hall, she could hear her provider saying, "Camila, I have great news," and she thought how interesting it was that there was another patient named Camila. At that moment, her doctor walked in and smiled. Camila knew that the good news was for her—she was the Camila who was pregnant!

Confirming That You Are Pregnant

Some Latinas seem to sense when they are pregnant. Others are not so sure. We may have carefully calculated our fertility cycles or used birth control devices, but because neither process is 100 percent effective, there is always a chance of pregnancy. What are some of the signs that you may be pregnant? You may be pregnant if:

- You miss your menstrual period.
- You have a relatively light period.
- Your breasts feel tender.
- You feel unusually tired or fatigued.
- You are vomiting or experiencing nausea.
- Your basal body temperature stays high when your period is due.

While these feelings and symptoms are important clues, to be certain you are pregnant you need to have a pregnancy test. As a first step, you may want to take a home pregnancy test before going to see your health care provider. Home pregnancy tests measure the presence of human chorionic gonadotropin (HCG). The concentration of this hormone in your urine increases when you are pregnant. Earlier versions of these tests required testing of morning urine. Today these tests are much more sensitive and can detect small concentrations of HCG. You can take the home pregnancy tests at any time during the day.

Although these kits are generally accurate, they sometimes indicate that you are not pregnant when you are. This is most likely to occur if you have miscalculated when you had your last period; it may be too soon to have detectable levels of HCG.

It is also important to note that women going through menopause sometimes produce high levels of hormones similar to HCG. As a result, their pregnancy tests may be positive when they really are not pregnant. This is known as a false positive.

If you still do not get your period and the results from the home-test kit are negative, you should see your health care provider. More sophisticated tests may be used to confirm whether you are pregnant. It may also be possible to determine that there is another cause for your missed period.

Pregnancy

Once I knew I was pregnant, I felt myself changing. It was great! I do not know what made it feel so great. All I knew was that I felt wonderful. We had not planned to have a baby now, but we knew we would make the adjustments in our lives to love and cherish this little one as he or she grew inside of me.

All of a sudden, I saw a different side of me. What can I say? I started feeling like a mom way before the baby was born.

—Ligia, 32

Pregnancy is not a science project. You cannot control the outcome 100 percent. Just enjoy it and have a positive attitude.

—Olivia, 22

The umbilical cord develops during the first month of pregnancy. This two-way lifeline brings nourishment and fluids to the growing baby and also carries away waste the baby produces. It is the beginning of the connection between mother and child.

Here are five things to remember for a better pregnancy:

1. Over 95 percent of pregnancies are normal.
2. The baby is exposed to whatever you are exposed to.
3. Each pregnancy is different.
4. There will be new experiences every day.
5. Be flexible given the likelihood that the unexpected will occur.

During pregnancy it is very difficult to know exactly how you will feel every day. The important thing to remember is to be flexible. Every day will be different. If this is your first pregnancy, keep in mind that although you may be prepared for many things, pregnancy and birth are often about the unexpected. You may have planned everything, but this is one time in your life where flexibility will serve you better. Your body is in control. To help you along, here are some of the things that may happen to you.

Living for Two or More

Whatever passes your lips or is absorbed by your body is also consumed by your baby.

Eating

Eating is the most important thing we do. Although vitamins are taken, food is the best way to feed your baby. You should eat in moderation and follow the guidelines your health care provider gives you. Pregnancy is not the time to diet or deny yourself food when you are hungry. It is important to eat well and healthfully so as to not gain more than the recommended amount of weight. You should avoid artificial sweetners.

Due to the methylmercury that is now found in some fish, you must be careful about the fish you eat. Some state health departments, e.g., Connecticut, and the Canadian Food Inspection Agency have set forth specific guidelines. These guidelines state that pregnant women, women planning to become pregnant, and children under six years of age should eat canned tuna no more than once or twice a week (light tuna is lower in methylmercury than white tuna), fresh or frozen tuna steak at most once a month, and no swordfish or shark. The Food and Drug Administration has emphasized that pregnant women, women planning to become pregnant, and children under six years of age should also not eat king mackerel or tilefish. Check with your local or state health department for information on whether it is safe to eat fish from local sources.

Drinking

You also have to be very careful about what you drink. Any alcohol you consume is also consumed by your baby. Keep in mind that while you may feel sober, small amounts of alcohol may be toxic to your baby, who is unable to metabolize it. Mothers who have more than two drinks a day may have babies who have fetal alcohol syndrome (FAS). Babies with FAS may have a deformed face and suffer from mental retardation and behavioral problems.

Breathing

What you breathe is also important. It is never good to smoke, but it is worse to smoke when you are pregnant because the baby is exposed to the same substances. Mothers who smoke have babies who are underweight and thus more likely to be mentally retarded or suffer from other problems. Just as you should not smoke during pregnancy, it is best to avoid being around smokers, toxic chemicals,

Warning

Check with your health care provider before taking any medicine (over-the-counter or prescription), herbal remedy, or treatment. If they are strong enough to create an effect on you they can also have an impact on the baby.

or other substances that emit fumes that could hurt the baby.

Drugs

Prescription and over-the-counter medicines, home remedies, natural products, illegal drugs—everything that passes your lips is also taken in by your baby, and although some of the products we use on a regular basis may be OK for adults, they may have a negative impact on a baby. Here is a list of the most commonly used substances and what you need to know about them.

- **Acetaminophen,** a nonaspirin medication found in Tylenol and other over-the-counter pain relievers, is the most widely used substance. Although it does cross the placenta, at present it is not known to cause any birth defects. If you use it in very high doses for a long period of time, however, the baby may develop liver and kidney problems.

- **Aspirin** should be avoided during pregnancy unless prescribed by your health care provider. For unknown reasons it seems to prolong pregnancy and labor. For women who take aspirin daily, it is also associated with excessive bleeding during delivery.

- **Ibuprofen,** found in Advil, Motrin, and other over-the-counter pain relievers, should also be avoided because it seems to prolong pregnancy. Although it is not known to cause problems to the baby, it does change the circulation in the heart of the fetus. Manufacturers recommend that it not be taken during pregnancy.

- **Antacids** are generally OK to take in low doses. There are no known negative effects on the baby, although you may experience diarrhea or constipation. Antacids with calcium (e.g., Tums) are believed to be beneficial.

- **Multipurpose products** that contain Cyclizine or pseudoephedrin should be avoided since there are data suggesting that they may produce congenital birth defects during the first three months of pregnancy.

Exposure to Other Chemicals

Read the labels and warnings of all the chemicals you use. Be particularly careful about the cleaning and gardening (including for houseplants) compounds that you use on a regular basis. Also avoid products that contain lead or mercury.

Exercising

It is good to engage in moderate exercise when you are pregnant. What is moderate has

Consejos

How to Do Your Kegel Exercises

The best way to identify the muscles you need to exercise is to become aware of the muscles that are working when you stop the flow of urine. These are the same muscles that are in your vagina, which you must work on.

At least five times a day, do twenty to thirty sets of contractions of the muscles in your vagina. Contract and hold for 3 seconds and then relax.

> **Warning**
>
> Do not go into hot tubs or saunas while pregnant.

to be judged by you and your health care provider. Be careful not to overdo it.

Whatever exercise you choose, you should make sure that you are comfortable. Wear the right bra and shoes. The temperature of the setting where you exercise should be comfortable. Make sure you have drinking water handy so that you can easily replace fluids throughout your exercises.

All exercise requires that you do some warm-up. As you build the intensity of your exercise, remember that exercise must be done in moderation—you should not get exhausted. Keep in mind that because you are pregnant you will be able to breathe less oxygen. This means that you will have to take it easier when you are doing aerobic exercises.

This may be a time to add Kegel exercises to your daily routine because they help build up muscles that are important for childbirth (the muscles that support the vagina, rectum, and urethra). These exercises can be done anywhere and do not require special equipment.

Many women are not aware of where these muscles are located or how it feels to flex them. Here are two ways to identify how it feels to flex these muscles: (1) practice stopping the flow of urine for 5 seconds at a time, (2) try to squeeze your partner's penis when it is inside your vagina (most men find this very pleasurable). The muscles you are working in both of these activities are the ones you want to build up.

Once you know which muscles you need to exercise, you can practice tightening them for 3 seconds and releasing them in sets of twenty to thirty at least five times a day.

Sex and Pregnancy

For some couples, sexual activity increases during the first six months of pregnancy; for other couples it decreases. Nearly all couples have decreased sexual activity during the last few weeks of pregnancy.

Except in rare instances, it is safe to have penile-vaginal intercourse during pregnancy. But while you may receive oral sex, your partner should not blow into your vagina, because this may force air into your bloodstream, resulting in a potentially fatal air embolism. During the last month of pregnancy, nipple stimulation may cause release of oxytocin—a hormone known to produce contractions of the uterus. The contractions will stop when the nipple is no longer stimulated.

Your comfort should be of the utmost concern.

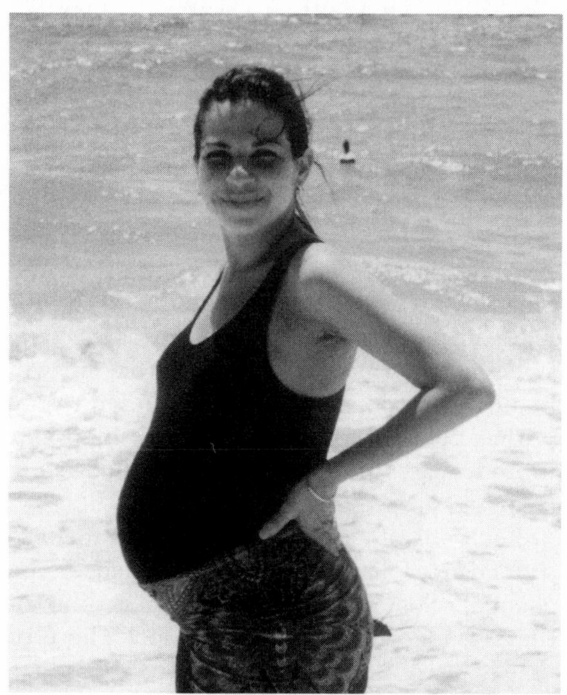

When you are pregnant you will get larger *and* be beautiful.

Hormonal Changes

At the physical level, the hormonal fluctuations that occur during pregnancy may change the texture of the skin, hair, and nails. Some women may get stretch marks, while others develop a distinct dark line from their belly button to their pubic hair. There are women who develop patches of pigmentation—some large, some small—all over the body.

At the psychological level, it is only natural for our moods to be more susceptible to change during this time. Some women become more emotionally sensitive during pregnancy.

What to Expect

Over 95 percent of women have a normal pregnancy. A normal pregnancy means that both you and the baby are healthy. It does not mean that everything goes exactly as planned or expected. In fact, very often what we know and expect is not entirely accurate or realistic. For example, although everyone talks about being pregnant for nine months, the fact is that pregnancy lasts approximately forty weeks. Each trimester lasts a little over twelve weeks.

What you should expect—and what is normal—is that during that time period your body will amaze you by the changes it undergoes. Latinas tend to be accepting of the physical changes in our bodies and try to maintain as many of our daily activities as possible, at the same time knowing that we will be unable to do all the things we used to do. Rather than fight the changes, it is important to understand the reasons why our bodies are changing in specific ways.

Each one of us will be different in the way we change and how we experience the changes. Some of us may experience all of these changes, but others may not. Those of us who have been pregnant more than once may find that each pregnancy is different from the previous one. The important thing is to be prepared for change. Here is some information about what to be aware of and what you should expect.

Your Baby's Father

There is very little research on the changes fathers undergo during a pregnancy. It is safe to say, however, that pregnancy will have a psychological effect on the father and in some cases a physiological effect too.

At the psychological level, pregnancy may be simplistically described as a magnifier of all the dynamics that are present in a relationship. Thus, loving couples often describe the period of pregnancy as a second honeymoon during which they feel particularly close and loving toward each other. When couples have severe problems, however, pregnancy may create a situation where the man physically or emotionally abuses the pregnant woman. It is important to remember that abuse is not acceptable at any time in a relationship. If abuse occurs during your pregnancy, it is dangerous for you as well as for the baby, and you should discuss this with your health care provider. (See the Resources on p. 14.)

Some men experience a physiological response during a woman's pregnancy. These symptoms, such as nausea, headaches, and vomiting, usually disappear as the pregnancy progresses. Although these symptoms have a psychological base, they are real and must be treated as such.

Pregnancy and Weight

It is natural and necessary for women to gain weight during pregnancy. Women who begin their pregnancy being underweight need to gain more weight than women who are overweight. If your weight is less than average, you should gain 28 to 40 pounds; women of average weight should gain 25 to 35 pounds; and those who are overweight should gain 15 to 25 pounds. The weight is gained gradually, so a woman of normal weight will

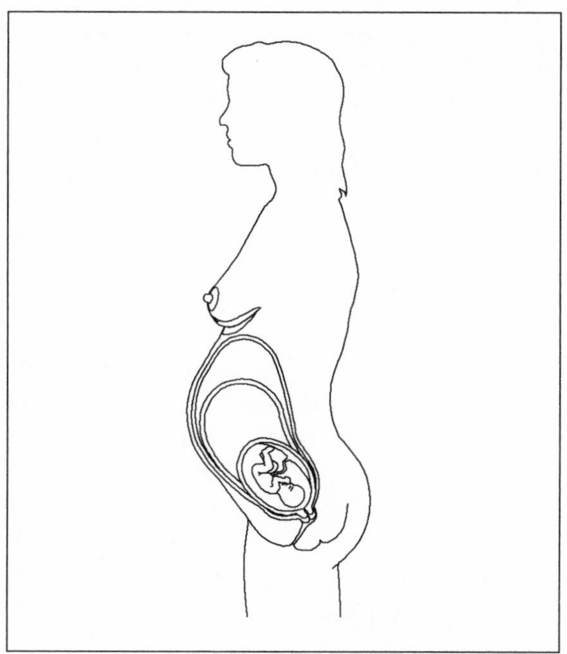

Growth During Pregnancy

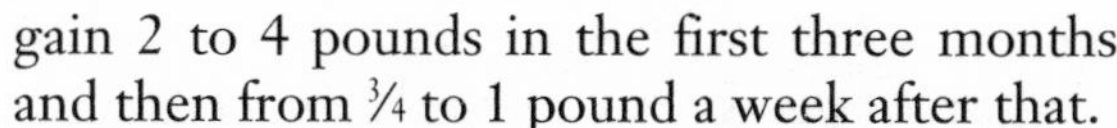

gain 2 to 4 pounds in the first three months and then from ¾ to 1 pound a week after that.

While it takes you about nine months to gain this weight, six months after giving birth most women have lost all the weight gained. For those women who do not, the average weight kept six months after giving birth is only 3 pounds.

Mood

It is natural to have an array of feelings as you prepare for the responsibilities of being a mother. Even if you are already a mother, adding another child to the family requires much thought and consideration. As if we did not have enough to deal with during pregnancies, the changes in our hormones make it even more likely that our feelings will fluctuate. Understanding our feelings is critical to making new arrangements, not only at home with our loved ones but also in our workplace.

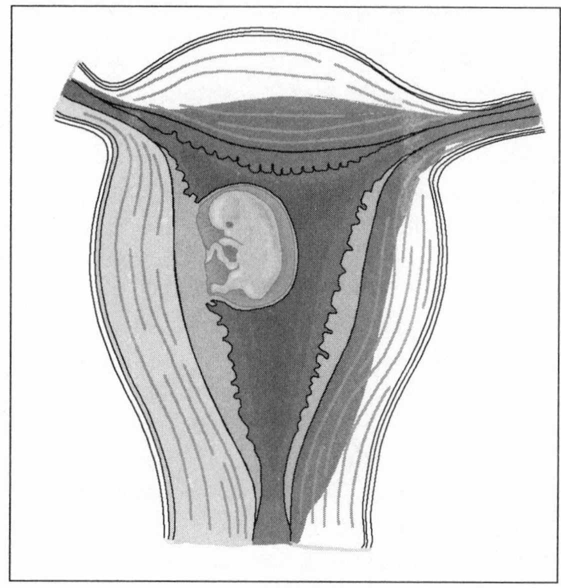

First Trimester

Most Latinas work throughout their pregnancy. If we are careful about what tasks we do at work (avoiding lifting or working with harsh chemicals or other toxic substances), we will be able to have a daily routine that helps us to maintain a positive attitude during pregnancy.

Months One through Three: The First Trimester

You

During this time period you will visit your health care provider at least once a month. What you feel will depend on you. Some women do not even notice that they are pregnant, while others have all sorts of symptoms.

For some, what they remember most about this time period is morning sickness—this means that when you get up you feel like vomiting. You may feel nausea at other times too. Remember that nausea is a sign of healthy pregnancy and is associated with

Consejos

Taking Care of Your Mind and Spirit During Pregnancy

1. Keep a journal of how you feel and record the baby's movements.
2. Get enough sleep. You may need more sleep.
3. Get regular exercise. If you were exercising before, you should probably do less; if you were not, you should probably do more.
4. Remember that it is OK to ask for help from others. You do not have to prove your independence.
5. Pray—you will feel better.

reduced risk of miscarriage. Some women report that things they normally like, such as perfume, may now make them want to vomit. The way to treat morning sickness varies with each woman. Bread, soda crackers, and tea seem to work for some. You may feel better if you eat small meals and do not let your stomach get empty. Keep in mind that the nausea and vomiting are usually limited to the first trimester.

Even if you are not experiencing any unpleasant symptoms, at the very least you need to be aware that your body is going through major hormonal changes. Some women describe their breasts beginning to feel full. Others may experience some spotting, which, as with any bleeding during pregnancy, requires that you let your health care provider know. Toward the end of the trimester, your pelvis changes shape as the joints connecting your bones become more flexible.

Some First-Trimester Tests

During your first visit to your health care provider, you will be given a pregnancy test to confirm that you are pregnant. Once your pregnancy is confirmed, you will be given a test to make sure that you have immunity to rubella (measles), as well as blood tests to assess your level of iron and other substances and to determine the Rh type of your blood cells. Your blood pressure, urine, and weight will also be monitored on a regular basis.

Ultrasound provides a relatively safe way to monitor the growth of the baby without having to insert anything into the womb or the placenta. The procedure begins with a lotion applied to your belly. A technician then moves a wand on your belly, and as the sound waves bounce off the belly, a picture appears on a

High Blood Pressure

Pregnancy-induced hypertension (PIH) ranges from mild to severe and usually occurs during the last thirteen weeks of pregnancy. PIH, also called toxemia or preeclampsia, is diagnosed in 6 percent of all pregnant women. High blood pressure is usually found in first pregnancies, teen mothers, women over forty-five, and women who are carrying more than one baby.

Some symptoms of high blood pressure are headaches, trouble with your vision (blind spots or blurred vision), and pain in your stomach. Preeclampsia that is left undiagnosed and untreated will deteriorate to eclampsia.

Eclampsia is diagnosed when the mother has seizures, convulsions, and/or coma. Eclampsia occurs in less than 0.1 percent of pregnancies and can be avoided by early diagnosis and treatment of preeclampsia. There is no way to prevent preeclampsia, but with good prenatal care it will not progress to eclampsia.

screen. The procedure is painless and produces minimal discomfort.

Ultrasound is a good way to see how the baby is growing and help determine how far along you are in your pregnancy. Usually the screen is positioned so that you and the technician can both see the image that is projected.

During the ninth to twelfth week of pregnancy, some women who are over thirty-five may choose to have chorionic villus sampling (CVS). CVS gives information about many congenital conditions and produces the same risk of miscarriage as does amniocentesis (1 in 200). The main advantage of CVS is that it can be done earlier in the pregnancy.

CVS is done in a hospital. Your physician will use ultrasound to monitor the location of the fetus and placenta and insert a needle through your stomach or vagina and cervix to draw out some of the chorionic villi, which are attached to the membrane that will become the placenta.

Once the fluid is drawn, it can take up to two weeks to get the results, depending on the test being done. Although CVS may be done much sooner than amniocentesis, there is still debate about whether the test itself may cause some deformities in the baby. Talk to your health care provider, and decide whether you should take this test.

Ongoing tests. Your blood pressure will be monitored on a regular basis. Some changes are all right, but if your blood pressure is too high, you may have pregnancy-induced hypertension (preeclampsia).

The Baby

This is a crucial time for the baby, during which much of its basic growth occurs. By the twenty-fifth day the heart begins to beat. At four weeks your baby is an embryo, approximately ½ inch long. The face begins to form, and the heart, lungs, and brain are developing. During the next few weeks, your embryo will become a fetus (which means "young one"), with all the major organs developing even more. Even the bones are starting to develop. By the end of three months, your baby is about 4 inches long, the fingers and toes have nails, and internal organs continue to develop.

Warning

See your health care provider if any of the following occur:

1. Vaginal bleeding/spotting
2. Pains in your belly
3. After the fifth month, the baby does not move for more than 24 hours
4. Continuous headaches (especially in months seven through nine)
5. Sudden swelling of eyelids, hands, or face
6. Problems with vision
7. Release of fluid from your vagina
8. Fever greater than 100.5

Months Four through Six: The Second Trimester

You

You continue to see your health care provider once a month. In most cases you will begin to feel better as your morning sickness goes away. Most of the other discomfort you experienced in the first trimester goes away with the beginning of the second trimester. Some women have constipation. This is when most of us begin to show a pregnant belly.

Some Second-Trimester Tests

Most health care providers will test you for hepatitis B virus (HBV) and diabetes. In most instances, both test results are negative. If you

Special Concern for Latinas: Gestational Diabetes

Only 3 of 1,000 pregnant women start their pregnancy as diabetics. During pregnancy, 30 more women out of 1,000 will become diabetic. Diabetes that develops during pregnancy is referred to as gestational diabetes and is much more common in Latinas than in the general population. Most health care providers do not screen for diabetes until women are in the twenty-fourth to twenty-eighth week of pregnancy.

It is very important to know when we are diabetic and to control the diabetes. Women with uncontrolled diabetes have babies that are malformed. Women diagnosed with diabetes are usually instructed to monitor themselves one to three times a day using a glucometer. With a healthy diet, appropriate medication, and exercise, women are able to control their diabetes and have healthy babies.

test positive for HBV, it means that you need to make sure you have good eating habits and rest during pregnancy. It is also likely that during childbirth you will pass HBV to your baby.

If you test positive for diabetes, your health care provider will put you on a special diet and monitor you closely to make sure that your diabetes is controlled. This is especially important for Latinas.

Every woman, regardless of age, may be offered a "Triple Screen" multiple-marker screening test. These tests are done at fifteen to eighteen weeks. The screening tests are to determine whether the baby has a neural tube defect and a risk of chromosomal defects. For example, if alpha-fetoprotein is too low, there is a possibility of Down's syndrome or other problems. These results may suggest a problem when there is none, and usually a second confirming test is done using amniocentesis. Amniocentesis is offered if a woman is over thirty-five years of age or if a couple has concerns about certain genetic disorders.

In amniocentesis, your physician needs to withdraw about an ounce of amniotic fluid to determine if there are any chromosomal abnormalities. The woman is asked to lie on a table while the physician views an ultrasound picture on a monitor to direct a long thin needle through her belly and uterus and into the amniotic sac, which surrounds the baby. It takes from several days to two weeks to get the results, depending on the number and types of tests requested.

Ultrasound will be used again to give a better picture of how the baby is growing only if the first one is questionable or if growth retardation is suspected.

The Baby

During the fourth month you may experience the first feelings of "quickening." This is the first movement you feel of your baby. For some women, it feels like a wave that is inside them; others describe a flutter or flurry they have never felt before; for others it is a sensation of "bubbles in the tummy." The movement will make you very much aware of the baby inside you. Over time, the movement will be a source of information about what the baby is doing.

Consejos

How to Reduce Swelling of the Ankles

1. Whenever possible, put your legs up.
2. Drink lots of water.
3. Do moderate exercise.
4. Wear support stockings (not knee-highs).
5. Watch salt intake

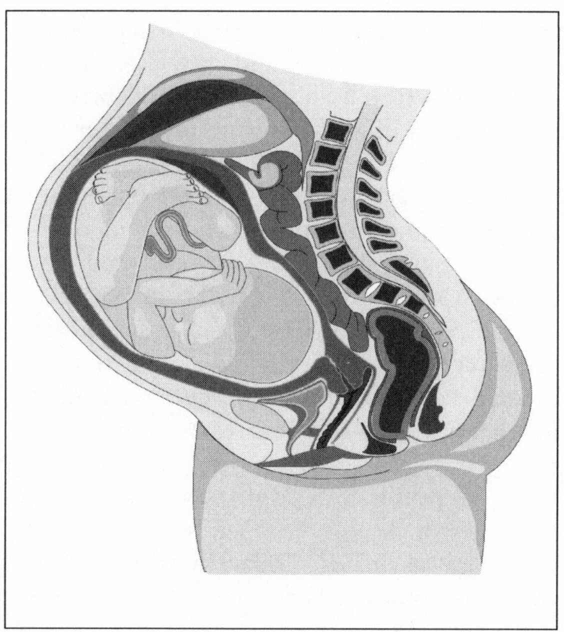
Side View of Last Trimester

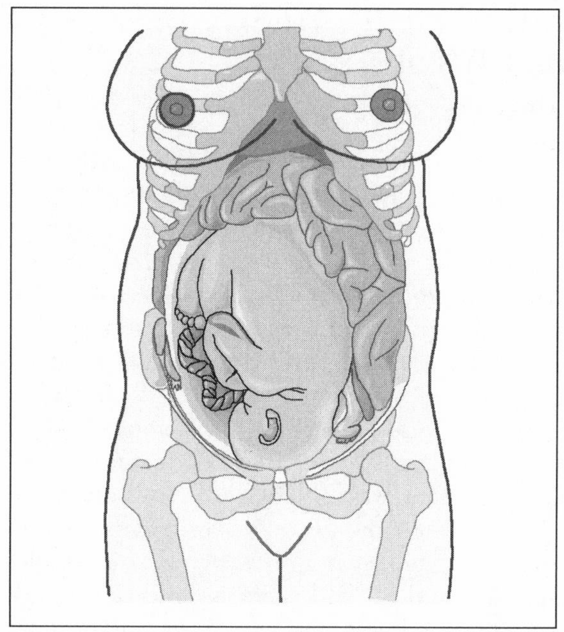
Front View of Last Trimester

During this time, the baby's nervous system and digestive system become more mature.

By the fifth month, the baby is about 12 inches long and weighs about 16 ounces. By the sixth month the baby is 14 inches long and weighs 1½ pounds. It is likely that your health care provider will use a Doppler or a fetoscope to hear the baby's heartbeat.

Months Seven through Nine: The Third Trimester

You

Now you visit your health care provider every two weeks. As the baby grows, your organs become more compressed. Most women feel more pressure on their stomach and bladder; some women begin to have backaches. Joints in the knees and hips also ache with the extra strain of the baby. You may have hemorrhoids, and varicose veins may begin to appear (in most cases these go away after pregnancy). It is common for ankles to swell and skin to stretch.

At the same time, women report that they feel the urge to nest and begin to prepare for having a baby in the home. For most women, it is advised to avoid heavy lifting.

Some women have to use breast pads because the breasts can begin to release a thick yellow substance called colostrum. Colostrum is a natural substance and is what your breasts will produce the first few days after you give birth (vaginal or cesarean) to nourish the baby. After three to five days, your breasts produce milk.

The Baby

There is a dramatic increase in movement—stretching and kicking. Babies may spend time in the breech position (tush down) until about the thirty-sixth week. At about that point, 97 percent turn upside down and prepare for delivery.

Giving Birth—Where, How, and When

Where to Give Birth

Most Latinas prefer to have their baby in a hospital. Others want to go to a birthing center, some of which are affiliated with a hospital. A few want to give birth at home. Whatever you choose, you should be well informed about the benefits and risks of each setting.

We have all heard of our *abuelas* (grandmothers) or *tías* (aunts) who gave birth at home. We also know the stories about how it was easier and simpler in a less technological and antiseptic world. Then we close our eyes and wish the same for ourselves. However, we must open our eyes and recognize that while our foremothers had *parteras* (midwives) and gave birth at home, there was also a high mortality rate among women and babies. The romanticization of home births fails to point out the risks involved. This is especially true when there are high-risk pregnancies or complications during birth.

Many of us feel that giving birth is a family event that needs to occur within a healthy and warm context. When our health care plan allows us to select where we can give birth, we must keep in mind what is important for most Latinas—a setting where our family is welcome. Our task is to understand our options and then make an informed choice.

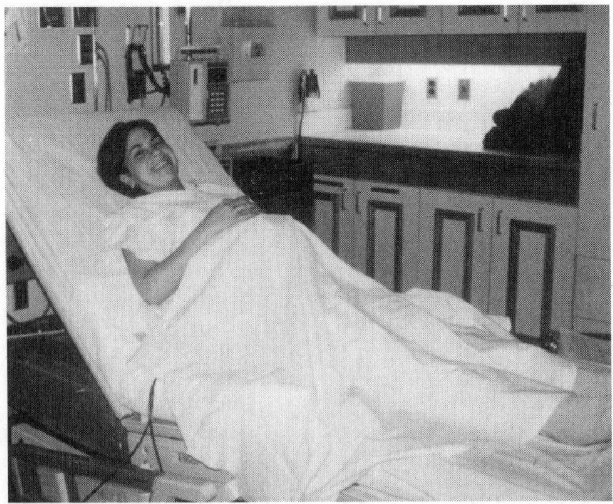

Each woman experiences her pregnancy in a unique way.

Until recently, the words *sterile* and *warm* seemed to be contradictory. Hospitals prided themselves on their sterility—not only in their procedures but also in the way patients were treated. Family members were not welcome in the labor area. The antiseptic treatment in hospitals, which may be credited for fewer maternal deaths, was contrary to the *personalismo* (personal, intimate, caring relationship) that a Latina needs. Today things are different, as hospitals strive to make delivery areas feel warm while maintaining even higher standards of sterility.

Insurance companies have sharply reduced the length of time a patient is covered for the postdelivery hospital stay, and there are increasing concerns that many women will not be given the time they need to fully recover in a controlled environment.

Remember that you do have choices about where to give birth. And the setting needs to be where you feel most safe and secure. While the experiences of *comadres* and *amigas* (family and friends) will help you understand different points of view, the choice of where you give birth and the type of provider you see is yours.

When you first know you are pregnant is a good time to think about the type of health care provider you want to see and where you want to give birth.

Each community offers different options. The regulations for each setting (hospital, free-standing birthing center, home, etc.) vary by locality, and because of that, while a free-standing birthing center may be ideal in one community, a hospital with a birthing center may be a better choice elsewhere. Consequently, it is essential that you call to get information and visit the different sites.

Whatever information you get about a setting should be in writing. Be sure to find out what your insurance covers and what your out-of-pocket costs will be. Additionally, make sure to visit the site and the health care provider. Listen to the conversations in the waiting room, and ask yourself if this is the kind of practice that you want to take care of you during your pregnancy. Most facilities will be happy to give you a tour. Take a good look at the rooms for labor and postdelivery.

What follows is a list of questions for you to ask the health care provider and the staff at the facility where you will give birth, along with some guidance to help you understand their responses.

1: How long can I stay after I give birth? Federal laws state that you must be able to stay in a hospital for 48 hours after a normal birth and 96 hours after a cesarean birth. Some settings are attracting more patients by offering an additional 24-hour stay at no cost. Make sure you know what coverage is offered by your health insurance plan, and make sure the setting you have selected for giving birth is included in the plan.

2: Will my family be allowed to be with me during labor? While many settings may say yes, some settings restrict family members to your legal husband. Make sure that you can designate who can be with you throughout childbirth and afterward.

3: What kinds of classes are offered before I give birth? Exercise classes, Lamaze classes, and classes on caring for a baby are good for most to attend. Even though you may have raised other children, there is always new information on the care of babies. It is good to be up to date with the latest treatments and warnings.

4: What kinds of classes are offered after I give birth? Exercise classes, breastfeeding classes, and other parenting classes are an important part of your support network after you give birth. It is very beneficial to become active in a total wellness program for you and your newborn baby. Most settings will use your pregnancy as a way to encourage you to become active in a program of health promotion and disease prevention.

5: What happens if my health care provider does not arrive in time? This may be a very important concern, especially for those women who have become attached to a specific provider. Even though you may be attended by one provider in a practice, it is good to know the other staff so that you feel comfortable with them and they understand what you will need. At the very least, be certain that your written records indicate any allergies you have and your preferences with respect to such matters as anesthesia and cesareans. Have a copy with you to take to the hospital.

6: What will be the procedure to decide if I need a cesarean? Of all births in the United States, 25 percent are by cesarean section. This number is often judged to be too high in comparison to other developed nations. You and your health care provider need to have a clear understanding of how a decision will be made with respect to a cesarean birth.

7: What happens if problems arise during labor? The answers to this question are very important when you are considering home births or using a free-standing birthing center. You need to know to which facility you will be taken and by whom you will be cared for if there are complications during your pregnancy or delivery. It is also important to know how you will be transported to a different facility in case of an emergency. Make sure that you feel comfortable with the answers you get. You do not want to have to address this issue when you are in the middle of labor.

How to Give Birth

Even if you have given birth before, you can never be fully prepared for childbirth. Latinas have indicated that each of their birth experiences has been different. Yet we know that if you know what to expect, it is easier to get through a difficult process.

We all know that giving birth is painful and that there is no glory in having excessive pain during childbirth. There is no way to totally eliminate pain, but we can learn to manage it. As a result of progress in accepting childbirth as a natural part of life and through medical research, there are a variety of methods to reduce pain during childbirth. These methods are discussed below.

Prepared Methods

These methods are sometimes referred to as natural childbirth or the Lamaze method. Until the 1960s the medical philosophy was to treat childbirth as a condition that had to be controlled. For many Latinas, this was unacceptable, because for us childbirth was not an illness but a wonderful part of a healthy adult life.

To counter the illness model of pregnancy, the trend toward natural childbirth, or prepared methods, evolved as a way for women to maintain control of the process of childbirth. The goal of these methods is to better prepare the woman and her family for the experience of childbirth. The underlying philosophy is that understanding the process helps in the relief of pain.

The Lamaze method is the most well-known system for preparing a woman and her family for childbirth. The Lamaze method developed from (1) research in Russia to condition women going through childbirth to relax when they felt a contraction; (2) the work of Dr. Lamaze, who in his clinic for metal workers in France added special breathing techniques to the conditioning work; and, (3) expansion in the United States of Dr. Lamaze's method to include the father or other family members in the birth process.

Overall, the Lamaze method seems consistent with the way Latinas view childbirth. There are some aspects that seem awkward to us, however. For example, in the United States it is common to refer to the person helping during childbirth as a birth "coach" rather than a birth assistant or supporter.

The implications of being a coach seem out of touch with the experiences of Latinas for two reasons. First, coaches are typically people who have actively engaged in the activity they are coaching, yet most birth coaches are men. Second, the birth coach is often encouraged to act like a coach, when in fact what the woman may want is support rather than direction.

On the whole, Latinas have enjoyed learning about the Lamaze method because it helps them understand the process of birth. But while we applaud the view of childbirth as a natural part of life, we acknowledge that there is no benefit to having excessive pain. In fact, what Latinas more often seek is a way to make childbirth healthy for the baby, supportive of the family, and as pain-free as possible.

I knew it was time for the baby to come soon. The pain was excruciating, and I was doing my best. My husband was trying to help, but when he said impatiently, "You're not breathing right. Focus on your breathing," I couldn't help but shout back, "Forget about the breathing! Be quiet and just hold my hand!"

—Dania, 38

Chemical Relief Methods

An epidural is the most common method of providing relief to a woman giving birth. A trained anesthesiologist inserts a small tube (catheter) into the base of the spine and carefully monitors how fast the anesthetic drips into your system. The anesthetic makes you feel numb from your waist down into your thighs. Some health care providers give an epidural during the beginning stages of labor (between 4 and 9 centimeters of dilation) and then let it wear away so that you will be able to push in the final stages of labor. Although you should not feel pain, you will be able to push. Modern pain medication can selectively block sensation but allow you to push. Most health care providers no longer let the epidural wear off.

Analgesics such as nitrous oxide (inhaled gas), morphine (by injection), and barbiturates are rarely used because of negative effects on the baby.

Combination Method

The most common method of giving birth involves a combination of chemical relief and prepared methods. This allows the woman to be as alert as possible during the birth process while alleviating the pain. The success of this procedure is based on the woman and the health care provider being flexible about how to proceed while keeping in mind the well-being of the mother and child.

Cesarean Method

In the United States, nearly 1 out of every 4 births is by cesarean section. The reasons for this high rate are not fully understood. Some health care activists attribute it to the reluctance of health care providers to take any risks when it comes to the health of the mother or child, and others attribute it to the sophisticated equipment available for monitoring when the baby is having problems. It is not known how many cesareans are scheduled in advance and how many are done based on factors that arise during delivery. Even Latinas who know they are going to have a cesarean do not always "schedule" their delivery.

When a cesarean is not done on an emergency basis, a woman may be given local anesthesia so that she can be awake to see the baby when it is born. A cesarean done on an emergency basis may require general anesthesia. Regardless, it is important to remember that a cesarean is major surgery and, depending on the fitness of the mother, requires three to six weeks for recuperation.

Myths and Facts

Myth: Anesthesia is not good for the baby.

Fact: Properly administered, anesthesia has no effect on the baby.

Myth: During pregnancy you can keep doing whatever sports you did before your pregnancy.

Fact: Generally it is OK to continue swimming, walking, and riding a stationary bicycle. Off limits during pregnancy are sports that involve changes in pressure (scuba diving, high-altitude sports) or are high impact (water-skiing, surfing, platform diving, high-impact aerobics).

Myth: When you are pregnant, you should take megadoses of vitamins.

Fact: Megadoses of vitamin A have been linked to birth defects. Before you take any vitamin, be sure to discuss it with your health care provider.

Myth: When your water breaks, you will release a lot of water.

Fact: Some women only release a trickle of water.

Myth: When you are retaining water, you should not drink water.

Fact: Ironically, you *should* drink water because it will help you release the water you are storing. You should also talk to your health care provider and make certain this is not a sign of something else.

Myth: You should not have children if you are over thirty-five.

Fact: Women over thirty-five can have children. There is, however, an increased risk of miscarriage and chromosomal abnormality (see table below). Also, women over thirty-five are more likely to have problems with fertility.

RISK FOR CHROMOSOMAL ABNORMALITIES

Age of Mother at Delivery	Risk of Down's Syndrome	Risk of Any Chromosomal Abnormality
20	1/1,667	1/526
24	1/1,250	1/476
28	1/1,111	1/455
32	1/769	1/322
36	1/289	1/156
38	1/173	1/102
40	1/106	1/66
42	1/63	1/42
44	1/38	1/26
46	1/23	1/16

Source: *The Harvard Guide to Women's Health.* Carlson, et al. Copyright © 1996 by the President and Fellows of Harvard College. Reprinted by permission of Harvard University Press.

Myth: You cannot have a cat if you are pregnant.

Fact: You can have a cat when you are pregnant, but you should not handle the cat's litterbox in any way. Toxoplasmosis is an illness caused by a parasite found in the feces of cats and other animals. Although the symptoms of this parasite are mild in adults, it can have a major impact on your baby by damaging its brain or eyes.

Myth: You must have an episiotomy.

Fact: While this used to be a routine procedure for all women giving birth, it is no longer considered routine. You do not need to have an episiotomy. Discuss with your health care provider your options with respect to an episiotomy. An episiotomy is done to prevent the tearing of the area between the vaginal opening and the anus (this area is called the perineum) during childbirth. Using scissors and a local anesthetic, the vaginal opening is cut toward the anus to make it larger. A disproven theory is that this is less painful than having the tissue torn as the baby comes out and is easier to sew together than a tear.

Recent experience indicates that the incision is rarely necessary. Moreover, women report that the healing process for the cut is very painful.

Consejos

As Soon as You Know You're Pregnant

1. Select your health care provider.
2. Select where you would like to give birth.
3. Identify who will be with you during childbirth.
4. Make known your preferences regarding anesthesia. This must be written down in case your doctor is not available.
5. Determine if you want an episiotomy (seldom avoidable for the first baby).
6. Since shaving the pubic hair is optional, make sure you make your preference about this known (most do not shave).

When to Give Birth

Only 5 percent of all women give birth on their due date. Although we know a lot about the development of the baby inside of you, we do not know what exactly makes childbirth begin. You will know it's time when the following takes place.

Contractions

The nature of these varies from woman to woman. While some women describe contractions as pain beyond words, others find that they are like very strong menstrual cramps. Your health care provider will tell you how long in duration and how frequent contractions have to be to signal that the birth process has begun. In early labor women may have contractions that are regular or irregular, lasting 30 to 45 seconds and 5 to 20 minutes apart. There is great variability in what women report in these early stages of labor. Usually, however, the time between contractions decreases.

It is common for some women to have "false contractions," or Braxton-Hicks contractions. These contractions are irregular and intense. They do not signal that labor has begun but rather that your body is preparing itself for labor. It is very hard to distinguish them from the early stages of childbirth.

Release of Liquid

Sometimes referred to as the water breaking, it is important to note that what is released will not look like water but merely be liquid in form and that the quantity of fluid released will vary by individual. Some women release a lot of fluid and others just release squirts. Once the fluid is released, you should see your health care provider because delivery must occur within 24 hours. If delivery is delayed, there is a risk that the mother or baby will get an infection.

After You Give Birth

This is a time of many adjustments—your sleep pattern is different as you respond to your baby's need to be fed; your hormones fluctuate as they try to return to previous levels; and your body begins the process of returning to the shape you want it to be. Some women may suffer severely from postpartum depression and need to see a mental health professional (see Chapter 13).

New logistics need to be negotiated—caring for other children in the home, setting things up at work, getting help from family and friends for cooking and cleaning in your home. You will also need to make sure you have adequate care for the baby when you need to shower, sleep, or just take a break.

Some Latinas find that they begin to feel amorous again. It is best, however, to wait for a few weeks after childbirth before you have vaginal-penile intercourse so that your cervix can close. This will reduce the likelihood of infection.

Now is the best time to start discussions about how many more children you want to have and how many years apart you would ideally like to space them.

Mind and Spirit

Throughout pregnancy, all of your activities should focus on bringing you mental peace and spiritual integrity. Pregnancy is a time when you should reflect on life and what it means to you and your family. You may want to educate yourself by reading about pregnancy, talking about child care issues with your partner and family, and trying to prepare yourself for the adjustments in life that a new child brings. Regardless of whether it is your first or fifth child, each new child requires a careful shift in the family. Some of us may see this as an opportunity to seek the support of a mental health professional.

Those of us who work outside the home may have to prepare ourselves and our coworkers for our new schedule. To make these changes thoughtfully and over time will create the least amount of disruption. Although the nine months of your pregnancy may have seemed very long, in fact, they were only the beginning.

Relaxation, prayer, and the loving support of those around you are critical during this time of change.

Summary

The way to get through pregnancy most successfully is to work with your body to prepare and support yourself through its many physical changes, make sure that you select a supportive environment for your care and childbirth, give yourself moments of relaxation, and finally, for Latinas who pray, to add to each day a special prayer of love and peace for their baby.

RESOURCES

Organizations

American College of Obstetricians and Gynecologists
P.O. Box 96920
409 12th Street SW
Washington, DC 20090-6920
(202) 638-5577 or (800) 762-2264
Resource Center
(202) 863-2518

National Healthy Mothers/Healthy Babies Coalition
121 N. Washington St. Suite 300
Alexandria, VA 22314
(703) 836-6110
www.hmhb.org

March of Dimes Birth Defects Foundation
1275 Mamaroneck Ave.
White Plains, NY 10605
(914) 428-7100 or
(888) MODIMES (663-4637)
www.modimes.org

National Center for Education in Maternal and Child Health
2000 15th Street North, Suite 701
Arlington, VA 22201
(703) 524-7802
www.ncemch.org

National Maternal and Child Health Clearinghouse
2070 Chain Bridge Road, Suite 450
Vienna, VA 22182
(703) 821-8955

National Women's Health Network and the Women's Health Network Clearinghouse
514 10th Street NW, Suite 400
Washington, DC 20004
(202) 347-1140
www.womenshealthnetwork.org

Hotlines

American Dietetic Association Consumer Nutrition Hotline
(800) 366-1655

American Institute for Cancer Research Nutrition Hotline
(800) 328-7744 or (800) 843-8114

National Hispanic Prenatal Hotline
National Alliance for Hispanic Health
(800) 504-7081 (Monday through Friday, 9 A.M. to 6 P.M., EST)

Su-Familia Family Health Helpline
National Alliance for Hispanic Health
866-SuFamilia (783-2645)

Books

Eisenberg, A., H. E. Murkoff, and S. E. Hathaway. *What to Expect When You're Expecting*. New York: Workman, 1996.

Lifshitz, Aliza. *Mamá Sana, Bebé Sano/ Healthy Mother, Healthy Baby.* New York: HarperCollins, 2002.

Publications and Pamphlets

"Alimentos Saludables/Bebé Saludable," 1991. In Spanish. Healthy eating during pregancy. Philadelphia Department of Public Health, Division of Maternal and Child Health, 1101 Market St. 9th floor, Philadelphia, PA 19107; (215) 875-5927.

"Blue Ribbon Babies: Eating Well During Pregnancy," 1992. Also available in Spanish. American Dietetic Association, 216 West Jackson Boulevard, Chicago, IL 60606-6995; (800) 745-0775 x5000.

"Getting Ready for Pregnancy: Things to Think about Before You're Pregnant," 1999. Pamphlet No. 1551. American Academy of Family Physicians, 11400 Tomahawk Creek Pkwy, Leawood, KS 66211-2672; (800) 944-0000. Other titles include "During Pregnancy: Taking Care of You and Your Baby." Pamphlet No. 1560.

"How Your Baby Grows," 1995. Pamphlet No. 09-345-00. Also available in Spanish. A monthly diary of your baby's development. March of Dimes, P.O. Box 1657, Wilkes-Barre, PA 18703; (800) 367-6630. Other English/Spanish titles include:

"Be Good to Your Baby Before It's Born." Pamphlet No. 09-002-00.

"Eating for Two: Nutrition During Pregnancy." Pamphlet No. 09-219-00.

"El Parto Prematuro." Pamphlet No. 33-205-04.

"Sound Nutrition for Your Pregnancy," American Institute for Cancer Research, 1759 R Street NW, Washington, DC 20009; (800) 843-8114
www.aicr.org

"Planning Your Pregnancy & Birth," 3rd Edition, May 2000.

"You and Your Baby: Prenatal Care, Labor and Delivery, and Postpartum Care," 1994. To order call the American College of Obstetricians and Gynecologists Resource Center, (800) 762-2264 or contact www.acog.org Other titles include:

"Pain Relief During Labor and Delivery." Pamphlet No. 6789/7654.

"Pregnancy Choices: Raising the Baby, Adoption and Abortion." Pamphlet No. 12345/76543.

"Vaginal Birth after Cesarean." Pamphlet No. 5678/7654, also available in Spanish as Pamphlet No. 23456/87654.

9

Menopause

De Mujer a Mujer . . .

From Woman to Woman

The relationship my mother and I had was very unusual as far as Latina relationships go—we were each other's best friend. So when I asked my mother about menopause, I was quite surprised at her response.

All Mom said was that hers came at a time in her life when all she noticed was that her period was less frequent. She knew she could not be pregnant, because she had not been with a man for years.

Mom did not worry that something could be wrong with her ovaries. She just assumed that whatever was happening was part of life. If she had cancer, then she would deal with that. If it was menopause . . . then her period would just go away. Consequently, when her period finally went away, she didn't think anything of it. For her it was a nonevent. She did not even remember when it had actually stopped.

Mom thought about all the drama that other women use to express what their menopause is about. For my mom, there had been lots of real drama in her life. So when it came to her period . . . well . . . it just went away and she kept on with her life.

For centuries in the past and even in our times, many women have defined their lives by their ability to have children. Historically, neither society nor medicine have responded well to the moment of life when women enter menopause. Some cultures have made women feel that menopause is the end of their womanhood, while others have tended to "medicalize" menopause.

Today things are different, and menopause needs to be viewed in a different way, not as the end point of a woman's life, but rather as part of the continuum of being a woman. Menopause should be seen as a positive change in our life. As Latinas live longer and healthier lives, most of us will spend nearly half of our adult years in the postmenopausal phase.

To talk about menopause in a new way means that we understand it as something we pass through. Sometimes referred to as the *cambio de vida* (change of life) or climacteric, menopause is the time of our lives when our ovaries stop releasing eggs (i.e., ovulating). This means that we can no longer have biological children, and sexuality can be fully enjoyed as an expression of intimacy without fear of pregnancy. Equally important to our health, however, is that we will no longer enjoy as many of the protections that estrogen (a key hormone) produced in our body, which reduced our risk of heart disease and osteoporosis. Similarly, we will no longer suffer from the problems created by estrogen.

Recently the term *perimenopause* has been used to capture the time when the process leading to menopause begins. This is in many ways an artificial concept. Perimenopause may stretch out for years for some women and last only a month for others. Some women have gradual changes leading up to the last egg, while others have a sudden and abrupt last period.

What Is Menopause?

"There are so many questions I have about menopause," said Anita. "I am glad that I have a friend to talk to about it," she added before going into her long list of questions. "What do you do about the dryness? How do I handle hot flashes? Does it get worse? What do I do so that no one notices? Am I too young?"

I just sat there, amazed at all her questions. "Dryness?" I thought to myself—I had no idea what Anita was talking about. All I could remember was being wet—sweating during the day, soaking my sheets at night with the perspiration that came from nowhere. The last thing I ever worried about was being dry. I had lived through my own menopause and thought that I could be helpful, but I realized that I really did not know what to say to Anita. Her experiences were very different from mine.

—Daisy, 54

In fact, menopause is a process that is different for every woman. Just as women experience their menstrual cycle in ways unique to each of them, menopause will also be unique to each. Although there may be common elements, the totality of menopause will be defined by the individual experiences of each woman.

When you ask Latinas about menopause, their responses range from a lot of smiles by the older women, to silence from the youngest members of the group, to a look from those who are currently experiencing it that seems to say, "Where do I begin?"

There is no exact instant when you enter menopause. Menopause is technically defined as the time when you stop menstruating for one year. This means that you stop ovulating and your ovaries also produce less estrogen. It is the time when your brain stops telling your body to prepare for pregnancy on a monthly basis. But this does not happen as a discrete event. For most of us, it is a series of physiological adjustments our body makes that culminate in the cessation of our menstruation.

There are several kinds of menopause: premature menopause, natural menopause, chemical menopause, surgical menopause, and stress menopause. In all cases the result is that the ovaries stop their monthly release of eggs.

- **Premature Menopause.** If a woman develops menopause before age of thirty-five the onset of menopause is considered premature. A complete evaluation should be done by your health care provider to rule out an autoimmune disease or a chromosomal problem. The cause of the premature menopause may be treatable.

- **Natural menopause.** Women are born with a limited number of eggs, and one day your body stops releasing eggs. This change may happen all of a sudden or it may occur over time. The time leading up to the change is called the perimenopausal phase. The time after menopause is called the postmenopausal phase.

• **Chemical menopause.** Some medications prescribed for the treatment of a variety of conditions, such as endometriosis, make the body believe that it is entering menopause. These medications alter the hormonal balance of the body and induce a chemical menopause. When you stop taking the medication, in most instances your ovaries begin to function again.

• **Surgical menopause.** Women who undergo removal of both ovaries are described as having a surgical menopause (see Chapter 6). The removal of both ovaries eliminates the possibility of releasing an egg. As a consequence of this kind of surgery, the body begins the process of menopause with a jump start. Sometimes medication is prescribed to ease the transition.

• **Stress menopause.** Sometimes women in their late thirties or older stop menstruating for several months due to some major emotional stress in their lives, such as illness, depression, or severe grief. When these are the reasons for the cessation of menstruation, the condition is called stress menopause.

Regardless of the type of menopause or the age of a woman, the symptoms are similar. In surgical and chemical menopause, the abruptness of the onset of symptoms may require greater adjustment for your body. Although women who have surgical or chemical menopause are told in advance that they will experience symptoms of menopause, it is often the case that they are not prepared for the symptoms when they have them.

What to Expect

The best way to understand menopause is to know what changes we may see in our body and to be prepared for their impact on our mind and spirit. According to the research available, some women report that they have no physical symptoms. It is very likely, however, that whether our symptoms are mild or severe, menopause will have some impact on how we feel about ourselves and on our spirit.

When I was in my late twenties, I had to take Danazol as the treatment for my endometriosis. It put me out of commission for a while. My ovaries went out of business and I stopped getting my period. Although not getting my period was nice, I had not been adequately prepared by my health care provider for all the symptoms I would experience as a result of this pseudomenopause.

I got the whole thing—I would get hot flashes and what I could at best call "arousal in the absence of anything." I would be writing some boring memo and all of a sudden I would feel very sexually aroused. I would look around and there was nothing. It had to be the Danazol.

Now I know before actual experiencing natural menopause what menopause will bring me: whatever strange feelings my body wants me to have, whenever it wants me to have them. It will definitely be out of my control.

—*Gabriela, 39*

Body

As women, our bodies thrive on hormones, including estrogen, progesterone, and androgen. When our ovaries start to produce lower levels of these hormones, our bodies are forced to find new ways to regulate themselves. A lot of what our bodies do during menopause is best described as trial-and-error attempts at adapting to these hormonal changes. The symptoms we have show the ways our bodies are trying to adjust.

Symptoms

Very often, to help our health care providers know what is going on with us, we become trained in using the same language they use. Some of the most common symptoms of menopause and descriptions of actual experiences are provided below. Keep in mind that once your body has adjusted to the reduction in hormones, most of these symptoms will go away.

• **Irregular periods.** One of the first symptoms noticed by women is changes in their menstrual cycle. Those Latinas who have always had irregular periods may have periods that are even more irregular or less frequent than usual. If your menstrual cycle was 27 to 33 days, you may find that you have cycles that are 21 to 38 days long. You may even skip a month or two.

• **Hot flashes.** This is one of the things about which it is true to say that when you have one you will know it. You will be doing whatever you are doing, and all of a sudden it will feel as if someone turned up your internal thermostat. The sensation will progress from hot to hotter and even hotter, even when objectively you know that the temperature around you has stayed the same.

You will probably look around to see if anyone else is experiencing discomfort and find that everyone is just going about their business. A hot flash can last for a few seconds or several minutes.

Some women have only one or a few hot flashes during their entire menopause, while other women have them several times a day. Some Latinas describe them as "hot waves" rather than flashes because of the way they seem to wash over them.

• **Night sweats** occur when you have a hot flash while sleeping. Some women just kick off the covers. Others wake up to bed linens wet with their own perspiration. The most troublesome side effect of night sweats is that they seem to disturb the amount of REM (rapid eye movement) sleep you get. Without sufficient REM sleep, you are likely to become irritable and have mood swings. You may have this experience for several months or not at all.

• **Vaginal dryness.** Some Latinas may find that a number of years after menopause, even though they are sexually aroused, they do not lubricate sufficiently to make intercourse comfortable. Using a vaginal lubricant (e.g., Astroglide), which can be bought in most cosmetic or drug stores (without a prescription), can alleviate this symptom. Some couples have found that use of a vaginal lubricant has contributed to their sexual pleasure.

• **Change in sexual desire.** Menopause often causes a change in sexual desire, and the changes can vary. Some women report that their sexual appetite increases; others report a complete loss of sexual desire. Each woman knows how much of a sexual appetite she is used to enjoying. When this appetite goes through a major change, it is difficult for us and for our partners. Usually couples adapt their lives to a certain amount of sexual activity; changes from the norm can place stress on us and our relationships.

The myth that there is never too much sexual desire is easily shattered when a Latina becomes a lot more demanding in her sexual needs. Some women experience what is called "inappropriate sexual desire," which means that they may feel aroused when there is no stimulation. There is no research that clearly identifies how much of this change in sexual desire is due to our bodies and how much is due to our feelings about our womanhood.

• **Early wakening.** Some women report that menopause affects their sleeping patterns, and in particular that they tend to awaken earlier in the morning. Whether you wake up on

> ***Consejos***
>
> Keep alert for news about the health consequences of the wild Mexican yam. From this yam, it is possible to produce a natural progesterone that has the same chemical structure as the progesterone produced in a woman's ovaries. To this point there have been no clinical trials on the impact of natural progesterone.

your own at 5 A.M. or 6 A.M. is less important than how different this is from the pattern you have had throughout your life. You are the best judge of what is happening.

• **Bladder problems.** Some women experience a mild loss of bladder control during menopause. The problem may not actually be your bladder or necessarily be related to menopause, but rather may be due to the muscles that control the outflow of urine. Sometimes when you sneeze or exert yourself in normal ways, you may release some urine. This is called mild stress incontinence. This weakening of the muscles that control urination may worsen during menopause. Muscle control can be helped by regular Kegel exercises (see Chapter 8). Hormone replacement will not correct this.

• **Feeling blue.** Since changes in our hormones can affect our moods, we need to recognize that at times it will seem that we are feeling blue for no reason. Women who have experienced symptoms of moodiness while premenstrual know that the rise and fall of hormones can affect how we feel emotionally as well as physically. Similarly, a menopausal woman might feel herself more sensitive to common stresses or more easily depressed.

Some of the other but less frequently reported symptoms that may be part of the menopause experience include difficulty concentrating, headaches, difficulty falling asleep, frequent urination, and sweating a lot more than usual.

No one can tell you exactly what combination of these symptoms you will experience. Some women have no symptoms; some have only a few symptoms; and others experience symptoms that make it impossible for them to follow their regular routine.

Menopause can occur when women are in their early thirties or in their fifties. Early menopause (including surgical and chemical) is defined as that which takes place before age forty-five. It is uncertain how many women have an early menopause; we do know that half of all women reach menopause before they are fifty-one.

Mind

Donna was in her late fifties now. For her, menopause came all of a sudden when she was in her early forties. She had always worked hard, but then one year she was asked to be part of a major political campaign. Donna knew that the added load would stretch her to her mental and physical limits.

She was not surprised when she stopped getting her period during the five months she campaigned. She just assumed that as soon as the campaign was over she would get her period back. But it never came back.

Donna laughs and says she was too busy campaigning to notice that she never menstruated again. Donna says, "Menopause was happening to me, but I was too busy to see it. I guess in some ways menopause passed me by."

It is a mixed blessing that Latinas seem to take menopause for granted. On the one hand it can prevent us from becoming unduly traumatized by this natural step in our adult development. On the other hand it can discourage

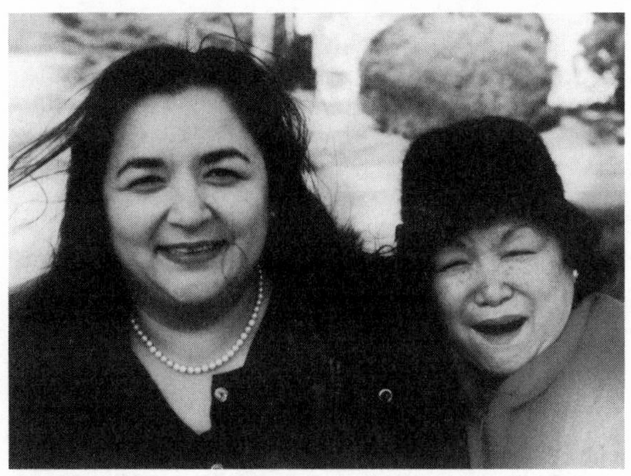

Mothers should share with their daughters what to expect as they grow older.

us from talking about our experiences, as if menopause is something to be kept hidden.

Perhaps the most important thing we can do for each other is to talk among ourselves about what menopause feels like, aside from what it does to our bodies. Too often younger women feel it is an insult or an invasion of privacy to ask older women they know about their experiences with menopause. This concern is not unfounded, because many women do feel uncomfortable talking about menopause—it means they have to acknowledge that they have gone or are going through this passage.

To explore how your menopause has affected you mentally, not just physically, ask yourself the following questions.

• **What does menopause mean to me?** It may mean nothing, and it may mean everything. The task is to honestly recognize your assumptions about this time of life. Is it a symbol of aging, or do you feel freed from the demands of childbearing or the concerns of pregnancy?

• **Does menopause make me less feminine?** Too many of us have been socialized with a definition of ourselves that equates womanhood with menstruation and fertility; that is, the existence of a high level of estrogen with being feminine. For many health care providers, Robert Wilson's 1966 book, *Forever Feminine*, which advocated that women should begin to take estrogen before menopause and continue to take it throughout their lives, contributed to the relationship between estrogen and femininity. The implicit message was that a loss of estrogen meant a loss of sex drive and thus a loss of our essential femininity. We know better now.

• **Do I feel bad that I can no longer have children?** Many women experience regret for the loss of reproductive function because they have been conditioned to see it as a large part of their definition as a woman. Latinas who have chosen never to have children as well as those who are infertile may experience sadness at the realization that with menopause they are now forever unable to have a biological child. Even women with children can feel a sense of loss when having children is no longer a choice—they feel as if the choice has been taken away from them.

• **How does menopause affect my life?** In many ways menopause should have no major impact on your life. It is not as if women leave their partners and start new relationships just because they have entered menopause. At the same time, because of the point in one's life when menopause occurs, some women may choose to see it as an opportunity to reorganize their life and to make desired changes. Now that they have freedom from pregnancy and contraception, they have the space and liberty to reevaluate their lives and to set new goals and priorities.

• **How will menopause affect those in my life?** The impact on the lives of others is determined by how much menopause affects our own life. If you are among the small group of women who experience severe mood swings, menopause will have at least a temporary impact on your relationships. Similarly, for those women who experience a loss of interest in sex, the nature of their relationships will also change. Talking about menopause to your partners, family, and friends will help them understand the transitions that you are experiencing in your life.

Spirit

Olivia had spent the last few decades defining herself by the three m's in her life: madre, mujer, y medicina *(mother, woman, and medicine). She had felt secure in who she was and in the choices she had made in her life. Her daughter had grown up to be a beautiful young woman, her son was doing well in college, she had a supportive and loving relationship, and she still saw some patients.*

Menopause did not come as a surprise to her. As a physician she felt she could easily handle the physical fluctuations produced by menopause. She knew that her hot flash was just a sign that her body was trying to regulate itself as its hormonal levels were shifting. The physical parts of menopause were straightforward. Her thoughts and spirit, however, seemed unsettled.

She was not sure how she wanted to spend the rest of whatever years she had left. Perhaps she would practice more medicine and focus more on the healing arts. She knew for sure that at the very least she would go back to church.

The experience of being in menopause may bring us closer to considering how we want to live the rest of our life. Depending on our age, our sense of life may be deeply affected by menopause. For those Latinas who believe in an afterlife, menopause is one more step in that journey. For other Latinas, menopause may help them become aware of the need for spiritual reconciliation. This phase of life brings new frameworks for old questions and the constant challenge to integrate our being with a higher, more spiritual world.

Getting Through It

The one thing we can all agree on is that menopause involves changes. What each one of us has to decide is how we want to address these changes.

Just as no one can predict the course menopause will take in any other person, no one can prescribe the best way for you to get through your menopause. For a substantial number of Latinas, getting through menopause is no different from anything else in our life. If we focus on our families and our work and add a little bit of our capacity for *aguantar*, we will pass through menopause better than ever. Most women experience few if any symptoms of menopause, and the passage is easily managed. But some women may have to take a more proactive approach to handling this stage in their lives.

There are things we can do to make the passage easier. We have to know what is the best medicine that is available for our various symptoms should they reach unmanageable levels. We have to develop mechanisms for talking about the difficult questions we are called upon to answer. And we must recognize that we are entering a new and greatly fulfilling part of our existence.

Body

The reason we experience so many physical changes is that our bodies are going through major hormonal fluctuations. There are a variety of options available to make it easier for our bodies. Some of these are described below.

Be Natural and Do Nothing

For the majority of women, this may be the best option. It may be that for these women menopause produces either no symptoms or tolerable ones. The onset of menopause may be sudden and not require medication for relief of symptoms.

The pros and cons of doing nothing are often debated in the absence of the long-term data that are necessary to make accurate and definitive statements about the best course of action to take. In short, we do not know for certain whether it is best to do nothing or to do something. Moreover, it is not known if there is any relationship between symptoms during menopause and increased risk of osteoporosis or heart disease. What we actually know about the impact of the symptoms of menopause on our bodies is very little.

We must decide with our health care provider what we should do. Sometimes, however, the decision to take medications is taken out of our hands because some health plans do not provide coverage for hormone replacement therapy (HRT).

While many of us may be enamored of things natural, we must understand that for some Latinas that course is not possible. In the 1990s Latinas who went through menopause early and were concerned about the early loss of some of the protection against heart disease and osteoporosis that estrogen provides were given HRT. Today some Latinas feel that it is better not to have the estrogen because of its relationship to endometrial cancer and breast cancer and increasing doubts about whether HRT provides protection against heart disease.

Nevertheless, it is your body, and the decision about how you want to address some of the physical symptoms of menopause should be yours.

Unfortunately, too often women have been encouraged to treat menopause as if it were a disease. In this model, menopause is not part of normal female adult development (which, in fact, it is) but rather a medical condition that must be treated. For women who see menopause as a disease or for whom the symptoms are very severe, medication, sometimes HRT, is prescribed to provide some relief.

Hormonal Replacement Therapy (HRT)

Cassandra had been worried about taking hormones to help her through her menopause. She had always felt it was better not to take pills. She preferred more natural ways to heal the body. So she asked her friend Cándida if she had taken any hormones during her menopause.

Cándida was quick to answer, "Hormones have been the most wonderful thing for me. I would never give them up. I was starting to have all the awful things you hear about menopause—hot flashes and night sweats. Then my doctor put me on the hormone replacement pills. I feel better than I did before menopause. They have made all these changes bearable for me."

Cassandra was surprised to hear such a glowing report from Cándida. Perhaps it would be all right to take some medication; maybe taking the pills would not be so bad. She would have to seriously consider it.

We know that estrogen is good for us. Estrogen is the hormone believed to provide the protective factors that delay onset of heart disease in women. Estrogen is also responsible for maintaining skin tone and vaginal lubrication. In the 1960s estrogen was routinely prescribed for all women who were going through menopause. In the seventies, data were starting to show that women who took estrogen had an increased risk for uterine cancer.

Research continued to investigate what combination of hormones would benefit women the most with the fewest risks. This became critical because mounting evidence documented the positive effects of estrogen—reduced risk of osteoporosis and possible reduction of heart disease.

Doctors soon found that hormone replacement therapy, which is a combination of estrogen and progestin (the synthetic form of the progesterone hormone) could make up for the hormones our bodies were no longer producing without increasing the risk of uterine cancer. We know that HRT reduces hot flashes, prevents osteoporosis, and in some cases may possibly prevent heart disease.

Although HRT is no longer new, the long-term effects of the treatment are still uncertain. For example, while estrogen is known to increase levels of good cholesterol (high-density lipoprotein, or HDL), progestins not only decrease HDL but also increase bad cholesterol (low-density lipoprotein, or LDL). Recent research questions whether HRT provides the protection against heart disease that we used to think it did.

Some women express concern about HRT and the increased likelihood of breast cancer. Current research suggests that the relationship is at best controversial. There are some studies documenting that HRT slightly increases the risk for cancer.

HRT is given in two ways: sequentially and continuously. Each method is tailored to the individual, based on discussions with the health care provider.

In the sequential method, you take estrogen for 21 to 25 days and add progestin pills around day 11 for 2 weeks. For the last 7 days of the month, no pills are taken. During this time, you have a pseudomenstrual cycle in which you bleed but do not release an egg. This is referred to as withdrawal bleeding. During these 7 days, some women also have a return of some of the symptoms of menopause, such as hot flashes.

In the continuous method, you take a combination of estrogen and progestin every day. Some women experience spotting when they start taking the medication, but this stops after a few months. Your health care provider may adjust the levels of estrogen and progestin so that you do not have any bleeding.

Good News: Women who are post-menopausal are less likely to be depressed than women who have not gone through menopause.

Synthetic forms of estrogen (those developed by combining chemicals in a lab) are used in birth control pills, while natural estrogen (collected from the urine of horse mares) is most often used for HRT. Although most women take estrogen in pill form, some women prefer the use of a patch, which slowly releases estrogen into the body. The patch is usually placed on the stomach and replaced once or twice a week. It is usually prescribed for women with liver or gallbladder problems because it allows estrogen to be absorbed directly into the body without having to be processed in the liver. The progestin is also given in pill form.

How much of each hormone you will receive must be determined by working closely with your health care provider. Since the menopause experience is so different for each woman, the treatment needs to be carefully tailored and monitored. Keep in mind that in order to maintain protection against osteoporosis, it is best to start HRT within the first three years of menopause and continue it indefinitely. For Latinas, who are known to have lower rates of heart disease and osteoporosis than the general population, the decision concerning HRT must be weighed carefully.

Although some women may benefit from HRT, there is increasing evidence that you should not have HRT if you have any of the following: breast cancer, clotting disorders, endometrial cancer, gallbladder disease, liver disease, undiagnosed abnormal vaginal bleeding, or a family history of breast, ovarian, or endometrial cancer.

Other hormonal treatments are also given during menopause to alleviate symptoms. Some women who complain about decreased sexual desire may be given testosterone, which might increase sex drive. For women who are concerned about vaginal dryness, a vaginal cream with estrogen is sometimes prescribed. Women who use this cream on a regular basis will probably also be given progestin pills to decrease the risk of uterine cancer. A new low dose estrogen ring that is placed in the vagina can substitute for the estrogen vaginal cream.

Hormonal therapies alleviate the physical symptoms of menopause. Whether they are worth the associated risks is a decision that you and your health care provider must make. HRT involves a long-term commitment and should be taken very seriously.

Exercise

Increasingly, research is supporting the notion that moderate exercise (none of this "no pain, no gain" compulsiveness), even strolling, has a lasting positive effect on women's hearts. For some reason, exercise seems to improve the way our body and our hormones function. In addition, the lack of estrogen's protective factors for the heart may be balanced by the benefits gained from even modest increases in exercise.

If you have been a couch potato most of your life, try walking three times a week for half an hour. When our estrogen level is decreasing, we have to take better care of our hearts. If you try it, you may find you like the way you feel.

Mind and Spirit

Much of what we think about menopause is mediated by what we experience physically. This is compounded by the fact that hormones have an effect on our mood. It may be that we are not experiencing some of the symptoms of menopause because we are taking HRT or antidepressants to alleviate them.

Whether or not we are taking medication, all of us who are going through menopause have questions, thoughts, and feelings. To better understand what we are going through, we must find ways to address these issues. Sometimes the answer is easy and obvious. At other times we have to search within ourselves. In most cases we benefit from sharing with other women and finding answers in the relationships that help define our days.

Myths and Facts

Myth: I will reach menopause at the same age as my mother.

Fact: There is no way to predict when a woman will enter menopause.

Myth: Once you go through menopause, it is not necessary to have pelvic exams or see your gynecologist.

Fact: Women need regular health care on an ongoing basis. Seeing your gynecologist and getting pelvic exams are key to prevention and early identification of health problems.

Myth: You do not have to worry about being pregnant when you go into menopause.

Fact: It is recommended that you wait one full year after your last period before you stop using birth control. Keep in mind that condoms should still be used to protect yourself from sexually transmitted diseases.

Summary

As Latinas, we do not usually talk about menopause, we just let it happen. While this may be our usual way of coping with it, we now have more options. We can choose to recognize the symptoms of menopause and decide whether we want to take medication, do Kegel exercises to address bladder problems, or just do nothing. Whatever we do, the choice is ours.

While most non-Latinas focus on what happens with the body during menopause, our focus is different. As our hormone levels decrease, we need to look at how our emotions and spirit are changing as our body is preparing us for the next phase of our lives. Where that will take us, we will decide.

RESOURCES

Organizations

American Association of Retired Persons—Women's Initiative
601 E Street NW
Washington, DC 20049
(202) 434-2277 or (800) 424-3410
www.aarp.org

American College of Obstetricians and Gynecologists
P.O. Box 96920
409 12th Street SW
Washington, DC 20090-6920
(202) 638-5577 or (800) 762-2264
www.acog.org

Association of Reproductive Health Professionals
2401 Pennsylvania Avenue NW, Suite 350
Washington, DC 20037-1718
(202) 466-3825
www.arhp.org

National Institute on Aging
9000 Rockville Pike
Bethesda, MD 20892
(800) 222-2225
Information Center
8630 Fenton St.
Silver Spring, MD 20910
www.nih.gov/nia

National Women's Health Network
514 10th Street NW, Suite 400
Washington, DC 20004
(202) 347-1140
www.womenshealthnetwork.org

National Women's Health Resource Center
120 Albany St. Ste. 820
New Brunswick, NJ 08901
(877) 986-9472
www.healthywomen.org

North American Menopause Society
PO Box 94527
Cleveland, OH 44101-4527
(440) 442-7550
www.menopause.org

Older Women's League
666 11th Street NW, Suite 700
Washington, DC 20001
(202) 783-6686 or (800) 825-3695
www.owl-national.org

Hotlines

Planned Parenthood Mid-Life Services
(800) 230-PLAN (800-230-7526)

Books

Greer, Germaine. *The Change*. New York: Alfred A. Knopf, 1993.

Henkel, Gretchen. *Making the Estrogen Decision*. New York: Fawcett Book Group, 1993.

Landau, Carol, M. G. Cyr, and A. W. Moulton. *The Complete Book of Menopause*. New York: G. P. Putnam's Sons, 1994.

Notelovitz, Morris. *Estrogen: Yes or No?* New York: St. Martin's Press, 1993.

Teaff, Nancy Lee, and Kim Wright Wiley. *Perimenopause: Preparing for the Change*. New York: Prima Publishing, 1999.

Utian, Wulf H., and Ruth S. Jacobwitz. *Managing Your Menopause*. New York: Prentice Hall, 1991.

Publications and Pamphlets

"Hormone Replacement Therapy," Pamphlet No. 3456/7654. American College of

Obstetricians and Gynecologists, P.O. Box 96920; Washington, DC 20090-6920; (800) 762-2264; www.acog.org. Other titles include "The Menopause Years," Pamphlet No. 456/765. Also available in Spanish.

"Menopause: What to Expect When Your Body is Changing," 1999. Pamphlet No. 1549. "Hormone Replacement Therapy" Pamphlet No. 1573. AAFP Family Health Facts. American Academy of Family Physicians, 11400 Tomahawk Creek Pkwy, Leawood, KS 66211-2672; (800) 944-0000

"Menopause and Perimenopause: A Guide for Patients," 1996. Patient Information series. American Society for Reproductive Medicine, 1209 Montgomery Highway, Birmingham, AL 35216-2809; (205) 978-5000.

"Perimenopause: Pathways to Change," 1994. Association of Reproductive Health Professionals, 2401 Pennsylvania Avenue NW, Suite 350, Washington, DC 20037-1718; (202) 466-3825. Available in Spanish.

"Menopause Talk," 2000. Solvay Pharmaceuticals, 901 Sawyer Road, Marietta, GA 30062; (770) 578-9000. Available in Spanish.

PART III

Enfermedades . . . Diseases

10

Alcoholism Is a Disease

Delia and Rodrigo were living together. Delia was madly in love with Rodrigo. Over time she found that she was jealous of every minute he spent away from her. And because his work required Rodrigo to travel a lot, they couldn't always be together.

One night Rodrigo's plane was delayed, and Delia sat home waiting for him. To calm her nerves, she began to pour herself some wine and drink it. And she did feel better. This began a pattern. The longer Delia waited, the more she drank. And the more she drank, the more certain she became that her Rodrigo was with another woman. By the time he arrived, she was wild with jealousy, and she attacked him—physically. She was out of control.

For many years, the conventional wisdom was that women did not drink, and that Latinas were less likely to drink than any other group of women. But the times are changing, and not necessarily for the better.

We should not be surprised. The alcohol and other advertising that we see suggests that someone who drinks has lots of fun, companions, and nice clothes. It is a sign of success to drink a certain brand of whiskey. To drink a beer and be happy and smiling gives you membership in the group of those who have made it. Thus, for Latinas too, drinking fine wine at a nice restaurant is now a sign of success.

Latinas today drink more alcohol than they did in the past. Most significantly, those Latinas who speak English and have better-paying jobs are more likely to drink. Latinas who abuse alcohol say they drink for relief, to get by, or to numb the pain from problems (which in fact the alcohol only exacerbates).

More so than in any other area of health, the diagnosis and treatment of alcoholism is based on the knowledge and experience of men. But women and men often drink for very different reasons, and when they drink they are judged in very different ways. Men drink because society says it is OK for men to drink, even to excess. Real men drink and hold their liquor, and when they do something wrong, it is often brushed aside with "Well, he just wanted to be one of the boys." For women the use of alcohol is viewed in a much less forgiving light. Generally society does not approve of women drinking to excess and considers that if a woman does so, whatever happens to her is her own fault.

As women and Latinas, the information we need about alcoholism is very basic—what it is, what it does, how to recognize its symptoms, and what to do about it. This knowledge will help us control the place we give to alcohol in our lives and in the lives of those we love.

How Much Alcohol in Each?

Drink	Percent Alcohol
Beer	5%
Wine	12%
80 proof	40%
150 proof	75%

How Our Body Uses Alcohol

Technically, alcohol belongs to a class of compounds that are fairly common in nature. Alcohol compounds have unique purposes, depending on their type; for example, isopropyl alcohol (rubbing alcohol), methanol (used in industry as a solvent), ethylene glycol (antifreeze), and ethanol (what we drink). The alcohol we drink is a product of the natural fermentation of sugar and grains.

When we drink alcohol, it travels to the stomach and intestines, where it is absorbed into our bloodstream. The bloodstream carries much of the alcohol to our liver to be metabolized. Our metabolism includes all the complex processes by which our body uses the substances we ingest, and it involves a variety of physical and chemical reactions.

The stomach and liver have special enzymes that help break down the alcohol into components more easily used by the body. Some of the alcohol is metabolized as soon as it enters the stomach. As alcohol accumulates, it can no longer be metabolized in the stomach and is instead absorbed by the stomach or the small intestine and transported to the liver. The small intestine is better prepared than the stomach to absorb alcohol. Most of the alcohol you drink is broken down in the liver.

The longer the alcohol stays in your stomach, the more of it will be metabolized in your stomach. When larger amounts of alcohol are metabolized in your stomach, less of it enters the bloodstream to go to the liver for processing. That is why when you drink on an empty stomach, you feel the effects of the alcohol faster than when you have a full stomach.

Blood alcohol concentrations (BACs) are a measure of how well the body is absorbing alcohol. For some reason, women do not seem to absorb alcohol into their systems as well as men. This means that women have higher BACs sooner than men and may be more vulnerable to liver damage.

The Impact of Alcohol on Our Body

People who are alcoholics drink more alcohol than their body can process. They become deficient in certain nutrients, especially vitamins A, B1 (thiamin), B6, D, E, and folate. Alcoholic women also have more irregular menstrual cycles and are more likely to have an early menopause. Women who are in the advanced stages of alcoholism also tend to lose more weight than men.

When you drink, your drinking has an impact on every part of your body. The more you drink, the worse the impact will be on your brain, liver, heart, and pancreas.

Effect on the Brain

Alcohol kills brain cells. This results in three categories of organic brain disease:

Warning: These Are the Risks You Face If You Are Pregnant and Drink

Quantity/Frequency	Risk
On occasion	Possible miscarriage, especially in the first trimester
2 drinks a day or less	Babies of low birth weight, born premature, with neurological problems
4 or more drinks a day	Babies with birth defects such as fetal alcohol syndrome, fetal alcohol effects, and alcohol-related birth defects
Binge drinking	Very dangerous to mother and baby

Wernicke-Korsakoff syndrome, alcoholic dementia, and nonamnesiac or non-Korsakoff disorders. These diseases are distinguished by whether there is loss of memory and by the extent of loss of intellectual ability.

Effect on the Liver

Alcohol is toxic to the liver, and although your liver may—up to a certain point—be able to handle it, alcohol does destroy it over time. Every time the liver is asked to process the alcohol contained in the blood, a part of the liver dies, never to be replaced. As the liver processes larger quantities of alcohol, it becomes more efficient at its work, with more of the liver dying in the process. When, as a result of alcohol, the liver can no longer function, the condition is known as alcohol-induced liver disease: fatty liver (alcoholic steatosis), alcoholic hepatitis, or cirrhosis.

In women, the effect of alcohol on the liver is magnified. Although women drink less alcohol than men, they are more likely to get alcohol-induced liver disease.

Effect on the Heart

Chronic alcohol consumption causes disturbances in the heart rhythm and diseases of the heart muscle.

Effect on the Pancreas

Alcohol is a causal factor in nearly two-thirds of all cases of pancreatitis. In this case also, the inflammation of the pancreas occurs sooner in women who drink than in men.

Warning: How Much Is One Drink?

One glass of wine	5 ounces (½ cup+)
One bottle/can of beer	12 ounces
One shot glass of liquor (80 proof)	1½ ounces

How Much Is a Drink?

We came from a family where it was considered very bad for men to drink alcohol in front of the women. It was just not allowed. This also meant that in a way it was OK for the men to go out and get drunk, but not in front of the women.

So when it was time for my new husband and me to have our first full family dinner at our house, I warned my husband about my family's attitude toward men drinking in front of women. He was still in medical school, so it was going to be a simple dinner. We decided to play it safe and save some money by not serving wine with dinner.

The dinner was very successful. Afterward, the entire family sat around that little space we called our living room to watch television. I noticed that my husband went to the kitchen. When he came

BLOOD ALCOHOL CONCENTRATION (%) WITHIN 1 HOUR

by Body Weight and Number of Drinks

Body Weight (lbs.)	1 Drink	2 Drinks	3 Drinks	4 Drinks	5 Drinks
100	.04	.09	.15	.20	.25
120	.03	.08	.12	.16	.21
140	.02	.06	.10	.14	.18
160	.02	.05	.09	.12	.15
180	.02	.05	.08	.10	.13
200	.01	.04	.07	.09	.12

Each drink is equivalent to 12 ounces of beer (5% alcohol), 5 ounces of table wine (12% alcohol), or 1½ ounces of 80 proof liquor (40% alcohol).

Note: .00–.04% Not legally under the influence; impairment is possible.

In 2000 the national limit was lowered to .08%. States have until 2007 to adopt this limit.

Source: National Clearinghouse for Drug and Alcohol Information, 1996.

out with a bottle of beer in his hands, I was speechless. And my mother—well, I knew what her look and silence meant.

Later, my husband asked me what had happened. I looked at him in disbelief and said, "I thought we had agreed that there would be no alcohol." His response was, "Yes, I know—I agreed to that. That's why I had a beer instead."

Beer is alcohol, and so is wine, and so is hard liquor. If, on an average, you drink more than two beers or two glasses of wine or two mixed drinks a day, you are damaging your liver.

Although the alcohol content of beer is less than that of hard liquor, the fact is that one typical serving of beer (12 ounces) has the same alcohol content as a 1½-ounce shot of hard liquor (80 proof). Similarly, when you drink 5 ounces of wine (a little more than ½ cup), you take in as much alcohol as in 1½ ounces of hard liquor.

The alcohol content indicated on the bottle or can gives you some information, but it is the number of ounces you drink that is important. Keep in mind that before-dinner drinks, after-dinner drinks, nightcaps, toasts, cordials, champagne, and "mimosas" are all drinks. Similarly, in terms of alcohol intake and the work your liver has to do to process alcohol, there is no difference between red and white wine.

How Much Is Too Much?

The quantity of alcohol consumed is the major factor. It does not matter whether it is beer, wine, or hard liquor. The risk for cirrhosis becomes a concern when men drink 6.2 ounces (80 grams) on average per day (e.g., four 12-ounce cans of beer or four 5-ounce glasses of wine or four drinks with 1½ ounces of 80 proof alcohol). For women, the comparable figure is 1.55 ounces (20 grams). While this pattern usually has to continue for ten to twenty years before the onset of cirrhosis, recent evidence suggests that women, and particularly younger women, may be having negative consequences much sooner than men.

The Occasional Drink

What does all this mean to those of us who have just "an occasional drink"? For women, it means that if you have a glass of wine or a beer at lunch *and* dinner, you are at risk for cirrhosis of the liver. Although much has been written about the benefits of wine, keep in mind that the benefits come from the grape portion of the wine and not the alcohol portion. You can have the same benefits by drinking grape juice.

All these warnings are based on data reflecting averages. You know yourself the best. If after one drink you feel that you lose control or act in ways that later you regret, you need to consider the wisdom of your decision to drink. At the very least, you should be careful about the company you keep when you drink.

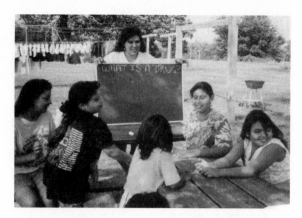

Too often we forget that alcohol is also a drug.

How to Recognize an Alcoholic

Start by looking in the mirror. An alcoholic in the early stages of the disease looks like you or me. The alcoholic we help could be our sister, our mother, our friend, our partner, or ourselves.

The table below may seem a bit simplistic, but it is accurate. Contrary to the stereotypes, alcoholism in the early stages may not involve mood changes or a pronounced need to drink at lunch or dinner. Some people do not become irritable or maudlin when they have a drink. In some cultures wine with dinner is a matter of course, but while not everyone in these cultures is an alcoholic, the rates of alcoholism tend to be higher. The facts are that some people develop the disease of alcoholism.

Many Patterns of Drinking Define the Disease of Alcoholism

Weekend drinker	4 drinks Friday, 4 drinks Saturday night, and 3 drinks Sunday
With meals only	1 drink with dinner every night and 1 drink with 4 lunches
Evening drinker	2 drinks every night

It is not a mystery why we drink. In our society there are many situations in which drinking is socially acceptable. Business meals (lunch or dinner), sports events, and celebrations are just a few of the times when alcohol is consumed. Alcohol is an acceptable, if not traditional, part of many events. It is all right for some people to have a drink some of the time. Some of us like the way alcohol tastes; others find that alcohol helps us to relax.

The problem is knowing when occasional alcohol use changes from being part of an activity to being the reason for participating in an activity. It is not easy to know when someone is in the early stages of alcohol abuse because each person shows different signs.

Having a drink may have started as a way to just take the edge off the day, deaden unpleasant feelings, or ignore whatever might be happening in one's life. After a while, however, all the alcoholic cares about is making sure there is access to another drink. When does a Latina change from looking forward to going to a family wedding to looking forward to the wine that will be served?

Initially the changes are often subtle and internal. The emotional scars that make the alcohol so necessary and soothing are typically hidden. Just as we hide the pain, we also get

Warning: Signs that Alcohol Is a Problem

1. Increased tolerance
2. Symptoms of withdrawal
3. Impaired control over behavior
4. Neglect of activities
5. Inability to fulfill roles
6. Hazardous use
7. Excessive time spent drinking

very good at hiding the symptoms.

In the early stages of alcohol abuse, a few drinks may give you a better feeling. As alcohol use progresses and your body becomes increasingly dependent on it, whatever good feeling there was is taken over by the craving for alcohol. That is what happens when a woman who drinks becomes a woman who has the disease of alcoholism.

So what are the symptoms of alcoholism? Some of them are described below.

1: Increased tolerance. Perhaps one of the greatest mistakes we make is to assume it is good to be able to "hold your liquor." Our bodies do not hold liquor; they process it.

While we may look at someone and be impressed at how much alcohol they can consume and still look fine, the reality is that they are not fine. Their liver is having to work extra hard to get rid of the toxins, and with each effort the liver makes to cleanse the blood of the alcohol, a little bit of the liver dies.

Moreover, in the vicious cycle of alcoholism, an alcoholic needs more and more alcohol to get the same effect. Getting sick, red-faced, or feeling nauseated after one or two drinks is the way the body warns you that it cannot metabolize alcohol well. Some have compared it to an allergic reaction. Consider yourself lucky if you drink and your body tells you to stop.

María took her mother on a trip to California. As her mother got dressed the first morning, María poured herself a beer. María's mother was surprised to see her daughter drinking so early. María said it was not early for her, because of the different time zone.

María's mother looked away. She wanted to believe that her daughter knew what she was doing, but she couldn't stop thinking about something. It was 9:00 A.M. in Los Angeles. Wasn't it then just 10:00 A.M. at home in Denver? It was still too early to have a drink. . . .

2: Symptoms of withdrawal. If you do not think you are an alcoholic, you should be able to give up drinking without having any physical symptoms. If you think that someone you love is an alcoholic, they should be able to go away on a trip and not drink for a while.

Unfortunately, persons who are alcoholic become irritable when they are not able to get alcohol. In the more advanced stages of alcoholism, withdrawal from alcohol is best done under medical supervision because of the severe physical reactions that may occur.

An alcoholic who has stopped drinking may want to drink again because a drink helps calm the feelings of physical and psychological discomfort they experience when they stop drinking.

3: Impaired control over behavior. "I drink because it makes me feel good, because then I can put up with whatever I have to put up with," explained Alicia, and added, "I drink because I want to. When I drink, I can have sex and not care. Drinking is the only thing that is good in my life, and it is mine. I control how much I drink."

Impaired control is when an alcoholic is unable to control the amount of alcohol she consumes or how long she spends drinking. Her intention may be to have only one drink, but once she begins she is unable to stop.

4: Neglect of activities. As alcohol takes over a person's life, they start to let themselves go. For Latinas, this means that a clean, well-groomed appearance becomes unimportant. Care of the home, work, or others may begin to deteriorate. Whatever sense of pride once existed seems to disappear in the alcoholic Latina.

5: Inability to fulfill roles.

Both my parents were alcoholics. I had to be raised by my grandmother because my parents could not take care of me. They could not even take care of themselves. And when I looked at them, I knew that I did not want to be like them.

When I got to college, I proved it to myself. Every day, for one whole year, I had three drinks and then I stopped. I never drank again. I knew that I did not have to become like my parents. I knew they drank because they wanted to. Drinking made them so mean.

—*Aida, 54*

Forgetting becomes a way of explaining the things the alcoholic is unable to control. An alcoholic has problems scheduling activities and keeping to that schedule. Over time alcoholics start to lose memories of what they have to do, and forgetting becomes a way of life.

After much covering up and denial, the alcoholic sinks to the point where she cannot do things that were simple before. The alcohol that she initially used to help her get by has now taken over to the point that drinking and looking for the next drink are all she can do.

6: Hazardous use. The alcoholic does not understand that driving while under the influence of alcohol is illegal and dangerous. Alcoholics may think they can do whatever they want and they end up in dangerous situations. It is this reduction of inhibitions that also results in risky sexual behavior.

7: Excessive time spent drinking. For some Latinas, the best way to think about alcohol in their lives is to see how much of their time they spend at events where alcohol is present. When a Latina starts attending events because it gives her permission to drink, alcohol has taken over her life. Similarly, a Latina who starts to pass up opportunities, or arranges her day, to allow for more time to drink (especially if it is to be alone and drink) may be an alcoholic.

Treatment

Overcoming Denial

I have no memories of my childhood. I do not know whether my mother drank, although I know my father had problems. I know both of my mother's parents were alcoholics, even that several of my mother's sisters and brothers were alcoholic. But I never remember my mother having a drink. I never saw her do anything like that.

Yes, sometimes she forgot things, but it was because she was absent-minded. And yes, her hands do have that trembling quality to them. But I never saw her drink.

Maybe she did. I do not know. Like I said, I have no memories of my childhood.

—*Marta, 36*

One of the greatest barriers to the treatment of alcoholism is denial. People who have problems with alcohol usually do not admit their problem. For Latinas, for whom *aguantar* is the cultural coping mechanism of choice and for whom depression is rampant, denial of alcohol abuse is an easy choice.

Alcoholics often live in the false belief that no one will notice as long as they drink when they are alone and continue to meet all their obligations. Since one of the effects of alcohol is to deaden the senses, alcoholics often cannot recognize when they do not meet their obligations. Moreover, while Latinas who drink may not admit to the consequences of their drinking, the situation is further obscured when persons around them mistakenly try to protect them by covering up for them and doing the things that they should have done.

It was nice to finally get away. Joaquín and I had been planning this vacation for a long time. We made a delicious lunch and toasted our weekend away with a fine bottle of wine. And it was OK when he said he wanted to watch the game. I went for a long walk.

By the time I got back, the game had been over for a while. Joaquín looked unhappy. It seemed that the star player for his team had gotten injured and would be out of the game for the season. Joaquín poured us both some more wine.

Then, out of nowhere, Joaquín became very amorous. I did not know what was happening as he kissed my body—it just felt different this time. As we made love, he was attentive, but—I don't know—it just was not the same. And it was obvious that it was more affection than Joaquín was used to sharing, because even though it was early in the evening, he seemed exhausted and went to sleep.

I got out of bed disappointed that he was so tired. I went to the kitchen to get some water. For some reason, the garbage can caught my eye. There, on top, were some crumpled papers that I did not remember throwing out.

I do not know what made me do it, but I moved those papers. Underneath, there were six empty bottles of beer. In the short time I was gone, Joaquín had finished most of the wine, had six beers, and hidden the bottles.

The next morning, Joaquín did not remember that we had made love. I knew then that there was a problem.

—Marisa, 38

The Alcoholic's Denial

If someone were to ask, "Are you an alcoholic?" one might answer, "Of course not"—sometimes a little too quickly. Ask a Latina what it means to be an alcoholic, and the response will most probably be stereotypical. Many Latinas will describe the behavior of a *borracho* (drunkard), someone who has a staggering walk, smells bad, and looks messy.

Our stereotype of the typical alcoholic also tends to describe male behavior—such as fits of rage and even physical violence, or even simply spending hours drinking beer and watching a football game. But women are very different from men, in what and where they drink as well as in how they act when they have a drinking problem. Latinas drink different drinks than Hispanic men do, metabolize alcohol in a different way, and also behave in a different manner. Of course, we may get wobbly and stagger and even get loud, but for many Latinas, alcoholism is a lonely, desperate course that is used to deaden the senses and numb the spirit.

To know whether or not you are an alcoholic, you must ask yourself and those around you how much you really drink. The answer is in the numbers.

The Support Network

In most cases, those people around an alcoholic mean well. They do not see the signs because they do not want to, or perhaps they do not know them. They may say it is *nervios* (nerves) or some other acceptable condition for a Latina to have. So the family and friends pick up and do what the alcoholic woman was supposed to do and didn't. The term *enabler* has been used to describe some of these support networks, but for Latinas, the concept has to be reinterpreted. If the family has had a history of coping and struggling, how are they to know that this is different? In most families, in fact, helping our relatives through difficult times is as natural as breathing.

To help evaluate whether your loved one is an alcoholic, stop doing things for them. Watch what they do. Ask them how they feel. It may be that through your lack of assistance, difficult as it may be for you, you force them to seek treatment.

Myths and Facts

Myth: There are no calories in alcohol, only in the mixers.

Fact: Alcohol has calories and no nutritional value.

Myth: You are not an alcoholic if you do not get drunk.

Fact: Alcoholics can usually "hold their liquor" better than nonalcoholics.

Myth: Beer is not considered an alcoholic drink.

Fact: A can or bottle of beer has as much alcohol as a shot of whiskey.

Myth: You can have up to three drinks and still be able to drive.

Fact: If you have three drinks, you are considered legally under the influence and should not drive.

Myth: Women have estrogen, which protects them from liver damage.

Fact: Women who drink damage their livers faster than men.

Myth: If you want to stop drinking, all you have to do is stop.

Fact: Alcoholism is a disease that needs ongoing physical and psychological treatment.

Myth: Taking aspirin helps you not to get drunk.

Fact: Aspirin makes it harder for your body to absorb the alcohol and will therefore produce a higher concentration of alcohol in your blood (BAC).

Myth: A blood test can show whether someone is an alcoholic.

Fact: Unlike most illnesses, whose diagnosis can be made through some objective test such as an x-ray or the results of a blood test, much of the diagnosis of alcoholism is based on self-report or the report of persons close to the alcoholic.

Body, Mind, and Spirit

Generally, women are still considered a special population in alcohol treatment centers. Although an estimated one-third of alcoholics are women, less than one-quarter of the alcoholics in treatment are women.

Research findings show that women do better in treatment that is specifically geared toward women. It follows that Latinas should seek treatment in institutions where the staff is culturally and linguistically proficient to meet their needs. Whether you go to a private clinic or stay at home with a supportive family, treatment will have to focus on your body, mind, and spirit.

Body

The most difficult part of having an addiction is to stop taking the addicting substance. All alcoholic treatment programs are similar in that they involve detoxification and psychological therapy. Treatment begins when you decide to stop drinking, at which point detoxification of your system begins. Some Latinas may decide to stay at home, while others would rather be in a facility where they can get medical care if needed. Sometimes medications are given to control the symptoms of withdrawal; to discourage alcohol consumption (when you take Antabuse and drink, you become sick); or to decrease desire for alcohol (e.g., antidepressants). Your health care provider will work with you to decide which is the best way to proceed.

The symptoms of withdrawal from alcohol show great variability from person to person and, on the mild end of the spectrum, can include jumpiness, anxiety, restlessness, difficulty sleeping, loss of appetite, physical tremors

Warning: Relapse Happens

An alcoholic may have to go into treatment more than once for it to be successful. Each attempt is important for the alcoholic and her family. If there is relapse, do not give up. The next treatment may be the last.

or shaking, and a craving for alcohol. Onset of symptoms usually occurs 24 to 36 hours after the last drink. Some persons (5 to 15 percent) hospitalized for alcohol withdrawal have epileptic-like seizures from 6 to 48 hours after their last drink.

In some instances, as part of treatment the drug called disulfiram (Antabuse) may be prescribed to discourage alcohol consumption. The drug has no effect unless the person drinks. If alcohol is consumed, the person will experience physical discomfort ranging from nausea to severe headaches, effectively rendering the alcoholic allergic to alcohol. However, the limitation of this course of treatment is that many alcoholics simply do not take their medication. In all cases, unless the alcoholic truly desires to stop drinking, medication alone will not help.

Once the alcoholic woman has gone through detoxification, she must abstain from all alcohol for the rest of her life. For a time some researchers claimed that alcoholics could learn how to drink socially (i.e., have an occasional drink). More long-term studies showed that the concept of "controlled drinking" did not work. For most people, controlled drinking was a step toward abuse. If you have successfully cleansed your body from alcohol, keep it clean.

Mind

For some Latinas, getting marital and family counseling is essential to the success of their alcohol treatment program. If a Latina has gone beyond the denial of her alcoholism, the opportunity may exist to engage her and her family in some constructive rebuilding of the family. Structural family therapy has been used with Latinas to help realign the family in a more balanced way.

Other Latinas may need the support that comes from 12-Step programs that are geared to women. Since men and women become alcoholics for different reasons, it is important to take part in programs that can address the issues of Latinas.

Latinas will also have to deal with feelings of shame, which are more profound than those experienced by non-Latinas because use of alcohol is considered more taboo for Latinas. Finding a therapist who can help you not just to stop drinking but to understand how you became an alcoholic in the first place will help you resolve what are usually misdirected feelings of shame.

Spirit

For some Latinas, turning to their faith has inspired them to stop drinking and given them the strength to continue abstaining from alcohol. Especially for Latinas who have had to deal with painful personal issues that they feel are beyond resolution, the reaffirmation

Alcoholics Anonymous (AA)

You may want to try it. If it does not work for you, it does not mean you are a failure or beyond treatment or that you do not have a "real" problem. You may want to try more professionally oriented interventions.

At present there is no controlled study confirming the success of AA. All that is certain is that AA works for some people some of the time.

of the spirit has provided them with the sustenance to continue. In addition, many churches hold special meetings for recovering alcoholics, to help them through the difficult times after treatment or especially to encourage them to return to treatment after relapse.

Summary

There are Latinas who are alcoholics or who live with alcohol in their families. The effects of alcohol on our brain, liver, and heart are sufficient to make us pause one moment before we have even that one glass of wine with dinner.

Understanding that one beer, one glass of wine, or a shot of alcohol are the same in terms of alcohol ingestion is very important. This helps us to better define when we are drinking in an acceptable manner and when we are drinking to excess.

The task for women who are alcoholic is to get past the denial that can shackle them to lives of solitude and to seek the best available treatment.

Treatment for the alcoholic Latina must include all aspects of their lives. The body must undergo detoxification, the mind must be healed by reestablishing new relationships with loved ones as well as with oneself, and the spirit must be nurtured so that it too can heal.

RESOURCES

Organizations

Adult Children of Alcoholics
P.O. Box 3216
Torrance, CA 90510
(310) 534-1815 (message only)
www.adultchildren.org

Al-Anon/Alateen Family Group Headquarters
1600 Corporate Landing Parkway
Virginia Beach, VA 23454
(757) 563-1600
(888) 4al-anon (meetings)
www.al-anon.alateen.org

Alcoholics Anonymous World Services Office
P.O. Box 459, Grand Central Station
New York, NY 10163
(212) 870-3400 or (212) 647-1680 (meeting referral for New York City)
www.alcoholics-anonymous.org

Children of Alcoholics Foundation
164 W. 74th St.
New York, NY 10023
(800) 359-2623 or (212) 595-5810 ext. 7760
www.coaf.org

Coalition of Alcohol and Drug Dependent Women and Their Children
Washington Office of the National Council on Alcoholism and Drug Dependence
1511 K Street NW, Suite 443
Washington, DC 20005
(202) 737-8122

Center for Substance Abuse Prevention's (CSAP) National Women's Resource Center for the Prevention of Alcohol, Tobacco, Other Drug Abuse and Mental Illness
515 King Street, Suite 410
Alexandria, VA 22314
(800) 354-8824

National Association for Children of Alcoholics
31582 Coast Highway, Suite B
South Laguna, CA 92677
(714) 499-3889
www.nacoa.net

National Association of Perinatal Addiction Research & Education
200 N. Michigan, Suite 300
Chicago, IL 60601
(800) 638-BABY (800-638-2229) (phone counseling) or (312) 541-1272 (publications)

National Clearinghouse for Alcohol and Drug Information
P.O. Box 2345
Rockville, MD 20847-2345
(800) 729-6686 or TDD (800) 487-4889
www.health.org

National Clearinghouse on Child Abuse and Neglect Information
P.O. Box 1182
Washington, DC 20013
(800) FYI-3366 (800-394-3366) or (703) 385-7565

National Council on Alcoholism and Drug Dependence
12 West 21st Street, 7th Floor
New York, NY 10010
(800) 622-2255 or (212) 206-6770 or (800) 475-4673
www.ncadd.org

Women for Sobriety
P.O. Box 618
Quakertown, PA 18951-0618
(215) 536-8026
www.womenforsobriety.org

Hotlines

National Drug and Alcohol Treatment Referral Hotline
(800) 662-HELP (800-662-4357) or TDD (800) 228-0427

National Help and Referral Line (Adcare Hospital)
(800) 252-6465

Publications and Pamphlets

General

"Alcohol and Health: Eighth Special Report to the U.S. Congress," 1994. NIH Publication No. 94-3699. U.S. Department of Health and Human Services, National Institute on Alcohol Abuse and Alcoholism, Washington, DC.

"Alcohol and Other Drug-Related Birth Defects: NCADD Fact Sheet," 1999. Information on alcohol and drug abuse relating to birth defects. National Council on Alcoholism and Drug Dependence, 12 West 21st Street, New York, NY 10010; (800) NCA-CALL (800-622-2255), a referral service, or (212) 206-6770. Other fact sheet titles include:

"Alcohol and Other Drugs in the Workplace," 1994. Information on alcohol and drug abuse in the workplace.

"Alcoholism and Alcohol-Related Problems," 1995. Information on alcohol abuse.

"Cómo Cuidar a Su Hijo Antes del Nacimiento," Information in Spanish on prenatal health care. National Clearinghouse for Alcohol and Drug Information, Center for Substance Abuse Prevention, Substance Abuse and Mental Health Services Administration, (800) 662-4357.

"Letter to a Woman Alcoholic," 1954. Alcoholics Anonymous Publications. Reprinted by *Good Housekeeping;* (800) 870-3400 or (202) 966-9115 (English) or (202) 797-9738 (Spanish).

Prevention

"Alcohol: What to Do If It's a Problem for You," 1999. A general overview of this topic. American Academy of Family Physicians, 11400 Tomahawk Creek Pkwy, Leawood, KS 66211-2672; (800) 944-0000.

"Does She Drink Too Much? From Men about Women in Their Lives," 1988. Information about alcohol abuse referral services. Al-Anon Family Group Headquarters, 1600 Corporate Landing Pkwy, Virginia Beach, VA 23454; www.al-anon.alateen.org. Other titles include

"Understanding Ourselves and Alcoholism," 1979.

"The Disease of Alcoholism." Information on how alcohol abuse leads to alcoholism. National Council on Alcoholism and Drug Dependence, 12 West 21st Street, 7th Floor, New York, NY 10010; (800) NCA-CALL. Other titles include:

"Facing the Challenge of Alcohol and Other Drugs." Information on how to identify alcohol and other drug abuse.

"Use of Alcohol and Other Drugs among Women: NCADD Fact Sheet," Information on the abuse of alcohol and other drugs.

"What Are the Signs of Alcoholism? The NCADD Self-Test," Test on signs of alcohol abuse and alcoholism.

"What Can You Do about Someone Else's Drinking?" Information on the signs of alcohol abuse.

"Healthy Women/Healthy Lifestyles: Here's What You Should Know about Alcohol and Other Drugs," 1995. DHHS Publication No. SMA 95-7094. Center for Substance Abuse and Prevention, Substance Abuse and Mental Health Services Administration, (800) 729-6686. Other titles include "If Someone Close Has a Problem with Alcohol or Other Drugs," 1992.

"Women and Drug Abuse: You and Your Community Can Help," 1994. Information about the signs of drug abuse. National Clearinghouse for Alcohol and Drug Information, P.O. Box 2345, Rockville, MD 20847-2345; (800) 729-6686 or TDD (800) 487-4889.

Treatment/Intervention

"AA for the Woman," 1976. Information on participating in an Alcoholics Anonymous program for women. Alcoholics Anonymous Publications, World Services Office, P.O. Box 459, Grand Central Station, New York, NY 10163; (212) 870-3400 or (202) 966-9115 (for English) or (202) 797-9738 (for Spanish). Other titles include "Information on Alcoholics Anonymous: Guidelines for Anyone New Coming to A.A. or for Anyone Referring People to A.A."

"National Directory of Drug and Alcohol Abuse Treatment Programs (2000)." SAMHSA's National Clearinghouse for Alcohol and Drug Information (NCADI), PO Box 2345, Rockville, MD 20847; (800) 729-6686.

11

Arthritis Is a Symptom

"Me Duelen los Huesos" . . . "My Bones Hurt"

I loved playing tennis, but when I was thirty-two I began having a pain in my right foot. I attributed it to the fact that now I was in my thirties and not as agile as I used to be.

At first everyone thought my injury had to do with the sports I played. Even my health care provider's diagnosis was that I had some sports-related injury. Then the diagnosis changed, and I was told I had a bone spur. The pain persisted on and off.

My next diagnosis was that I had a neuroma on my foot. I never really found out what that meant, because fairly soon it was ruled out. Then, with certainty, I was told that I had gout.

As the months passed, the pain seemed to spread, and soon it went into my shoulder. After a while one knee began to hurt, and in a few weeks the pain had spread to both knees.

My knees got very swollen. When my right knee nearly reached the size of a basketball, my provider inserted a long needle in it to extract the liquid. They analyzed the liquid and came back with the results: I had rheumatoid arthritis.

It took a year and five specialists after that initial pain in my foot to finally determine that I had rheumatoid arthritis.

—Tensia, 34

Very little is known about arthritis in Latinas. For instance, we do not know how many Latinas have arthritis. The reason for this is that we often use the word *arthritis* very loosely. The word means "joint inflammation" and thus describes only a symptom and not the cause of the condition.

We mistakenly use the words *arthritis* and *rheumatism* interchangeably as catchalls for what in reality is over a hundred different types of diseases. What these diseases have in common is that often the first indication you have that something may be wrong is a symptom—pain in your joints. That pain is due to the inflammation in your joints and is what is called arthritis. This symptom suggests that you have a problem with (1) your muscular and skeletal system or (2) the connective tissue of the body. For simplicity, it is acceptable to talk about joint disease when referring to either of those problems.

Whatever the cause, arthritis is inflammation in the joints (i.e., the area that connects bones). This inflammation is due to either too much friction or the inability of the joint to

Do You Know the Impact (Weight Plus Power of Movement) on Your Joints?

- When you walk, three to four times your body weight goes through each knee joint.
- When you do a deep knee-bend, up to ten times your body weight goes through your knees.
- When you stand, your hips support six times your body weight.

evenly distribute stress. Although in some cases cartilage may be damaged, the primary problem often resides in bone, ligaments, surrounding nerves, and muscles.

Joint diseases fall into a variety of categories. A few of the most common are:

- Osteoarthritis
- Diffuse connective tissue disease (e.g., rheumatoid arthritis or systemic lupus erythematosus)
- Arthritis associated with spondylitis (e.g., psoriatic arthritis)
- Infections of bones and joints (e.g., infectious arthritis)
- Crystal-induced conditions (e.g., gout)

Although many of these diseases have similar symptoms, the extent of the symptoms varies. Moreover, it is likely that they are each caused by different combinations of factors—genetic, environmental, work-related, and infectious factors. In other instances, arthritis may be due to more than one disease.

This chapter focuses on the kinds of joint diseases that are more common in women—osteoarthritis, rheumatoid arthritis, systemic lupus erythematosus, and gonococcal arthritis.

As a first step in understanding arthritis or joint diseases, we need to understand what joints do.

What a Joint Does

Wherever two bones meet, you have a joint. For example, your wrists, knees, hips, and elbows are joints. The joint is a wonderful mechanism of the body that allows movement of one bone over another without friction and with relatively little stress.

In order to do its work, the joint area is made up of two major types of material: (1) cartilage, which is the cushioning, or shock absorber, for all the weight and power that travels between two bones, and (2) synovium, which surrounds the cartilage and contains a lubricant to reduce friction.

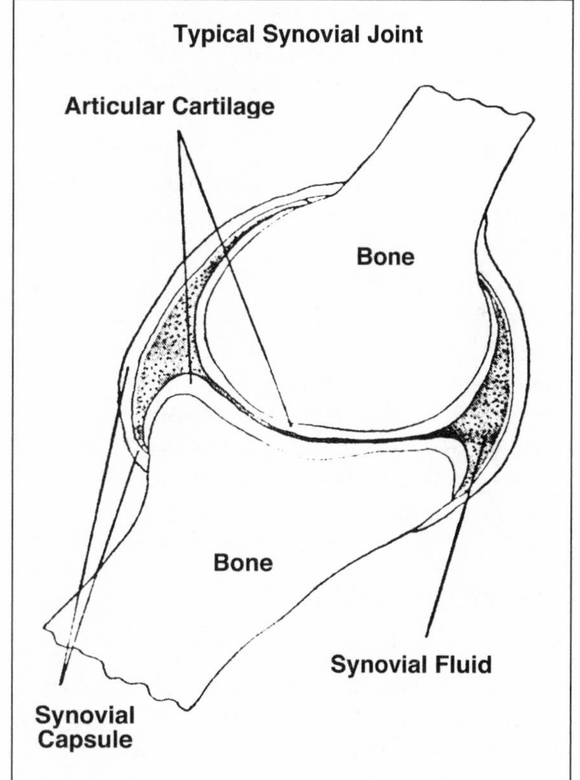

Arthritis

How Do I Know If I Have Arthritis?

The Arthritis Foundation lists the following as the warning signs of arthritis:

- Pain
- Stiffness
- Occasional swelling

Cartilage

Cartilage is a dense, flexible, rubbery connective tissue. Since it has neither nerves nor its own blood supply, it is not the cartilage but the nerves in the surrounding matter that give us the feeling of pain. For the same reasons, cartilage cannot heal itself as well as other tissue. Moreover, the new cartilage that sometimes appears after an injury is not as strong or resilient as the cartilage it replaces.

Synovium

The synovium is a capsulelike membrane filled with a substance called synovial fluid, which acts as a lubricant between the bones. Synovitis is the inflammation of this membrane.

If you have pain, stiffness, or occasional swelling in or around a joint for more than two weeks, you should see your health care provider. Sometimes the symptoms come on slowly and at other times appear suddenly. Remember that only your health care provider can tell you whether you have arthritis.

Osteoarthritis

The most common type of arthritis is osteoarthritis (OA), and we know that OA is particularly hard on women. For unknown reasons, women are twice as likely to have OA as men, although in certain areas of the body, such as the hip, it is equally likely in males and females. Although there is some recent research on African-American women, there is no information on Latinas and OA. All we know is that African-American women are twice as likely as non-Hispanic white women to have OA.

Causal Factors

OA is typically due to loss of cartilage at the joint. Given the specific functions of the joint, OA seems to occur as a result of continuing friction across damaged cartilage. Not surprisingly, the joints that take the greatest load on a continuous basis, such as the knees, seem to wear out most frequently.

Recent evidence suggests that the repetitive stress involved in some jobs (factory work, keyboarding) may contribute to the likelihood of getting OA. Prior injury to a joint is also a risk factor for early arthritis.

Diagnosis

It is not possible to give a precise time for the onset of OA, although we do know that the chances of a diagnosis of OA increase with age. By the time most of us are forty, our weight-bearing joints will have undergone some degree of deterioration, even though we may not have symptoms. Over time our joints wear out even more, with most people over sixty-five having OA in one of their joints and 4 out of 5 persons over seventy-five having OA in at least one joint.

For many years the main way to diagnose OA was to look at x-rays. But since x-rays show only the bones, very often the x-ray findings do not seem to reflect what a person says they feel. For example, over 50 percent of people with OA diagnosed from x-rays do not have symptoms. Typically, the deformity shown in the x-rays is more severe than the pain experienced in the joint.

More recently, the tendency has been to diagnose OA through the use of magnetic resonance imaging (MRI). MRI provides more information than x-rays because it depicts the bones, joint lining, and cartilage in much greater detail.

The signs of OA usually begin to emanate from a specific area (hand, knee, hip, foot, spine, or other joints). Some types of OA affect joints such as the elbows, shoulders, or those between toes. OA of these joints is often related to either work factors or a metabolism problem. When there are signs throughout the body, a different diagnosis is given, reflecting a more systemic problem.

Stages

In the early stage of OA, the cartilage has become thicker than normal. Typically there is pain when using the joint and relief when resting. In later stages, the thickening is reduced because there is more loss and softening of cartilage. At this advanced stage, there is pain with the slightest motion—even when resting. Some sufferers report feeling pain even while sleeping.

Prevention

Since there is no specific causal factor for OA, there is no one thing you can do to definitively prevent onset of the disease. What is known is that for persons who are overweight, a loss of 11 pounds (5 kilograms) results in a 50 percent decrease in the chances of developing OA in the knee. The loss in weight reduces the amount of force which passes through the knee during normal daily activity.

Treatment

There is no cure for OA, but there are treatments and ways to organize your life that can make OA more tolerable. In order to do the things that we must do in our lives, many Latinas learn to shift their weight around or use a different part of the body than the one that hurts. For example, when one of our knees is hurt, we shift our weight to our hip to get in and out of a chair. Although this provides some short-term relief and the ability to complete tasks, over the long run we wear out the part of the body that is not structured for carrying the extra load of the joint that is no longer working well. Thus training people to shift their weight properly becomes an important part of treatment.

There are, of course, different things that you can do to reduce the discomfort, depending on which joint is affected:

- Hands: Hot soaks, paraffin wax applications, and avoiding activities that aggravate the pain. A temporary splint may be helpful to keep the joint from moving when it is most painful.
- Spine: Sometimes your health care provider may recommend use of a collar or traction. In some instances you may be given a special corset to support your abdomen.

Treatments focus on three broad areas: physical therapy, medication, and in some instances surgery.

Physical Therapy

The major goal of physical therapy is to prevent overuse of joints while at the same time encouraging activities that maintain your ability to move your joints as much as possible. Walking or using a stationary bicycle (without tension) is recommended. If necessary, using a cane for walking is helpful in reducing the force on lower extremities. If you use a cane, it should be held in the hand opposite the injured knee.

Rest and exercises recommended by your health care provider may help maintain your range of motion. Knee exercises that strengthen upper thigh muscles may be part of regular physical therapy.

In addition, some patients have found pain relief with acupuncture or through going to a chiropractor. Whatever you decide to do, be sure to discuss it with your health care provider. Keep in mind that the best physical therapy is consistent and slow.

Medication

Medication is an important component of the treatment plan. There are three major groups of medications used in treatment of OA: acetaminophen; aspirin; and non-steroidal anti-inflammatory agents (NSAIDs). Aspirin and NSAIDs work well against pain and inflammation while acetaminophen works best against pain. Since inflammation is not the dominant feature of OA, it is always best to start therapy with acetaminophen as it has much fewer side effects than NSAIDs. Acetaminophen is also much less expensive.

If your health care provider initially recommends NSAIDs, ask if you can try acetaminophen first. If that does not work, then you can move on to NSAIDs or aspirin. The major side effect from aspirin and older NSAIDs is irritation of the stomach that can sometimes lead to ulcers and bleeding.

There is a new class of NSAIDs called COX-2 inhibitors (Vioxx and Celebrex). COX-2 inhibitors cause much less stomach irritation. Because they are much more expensive, they will usually only be used if your health care provider thinks you are at a higher risk for stomach irritation, e.g., you have a history of ulcers.

In extreme cases, corticosteroids can be used to give a temporary measure of relief. When these drugs were first discovered, they seemed to be a miracle cure. Like cortisone, which is one of the hormones produced by the body, they seemed to boost patients' strength and vitality. However, as the use of corticosteroids spread, it became clear that long-term use produced significant negative consequences, such as Cushing's syndrome (weight gain, moon-face, thin skin, muscle weakness, and brittle bones).

The current recommendation is that if corticosteroids are called for to relieve pain, the medication should be administered infrequently and in the form of a localized shot in the affected area.

All medications have some side effects. Your health care provider will work with you to determine which one works best for you.

Surgery

Depending on your health and age, your health care provider may suggest hip or knee replacement if you have such severe OA in those joints that you are barely able to walk without constant pain. Two things that should be considered with regard to the replacement of the hip or knee are (1) the risk of complications from surgery and (2) the probabilities that the device will not function properly. Generally speaking, joint replacement is more successful in less active people; active people can experience more loosening of the artificial joint over time.

Another complication of this treatment is that usually, ten years after surgery, the cement that holds the implant in place breaks into tiny particles that can only be seen by a

Do You Know Your Nonprescription Nonsteroidal Anti-Inflammatory Drugs (NSAIDs)?

Brand Name	NSAID
Advil, Motrin IB, Nuprin	Ibuprofen
Aleve	Naproxen sodium
Anacin, Ascriptin, Bayer, Bufferin, Ecotrin, Excedrin	Aspirin (salicylate drug subset of NSAIDs)

microscope but that cause inflammation in the area. To alleviate this problem, in the early 1980s new procedures were developed that do not use joint cement. Instead, the expectation was that your bone would grow into the porous surface of the joint. Unfortunately, this process is not as successful in women with osteoporosis. Currently, new processes are being investigated to make cement that holds implants in place and lasts longer.

As with any surgery, hip or knee replacement is an invasive procedure, and complications can occur. Given the potential risks, this is a solution best relied upon only in the most serious cases, when mobility has been severely curtailed.

Rheumatoid Arthritis

For as long as I can remember, my mother was proud of her beautiful hands. She told the story so many times of how once she had sat waiting for a bus when a young man approached her. He told her that she had the most beautiful hands he had ever seen, and then he asked her permission to sketch them. Those were the hands she remembered, and when she looked at her hands, those were the hands she looked for.

But Mom had to do all sorts of work to support us, and as she grew older she would look at her hands with great sadness. She could not straighten her fingers. She would drop things as she felt the strength leave her hands. Her hands were not the same. Somehow arthritis had taken over.

Yet as the years pass, whenever I look at her hands, I still find them so beautiful. . . .

—*Marta, 53*

Rheumatoid arthritis (RA) is two to three times more common in women than in men, occurring in 4 percent of all women. Most women have their first symptoms between the ages of twenty-five and fifty, although the illness may occur at any age.

While OA usually affects only one or two joints, RA is a disease that can affect the entire body. RA results in progressive inflammation, destruction, deformity, and disability of multiple joints in a symmetric fashion. We do not understand what causes it.

The severity of the symptoms of RA varies greatly. There may be periods when sufferers experience very serious effects, immediately followed by a time of remission, which can last for the rest of your life or for a few months.

Causal Factors

There is no single known cause of RA. Although research is in the early stages, it is hypothesized that causal factors are a combination of infectious agents, genetics, and autoimmunity problems. There is also some hormonal influence, as shown by the fact that symptoms go away with pregnancy. Also, women on oral contraceptives are less likely to get RA.

Diagnosis

No one test will tell your health care provider whether you have RA. Instead, your health care provider will rely on clinical findings (looking at you, asking you questions, checking how much movement you have without pain) and the results from specialized blood tests.

Health care providers have a difficult time diagnosing RA because it does not look the same in every person. For some people RA produces symptoms throughout the body all at once, causing fever and fatigue while in others the symptoms start initially in just the small joints of the hands. The most common complaint is that the joints affected feel tender even without being touched, and stiff.

Treatment

I thought my whole world had crashed when I was told that I had arthritis. Luckily I had a lot of love and support.

And I tried everything. I went to the curanderos *(healers) in the community, and they told me my arthritis was treatable. They said that first I had to make my peace with God. It seemed that they felt God had sent me a signal to slow down. Yes, I still had to do all the things I had to do in my life, but I had to take it easier.*

So, I tried hard to slow down.

Now I do everything I can for my family, my work, and myself. That means I take my medicines, mainly the one with the long name I can never remember. It also means that to keep myself in balance I get massage and acupuncture.

I know that because of the type of condition I have, I will have to be monitored for the rest of my life. Maybe I will be lucky and go into remission.

—Yolanda, 36

At one time, health care providers thought that the most important part of treatment was the control of pain. But although control of pain is important, most Latinas with rheumatoid arthritis are concerned most about being able to perform their day-to-day tasks. Thus they want to receive treatment that takes this into account.

Treatment needs to focus on finding ways to slow down the degeneration of cartilage and reduce inflammation. This will enable us to improve or maintain the level of activity in our lives. When it comes to RA, treatment must be tailored to the individual.

Physical

RA treatment requires that you become a well-informed consumer. If you are experiencing very severe and painful RA, you may be instructed to rest in bed for several days. For other, less severe cases, use of a splint on the affected joint may provide all the necessary rest.

A combination of exercise (prescribed by your health care provider), rest, and, where necessary, occupational therapy is usually recommended. Exercise should be limited to the noninflammatory periods and emphasize maintaining good range of motion in the joints by restoring muscle mass. Exercising should not make you feel exhausted or fatigued. For some Latinas with RA, rest periods are redefined as the time when they are not using their joints and can have quiet time to read, think, or pray.

Medication

The specialists who take care of rheumatoid arthritis have long known that the major problem in RA is that the initial inflammation of the joints will lead over time to irreversible destruction of joints and disability. The aspirin and NSAIDs that were discussed in the treatment section of OA can reduce inflammation and pain in RA but they do not prevent joint destruction.

Fortunately, there are many new drugs now available known as disease-modifying anti-rheumatic drugs (DMARDSs). DMARDs are much more effective in slowing down and preventing joint destruction. Some of these drugs are sulfasalazine, hydroxychloroquine, methotrexate, and tumor necrosis factor inhibitor (Etanercept). These medicines work best when given in combination and work better when given early in the course of RA. If you have a diagnosis of RA and your health care provider is not familiar with DMARDs, ask to be referred to a specialist.

Surgery

Since RA is an autoimmune-related disease, its treatment focuses on medication and not surgery, although sometimes surgery is of value in modifying some of the more severely damaged joints.

Myths and Facts

Myth: It is best to exercise the joint when you have arthritis pain.

Fact: It is best to rest and not overuse the joint.

Myth: Arthritis pain is best treated with cold compresses.

Fact: Hot compresses and warm baths may be helpful.

Myth: OA is not related to weight.

Fact: Persons with greater weight have an increased likelihood of OA of the knee, hips, spine, foot, and ankle.

Myth: It is always easier for your body to handle a small load.

Fact: A small load that is unexpected (e.g., when you trip on an uneven surface) may cause more damage than a larger load for which you are prepared (e.g., when you jump down three steps).

Myth: Joint replacement is best for those individuals who are active.

Fact: Joint replacement is more successful in persons who are less active.

Myth: There is no treatment for arthritis that is due to Lyme disease or gout.

Fact: Lyme disease can be treated with antibiotics, and gout can be completely controlled with drugs.

Myth: People with OA have shorter lives.

Fact: OA does not seem to affect life expectancy.

Myth: Gold injections are the best new treatment for arthritis.

Fact: Gold injections were first used in the 1930s. Since then, a variety of other medications have also been used, including penicillamine, hydroxychloroquine, methotrexate and sulfasalazine.

Systemic Lupus Erythematosus

Systemic lupus erythematosus (SLE) is an autoimmune disease. Young adult females have the highest incidence, and 9 out of 10 persons with SLE are female. SLE is twice as common in Latinas and African-Americans as in the general population. SLE is commonly known as lupus.

If you ask your Latina friends about lupus, you may be surprised to find how close this disease is to you. And lupus is not "just arthritis," but a serious illness that can cause death if left untreated because it may result in long-term complications such as end-stage renal disease or chronic lung disease.

Causal Factors

We have no idea why people get lupus. The best guess is that genes and the environment play significant roles. Part of the difficulty in studying lupus is that although it is a chronic disease, its effects come and go, sometimes with long periods of remission. Studying people at the same stage of the disease is often difficult. Researchers are still trying to determine whether lupus is caused by one factor or multiple factors.

Diagnosis

During the early stages, lupus is very difficult to diagnose because it can easily be mistaken for rheumatoid arthritis. Women with lupus may describe themselves as tired, depressed, and losing weight without even trying. They are often sensitive to sunlight.

At a more advanced stage of the disease, for unknown reasons, most patients develop a butterfly-shaped skin rash across the middle of their face. Again, most of the diagnosis will depend on your health care provider's clinical assessment of your symptoms and what your blood tests reveal. The diagnosis is usually made after eliminating other similar illnesses.

Treatment

For purposes of treatment, lupus is classified as either mild or severe. In mild cases the symptoms include fever, arthritis, headaches, and rash. It is not usually necessary to treat mild cases. It is not known whether all mild cases will stay mild or become severe. Severe lupus is a life-threatening illness because of

Think Again: Copper Bracelets, Magnets, or *Uña de Gato* (Cat's Claw) for Arthritis?

When it comes to arthritis, it seems that everyone has a cure. And that is partly because arthritis is an illness that comes and goes. That is why many of the bracelets, potions, special juices, jewelry, and other objects seem to work.

If we put on a bracelet and the arthritis pain goes away, we think it is because of the bracelet. The reality is that in the natural course of the illness, it gets better and it gets worse with no predicting where in the cycle you are. Many special elixirs for the cure of arthritis are just very expensive sugar water.

The mind is the most powerful part of our body, and if we believe that the magnet or bracelet made the pain go away or that the elixir is special, perhaps it is because our mind wanted to believe that and made it happen. Perhaps folk medicine and folk remedies provide a special key for unlocking our ability to heal ourselves.

The challenge is to get to the point where we can do without the bracelet and all we need is our mind.

complications that involve the blood, kidneys, stomach, or lungs. In severe cases, therapy usually requires an immediate injection of corticosteroids.

Lupus can be controlled with two major kinds of medication—drugs that reduce inflammation of tissues (anti-inflammatory drugs, cortisone, antimalarial drugs) and cytotoxic chemotherapies (used to suppress the malfunctioning immune system that is believed to cause tissue to become inflamed).

Gonococcal Arthritis

The highest incidence of gonococcal arthritis is in young adult females. The good news is that 95 percent of those affected are able to fully recover the functioning of their affected joint. As with most gonorrhea, there may be no symptoms (see Chapter 18) except for the joint pain. The infection seems to move around and settle in one or two joints. Usually the tendons around the wrist and ankle seem to be most vulnerable.

Causal Factors

In most cases, this type of arthritis is a result of having been involved in sexual activity with someone who has gonorrhea.

Diagnosis

If someone has gonorrhea and it is not treated, it may progress and become gonococcal arthritis. The symptoms will appear quite suddenly—fever, severe pain, and inability to move selected joints. The joints that are affected will be swollen, tender, warm, and red.

Treatment

The first course of treatment is medication to treat the gonorrhea. Anti-inflammatory drugs are then added to reduce the pain of arthritis. Although gonorrhea induced arthritis can be totally cured with antibiotics, if it is not treated early enough irreversible joint damage can occur.

When gonococcal arthritis is first diagnosed, it is common to keep the joint immobile. As soon as possible, passive range-of-motion exercises should begin. If the knee is the joint affected, exercises to strengthen the upper thigh are usually added to the physical program. When there is no pain, the exercises are done twice a day to strengthen the joint.

Mind and Spirit

At some time, 20 percent of all persons with arthritis get depressed.

The consequences of various types of arthritis are pain and often an increasing inability to meet our daily obligations. This has a major negative impact on our mind and spirit. It is not surprising then that some of the research shows that psychosocial stress may cause the worsening of many rheumatic disorders.

What can we do when we have a body that feels waves of pain that seem to come from nowhere? What some of us do is start to listen to our bodies and keep track of when the changes seem to come.

Sometimes what seems to be a random event is not as random as we would like to imagine. Given the important but undefined role that hormones play in rheumatoid arthritis, we have to see how our emotions may directly affect how we feel.

What can we do to function better when we have arthritis? Here are a few simple things.

1. Accept our limitations. When we have arthritis, this translates into sometimes not being able to do the things we once enjoyed. To accept these changes means that we can move on to the next part of our life.
2. Accept new ways of doing things. Although we may be unable to do all the things we used to do, we can still find new things to do and different ways to do what we did before. Perhaps instead of running you may choose to walk. And when you walk, you may actually be able to look at the people you pass and smile. When you cook, you may find that you need help in lifting pots and heavy items. Perhaps now is an opportunity for you to share the kitchen with a loved one and teach others in the family how to cook.
3. Create a new time frame for living. Many Latinas get into the habit of doing everything on a schedule set up by some vicious taskmaster—usually ourselves. Now we have to think of not doing it all, but doing what we can when we can.
4. Ask for help. The nicest words are sometimes "Can you help me?" It is OK to ask, and it is OK for people to say no. All we have to do is ask somebody else. And we might even be surprised at how eager people are to help.
5. Be patient. For our minds to be healthy and for our bodies to heal, we have to learn to let things unfold at their own speed. That means it is OK if things take a little longer, it is OK if people make mistakes, and most of all, it is OK if we make mistakes too.

Spirit

I couldn't help but smile when I saw the March-April 1996 issue of *Arthritis Today* magazine. The cover news and feature story was "The Faith Factor—Surprising Evidence of Spirituality's Power over Illness."

For some reason, it seems that in at least one area there is increasing awareness that praying and working with God are part of the healing process. When it comes to our autoimmune system, very little is known. Slowly new evidence has accumulated that faith and positive feelings seem to have a strengthening effect on the autoimmune system. The subject is very new, and because our research tools are not sophisticated enough to measure the complexities of the immune system, we are still learning about how to maximize the benefits of prayer.

In the interim, each one of us has to pursue this spiritual course in the way we see fit. For some of us it may be joining a prayer group at our local church; for others it may be volunteer work at a local agency helping others less fortunate than ourselves; and for others, just getting out of bed and facing the new day may be our act of prayer to God. Each one of us, in her own way, looks inside her heart to find the best way to pray. With the pain that is part of arthritis, we find that prayer is often a major tool for helping us manage a situation that seems out of our control.

Summary

Arthritis is a symptom and not a disease. Of the different joint diseases, osteoarthritis, rheumatoid arthritis, lupus, and gonococcal arthritis are the most likely to affect women. Each one has its specific course of diagnosis and treatment.

What is certain is that in all these diseases, with all their fluctuations of disease and remission, maintaining a sound mind and a committed spirit is essential. And who better to lead the charge on this than ourselves, as Latinas who for generations have made mind and spirit essential keys to our health.

RESOURCES

ARTHRITIS

Organizations

American College of Rheumatology
1800 Century Place, Suite 250
Atlanta, GA 30345
(404) 633-3777
www.rheumatology.org

Arthritis Foundation
1330 Peachtree Street
Atlanta, GA 30309
(800) 283-7800 or (404) 872-7100
http://www.arthritis.org

National Arthritis and Musculoskeletal and Skin Diseases Information Clearinghouse
National Institutes of Health
1 AMS Circle
Bethesda, MD 20892-3675
(301) 495-4484 or (877) 22-NIAMS
www.nih.gov/niams

Books

Brewerton, Derrick. *All about Arthritis: Past, Present, Future*. Cambridge: Harvard University Press, 1995.

Lorig, Kate. *The Arthritis Helpbook*. Reading, MA: Addison-Wesley, 2000.

Publications and Pamphlets

"Arthritis and Employment: You Can Get the Job You Want: Information on Meeting Employment Challenges," October 1994. Pamphlet No. 9070. Arthritis Foundation, 1800 Peachtree Street, Atlanta, GA 30345; (800) 283-7800. Internet: www.arthritis.org. Other titles include:

"Fast Facts About Arthritis," Information about how to handle discomfort caused by arthritis.

"Back Pain: Advice, Information, and Guidance," May 1995. Disease series.

"Diet and Arthritis," February 1995. Information about a healthy diet for arthritis sufferers.

"Exercise and Your Arthritis," June 1995. Disease series. Information on how to exercise for those suffering from arthritis.

"Arthritis Answers," January 1991. Bilingual (English/Spanish) information for those suffering from arthritis.

"Fibromalgia," July 1995.

"Using Medications Wisely." Serie en Español.

"Infectious Arthritis," February 1988. Medical Information series. Basic facts on infectious arthritis.

"Guide to Intimacy," Facts about sexuality for arthritis sufferers.

"Managing Your Activities: Using Your Joints Wisely," July 1995. Self-Management series. Information on how to live with arthritis.

"Managing Your Healthcare," August 1995. Self-Management series. Information on how to live with arthritis.

"Managing Your Pain," March 1995. Self-Management series. Information on how to live with arthritis.

"Managing Your Stress," August 1995. Self-Management series. Information on how to live with arthritis.

"Rheumatoid Arthritis," March 1995. Disease series. Information on how to deal with the condition of rheumatoid arthritis.

LUPUS

Organizations

American College of Rheumatology
1800 Century Place, Suite 250
Atlanta, GA 30345
(404) 633-3777
www.rheumatology.org

Lupus Foundation of America
1300 Piccard Dr., Suite 200
Rockville, MD 20850
(800) 558-0121 (English), (800) 558-0231 (Spanish), or (301) 670-9292
www.lupus.org

National Arthritis and Musculoskeletal and Skin Diseases Information Clearinghouse (National Institutes of Health—NIH)
1 AMS Circle
Bethesda, MD 20892-3675
(301) 495-4484 or (877) 22-NIAMS

Books

Dibner, Robin, and Carol Colman. *The Lupus Handbook for Women.* New York: Simon & Schuster, 1994.

Wallace, Daniel J. *The Lupus Book.* New York: Oxford University Press, 2000.

Publications and Pamphlets

"Lupus: Advice, Information and Guidance." Pamphlet No. 9052. Arthritis Foundation, P.O. Box 7669, Atlanta, GA 30357-0669; (800) 283-7800. www.arthritis.org

"Lupus Erythematosus: A Handbook for Physicians, Patients, and Their Families." 2d ed. Lupus Foundation of America, 1300 Piccard Dr., Suite 200, Rockville, MD 20850; (800) 558-0121 or (301) 670-9292. Available in Spanish.

"Arthritis: How to Stay Active and Independent." Pamphlet No. 1511. American Academy of Family Physicians, 11400 Tomahawk Creek Pkwy, Leawood, KS 66211-2672; (800) 944-0000.

12

Cancer

Ana knew everything there was to know about health and made sure to use the facts to guide what she would do. She was pleased with her own self-discipline because, even though it was a hassle when she woke up every morning, she exercised for half an hour.

Her breakfast was modified-traditional—she still ate chorizo *with eggs, but limited it to once a week, and when she had cereal, she used low-fat milk. She knew it was important to watch what she ate and to be active.*

As Ana quickly read over the self-help articles in the newspapers, she was relieved that she did not have to worry about cancer, because no one in her family had cancer and she had read that Latinas had lower rates of cancer than other women. That, of course, was good news because it gave her one less thing to think about.

There is good news about cancer. With early detection and treatment you *can* survive it and have a full and active life. This is what we, as Latinas, have to know. Too many of us are immobilized by the fear that a diagnosis of cancer means no cure. And thus, when it comes to cancer, we seem to see it as an automatic death sentence and do not respond to the signs that tell us there is something wrong with our bodies when it is still early enough to fix it. We also falsely assume that just because none of our family members have cancer, we won't get cancer either. Instead of remaining vigilant to the warning signs, we prefer to believe that if we just focus on having a healthy mind and spirit, our bodies will come along.

We need to understand what cancer is, how it is diagnosed, and what options we have for its treatment.

Cancer—The Basics: Risk Factors, Early Detection, Diagnosis, and Treatment

Cancer is defined as the unrestricted growth and division of cells, resulting in a mass of cells called a tumor. As the tumor grows, it may invade and destroy nearby cells, tissues, and organs.

There are two kinds of tumors: benign and malignant. A benign tumor is not cancer. Some of the more common types of benign tumors are polyps (small growths) and cysts (liquid-filled sacs). Neither cysts nor polyps spread to other parts of your body. Keep in mind that most women have cysts in their reproductive systems (see Chapter 6). The natural variations in the menstrual cycle can make some cysts appear and then disappear. Depending on the kind of cyst, in most instances it is up to you to decide whether you want to have the cysts removed. If you do have a cyst removed, there is always the chance that it will grow back.

If a tumor is made up of cells that divide rapidly in ways that are not normal, it is a malignant tumor. A malignant tumor is cancer. Much of the concern about cancer is related to whether cancer cells in the tumor have traveled to other parts of the body.

Cancer cells can spread to nearby lymph nodes, organs, and other structures. Cells may spread further throughout the body by using the bloodstream or the lymphatic system as a freeway. *Metastasis* is the word used to refer to the stage when cancer cells are found in other parts of your body. For example, if you have cervical cancer and it spreads to your intestines, it is not intestinal cancer but metastatic cervical cancer.

The challenge for medical researchers is to find out what causes the cells to divide in this disruptive manner. Most researchers assume that understanding the cause of the disruption in the production of cells will point the way to a cure. However, the possibility that any one factor causes all cancers is considered unlikely.

There are many theories that attempt to explain what causes the change in the way the cells divide. A number of factors are suspected or identified: tobacco, exposure to environmental hazards, biochemical changes in our body due to stress, the presence of a virus (HPV, discussed in Chapter 18), genetic defects, and many more. Future research will probably show that for each woman, there is a unique combination of causal factors that encourages cells to divide the wrong way.

Risk Factors

The study of risk factors identifies those conditions commonly found among persons who have a disease, in this case cancer. In most instances, all that can be established with risk factors is that they might produce a predisposition or tendency toward the disease; that is, there is a greater likelihood of the disease occurring. A risk factor is not something that causes the disease but instead is associated with the disease. For example, although smoking is a *risk* factor for lung cancer, the *causal* factor in lung cancer is not the smoke but the nicotine in the tobacco being inhaled.

Early Detection

Regardless of the area of the body where cancer develops, the earlier the cancer is detected, the greater the chance of successful treatment with less toxic methods. Scientific advances have also increased the survival from cancers that are diagnosed at later stages.

Diagnosis

In most cases, the first step involves getting a small sample of the material that forms the cancerous area or tumor so it can be carefully examined. This is referred to as a biopsy. Biopsy requires removal of part of the cancerous material or tumor. This material is sent to a laboratory to determine whether cancerous cells are present. If they are present, the pathologist examining the material will also be able to specify:

- The type of cancer
- Whether it is found in other tissue

- Whether hormones encourage its growth (This important information helps determine the type of medication you may receive to decrease the size of the tumor.)
- Its rate of growth (If the cancer is growing rapidly, it may be important to do all that can be done to stop it from growing.)

After the biopsy, your health care provider will tell you what was found. If the tumor is benign (not cancerous), your provider may still want to continue monitoring you closely as a precautionary measure. If the biopsy indicates that the tumor is malignant, it is important to know the stage of the cancer.

The stage of a cancer is determined by the size of the tumor and by performing imaging studies (e.g., x-ray, magnetic resonance imaging) and possibly other surgical biopsies to determine the extent to which cancer cells are found in surrounding areas. For example, the surgeon might take samples from the nearby lymph nodes as well as other parts of the body. It is important to determine if the cancer has spread to the lymph nodes—small, bean-shaped structures found throughout the body, which produce and store cells that fight infection. For each type of cancer, the stage or extent of disease has its own implication with respect to the choice of treatment and the likelihood of its success.

If you are found to have cancer, remember to allow time to organize your thinking about your situation, as well as to consult other health care providers (for second opinions), family, and friends, before you proceed with treatment. You may also want to contact some of the organizations listed in the resource section of this chapter. It is essential to get a second opinion about your treatment so that you can have a broader perspective about your treatment options. Sometimes you will need a third and fourth opinion. You will have to weigh all the pros and cons based on each opinion. Remember in doing so that to take good care of yourself you must have the best information possible. If you seek a second opinion, you are not being disloyal to your health care provider or showing disrespect to his or her opinion. You are checking to make sure that what happens next is what ought to happen *for your own good*.

Key Questions About Treatment

1. What are the side effects of the treatment?
2. How long will the treatment last?
3. How long will it take to return to my normal schedule?
4. What do you recommend I do after treatment?

Treatment

Treatment for cancer may involve surgery, medication (chemotherapy or hormonal therapy), and/or radiation therapy. The term *adjuvant therapy* is used to describe the additional therapy that may be given after successful surgery. Adjuvant therapy destroys cancerous cells that may not be detected by any existing diagnostic test.

The most important things to do are (1) get a second opinion, (2) make sure you know the stage of the disease, and (3) understand the pros and cons of different treatments.

The grade or stage of the cancer will determine the type of treatment. Remember that the decision about type of treatment should be made jointly by you and your health care provider. Some of the factors that will be taken into account are your age and general health and whether you want to have children.

There is great variability in the side effects produced by each of the treatments. Each woman will show a different combination of side effects, with considerable variability in their intensity.

Surgery

Depending on how widely the cancer cells have spread, surgery may be limited or more extensive. Sometimes your surgeon may have to remove some nearby lymph nodes to make certain that they do not contain cancerous cells.

Medication

Most cancer treatment involves medicines that fit into one of three categories:

1: Hormonal therapy. Since some tumors grow faster in the presence of hormones, these tumors can be reduced in size by decreasing the amount of hormones available. Hormonal therapy blocks the access of hormones to the cancer cell.

2: Chemotherapy. These medicines work on the rapidly dividing cancer cells. They also work on normally dividing noncancer cells, which explains their capacity for side effects. When something has such an extensive impact, it is referred to as systemic treatment.

The good news about systemic treatment is that cancer cells will be destroyed throughout the body. The bad news is that other cells that divide rapidly (blood cells, hair follicles, cells that line the digestive tract) but are not cancerous may also be damaged. This damage is serious but temporary and may include, for example, hair loss and a decrease in the body's ability to fight disease as a result of a decrease in white blood cells.

Typically the pattern of medication involves treatment, recovery, treatment, recovery, and so on. It is important to eat well during treatment because patients who eat well are better able to withstand the effects of treatments. This is not a time to go on a diet.

3: Biological therapy. This type of therapy boosts the body's immune system. As an example, the use of interferon is the most common way to treat cervical cancer on an outpatient basis. Some patients experience flu-like symptoms, which can be severe, but at the end of treatment these symptoms disappear.

Survival rate is a unit of measurement used by researchers to compare the value of one treatment to another. It usually means that the patient is alive at least five years after treatment. It does not include information on quality of life.

Radiation Therapy

Radiation stops the growth of cancerous cells by reducing their ability to reproduce. Radiation may be given in two ways—externally or internally. In the external method, you are treated as an outpatient for up to six weeks, five days a week. Each session lasts approximately 1 hour, during which the cancer site is exposed to radiation. Special care is taken to limit the area of exposure because radiation can damage other areas of the body.

The internal method is relatively new and spares healthy tissue. In this inpatient treatment, a capsule with radioactive material is implanted at the site of the cancer and left for a period of time. During this time, you may stay in the hospital.

During radiation treatment, it is common to feel tired. The tiredness may increase as treatment progresses, and it is important to match your activity to your energy level. It is also common to lose hair and have some skin irritation, but these symptoms are usually reversible when treatment is discontinued. In order to feel more comfortable in the short

LATINAS AND CANCER

Five Most Frequently Diagnosed Cancers		Five Most Common Types of Cancer Deaths	
(Rates Are Average Annual per 100,000)		(Rates Are Average Annual per 100,000)	
Breast	69.4	Breast	15.27
Colon and rectum	24.0	Lung and bronchus	11.01
Lung and bronchus	19.6	Colon and rectum	8.36
Cervix	15.8	Pancreas	5.43
Uterine	13.3	Ovary	4.92

Source: National Cancer Institute SEER Program, 1990–1996 data.

term, it helps to wear light clothes that do not rub the treated area.

After Treatment

We are learning more about cancer every year, and as a result the chances for recovery keep getting better. The resources section of this chapter lists many organizations that provide help in the transition back to the way you used to spend your time.

You will need to take care of yourself and go for regular checkups. For some, the experience is a reaffirming call to live life fully and to love those around them; for others, a time of more painful change may ensue. The important thing is to recognize that your treatment was a major step—and that there are many more positive ones to take.

The Facts: Lung, Colorectal, Breast, Cervical, Uterine, Ovarian, and Pancreatic Cancer

Now, having a basic understanding of cancer, we can discuss those cancer sites that are most likely to be of concern to Latinas—breast, colon and rectum, lung and bronchus, cervix, uterus, ovaries, and pancreas. Regardless of the cancer site, the most important factor to remember is that early detection is essential. The earlier treatment occurs, the more lives are saved.

Lung Cancer

Elisa had been smoking for thirty years. She thought nobody knew because she never let people see her smoke. When her friend Ana complained about the cigarette smoke that clung to her, Elisa was surprised. Elisa figured that maybe Ana had a delicate nose. What had Ana meant when she said Elisa's hair and clothes and even the jacket she took off smelled like cigarettes?

But to Elisa it really did not make much difference. Elisa knew that smoking would kill her, but she didn't care—at least she knew what would kill her.

Since 1987, each year more non-Hispanic white women have died of lung cancer than of breast cancer. Latinas, who are the group least likely to smoke, are still more likely to die of breast cancer than lung cancer. But we are losing our good health habits. With aggressive advertising aimed at Latinas by the tobacco industry, we are experiencing a fatal shift in our behavior. Today young Latinas are the group most likely to smoke.

Unless this trend is stopped, we will see premature deaths of Latinas due to lung can-

Remember—

- More non-Hispanic white women die from lung cancer than breast cancer.
- Smoking cigarettes is the major cause of lung cancer.
- Not smoking is the most effective way to reduce your risk of lung cancer.
- Precancerous cells usually return to normal if a person stops smoking.

cer surpass deaths due to breast cancer. Already there is evidence of this changing trend. According to the American Lung Association, from 1958 to 1988 the lung cancer death rate for Latinas rose from 4.8 to 10.8. The tragedy is that the majority of lung cancers may be avoided simply by not smoking.

Other causes of lung cancer include exposure to radon, asbestos, environmental tobacco smoke (ETS or secondhand smoke), air pollution, and radiation from occupational, medical, and environmental sources.

Early detection of lung cancer is usually not possible because symptoms do not appear until the disease is at an advanced stage, making treatment less effective. The combined survival rate for all stages of lung cancer is 14 percent. When the cancer has not spread and is in only one location, improved treatment has increased the survival rate to 49 percent of cases.

The most important fact to remember about lung cancer is that smoking causes most of it.

Colorectal Cancer

Our digestive system begins with the mouth and ends with the rectum. The purpose of this system is to remove from food the substances the body needs and eliminate what is not used. Food is broken down in the stomach and small intestines. It then travels through the colon (which is 5 to 6 feet long) and rectum (the last 6 to 8 inches of the colon), which absorb whatever water is left. The leftover waste material is a solid product (stool), which is eliminated through the anus. Cancer cells that originate in the colon or rectum are called colorectal cancer.

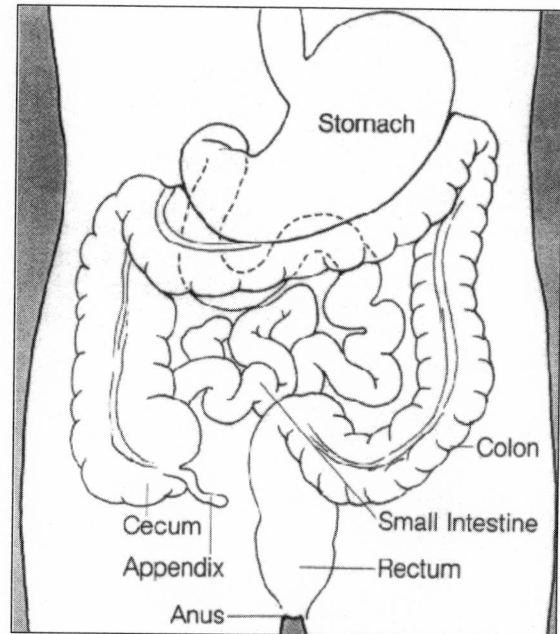

Digestive System

The major risk factors associated with colorectal cancer are being over fifty years old; having a sibling, parent, or child with colorectal cancer; having the inherited condition known as familial adenomatous polyposis; diets high in fat and low in fruits, vegetables, and high-fiber foods (breads and cereals); a history of polyps; excessive alcohol intake; sedentary lifestyle; and having ulcerative colitis or inflammatory bowel disease. With the exception of the age factor, at least three-quarters (75 percent) of all persons with new cases of colorectal cancer have no known risk factor.

Early Detection

As always, you are the best person to notice changes that need to be brought to the attention of your health care provider. Make sure that you recognize the symptoms below and that you see your health care provider to obtain a diagnosis because these symptoms may also be caused by ulcers, inflamed colon, or hemorrhoids.

- A change in bowel habits
- Diarrhea or constipation
- Blood in or on the stool (either bright red or very dark in color)
- Stools that are narrower than usual
- General stomach discomfort (bloating, fullness, and/or cramps)
- Frequent gas pains
- A feeling that the bowel does not empty completely
- Weight loss with no known reason
- Constant tiredness

Diagnosis

Early detection is usually accomplished with some combination of the following tests. Your health care provider should discuss with you the physical exams and tests that you will undergo.

- Digital rectal exam. In this exam your health care provider inserts a lubricated gloved finger into the rectum to feel if there is anything unusual.
- Fecal occult blood test (FOBT). This test determines whether there is hidden blood in your stool. Blood in the stool may be caused by several conditions. For most of us, beginning at age fifty this test will be part of our regular annual exam. In this test, a small sample (smear) of your stool is collected, placed on a plastic slide, and analyzed by a laboratory.
- Flexible sigmoidoscopy (FlexSig). In this test your health care provider uses a special instrument (sigmoidoscope) to look into your lower colon and rectum to see whether they can see any polyps, tumors, or other abnormalities.

  The sigmoidoscope is a thin, flexible plastic tube, which is inserted through your rectum and into your colon. Within the tube are a fiber-optic light and magnification device. Often if a polyp is found, your health care provider will be able to remove it using instruments passed through the tube, and you will not have to undergo abdominal surgery. Most growths that are removed are sent to a lab for biopsy.

  You will experience discomfort and even pain during this procedure, but it usually lasts only a few minutes. After age fifty, your health care provider will want you to have this exam every three to five years.

If any of the above tests raise concerns, the following tests may be recommended.

- Lower GI series or double contrast barium enema (DCBE). This test involves a radiologist taking x-rays of your colon and rectum (i.e., the lower gastrointestinal area). Getting the best picture of this area requires that your colon and rectum be as clean as possible. You will be advised to follow a special diet (low-residue or liquid diet) for 24 hours, followed by a laxative and enemas. Throughout this time you will be encouraged to drink lots of water and clear liquids.

  The test takes 20 to 30 minutes. While lying on your side, you will be given a barium enema, gently rolled to the left and right, then asked to stand so that the barium will fill the colon and rectum, permitting them to be outlined on the x-ray. When most of the barium has been removed, air may be pumped into the colon so that it is easier to see lesions in the lining. When air is added, it is called an air contrast or double-contrast barium enema.

This procedure is uncomfortable, especially if air is pumped into your colon, but the pain will last only a short time.

- Colonoscopy. This test is increasingly replacing a lower GI series as a diagnostic test for colorectal cancer. You will be given some combination of laxatives and enemas to prepare you for this important but unpleasant procedure. It involves using an instrument that is similar to the flexible sigmoidoscope but longer in order to see more of the colon. You will be sedated but awake throughout. If a growth is found, it may be removed using the same instrument and sent to a lab for biopsy.
- Virtual colonoscopy. This is a relatively new technique in which data from computed tomography (CT) scans are combined to produce an image of the colon lining. While you still need laxatives and enemas to prepare the colon, you will not have to be sedated for this procedure, which takes less than a minute. The effectiveness of this method needs to be tested through more widespread use.

In colorectal cancer, determining how advanced the cancer is—that is, the stage of the cancer—may be done by using a variety of imaging techniques to see if the cancer has spread to the lungs or liver. X-rays, CT (or computed axial tomography, CAT) scans, and ultrasonagraphy are used to determine if colorectal cancer is found elsewhere. Some health care providers also ask that a special blood test (carcinoembryonic antigen, or CEA, assay) be performed. Some people with colorectal cancer that has spread have higher than normal levels of CEA.

> **Remember—**
>
> Colorectal polyps should be removed because they can become cancerous.
>
> Only a small percentage of persons with rectal cancer will require a colostomy where the upper portion of the colon is brought out to the skin and the entire rectum is removed.

Additional Facts about Colon Cancer

If you have colorectal cancer, it is likely that you will undergo abdominal surgery.

The stages of colorectal cancer are:

Stage 0	Carcinoma in situ. Cancer is found only in the innermost lining of the colon.
Stage I	Cancer has spread to the second and third layers but still involves only the inside wall of the colon. Sometimes called Dukes A colon cancer.
Stage II	Cancer has spread to the outside wall of the colon but not to the lymph nodes. Sometimes called Dukes B colon cancer.
Stage III	Cancer has spread to nearby tissue and the lymph nodes. Sometimes called Dukes C colon cancer.
Stage IV	Cancer has spread beyond nearby tissue and lymph nodes to other parts of the body. Sometimes called Dukes D colon cancer.
Recurrent	The cancer has returned after treatment and is in the colon or some other part of the body, often the liver and/or lungs.

There are several possible kinds of surgery, depending on the stage of cancer. Here are some of the key words to help you understand what may happen in surgery.

Colectomy	Removal of the part of the colon and rectum with cancer and some of the surrounding healthy tissue.
Anastomosis	Reconnecting the healthy parts of the colon or rectum.
Colostomy	When the healthy sections cannot be connected, the surgeon creates an opening (stoma) in the abdomen through which stool may be eliminated. Sometimes this is done on a temporary basis to allow the lower colon or rectum to heal before reanastomosis is attempted.

If you have a colostomy, you will wear a special disposable bag to collect body wastes. The United Ostomy Association has support groups that help people adjust to a colostomy.

When colorectal cancers are detected in an early, localized stage, the survival rate five years after diagnosis is 90 percent. Unfortunately, only 37 percent of colorectal cancers are discovered in the early stages. However, even the survival rate for stage III colorectal cancer is 65 percent with appropriate surgery. The key is early detection.

Breast Cancer

Nearly 50,000 women die each year from breast cancer. Despite these high numbers, the reality is that our knowledge about breast cancer is growing, as is our optimism about its treatment.

Latinas are often not concerned about this kind of cancer because they have read that compared to other women, Latinas have lower rates of breast cancer. While this is accurate, the sad fact is that for Latinas diagnosed with breast cancer their five-year survival rate is lower than that of non-Hispanic white women with the same diagnosis.

Many Latinas think they do not have to worry about breast cancer because no one in their family has had breast cancer. However, over 80 percent of women with breast cancer do not have a relative with breast cancer. These facts need a bit more explanation.

The research clearly shows that women with breast cancer in their families are more likely to get breast cancer. It is also true, however, that the bulk of women who have breast cancer do not have it in their family. Moreover, even when someone in the family has had breast cancer, it is likely that many family members will be unaware of it.

Much has appeared in the popular press about the genes you get from your family being a risk factor. Unfortunately, when we hear that breast cancer "runs in families," most of us jump to the wrong conclusions. It sounds as if something in the family gene pool will make everyone in the family have breast

Women who are at highest risk for breast cancer are those who:

- Have a mother, sister, or daughter with breast cancer
- Have a personal history of breast cancer (have had breast cancer before)
- Are over fifty years of age
- Have never been pregnant
- Had their first full-term pregnancy after age thirty
- Had their first menstrual period before age twelve
- Began menopause after age fifty
- Are more than 10 percent overweight
- Have more than two alcoholic drinks per day.

cancer. In fact, in most instances, all we are implying is that the women in a given family are more likely to get breast cancer. It does not mean that every female member of that family will get breast cancer.

The focus on risk factors helps us identify those of our behaviors that we can change in order to be healthier. For example, limiting our exposure to radiation is a good way to reduce our risk of breast cancer. There are also risk factors that are an uncontrollable part of a normal life, such as age (i.e., being over fifty years old). There are other risk factors that we cannot change, such as the number of children we gave birth to. The important thing to keep in mind is that risk factors should be considered guideposts not predictions.

How these risk factors apply to Latinas is unclear. What we are certain of is that while breast cancer still occurs less frequently in Latinas, the incidence of breast cancer is increasing faster among Latinas than among other women.

Early Detection

As I looked up at my shower head, I could see the card I had hung there that instructed me on the proper way to do a breast self-exam. Every day I saw the pictures that told me what I had to do. They had arrows pointing in all the directions I was supposed to touch my breasts and feel myself in order to properly examine my breasts.

And I always did the same thing. I looked at the shower card, patted my breasts firmly, and sighed a breath of relief that I had not felt anything. I reassured myself that I had nothing to worry about because I hadn't found anything.

—*Milena, 35*

As Latinas, just looking at our breasts is often difficult. Even when we bathe or shower or put on a bra, too often we do not actually look at our breasts. And then when we do look at our breasts, we complain about their size or shape or the way they hang.

If, as Latinas, we find it difficult to look at our own breasts, it is doubly difficult to touch them. It is probably safe to say that most Latinas have had their breasts touched by others more than by themselves. The reasons for this are complex. For some, touching breasts is sexual, and women have been taught not to touch their sexual organs. For others, the fear of finding "something" immobilizes them and makes it impossible for them to touch their breasts.

Yet knowledge is essential, especially when there is something wrong. The earlier we find a problem, the less extensive the treatment (lumpectomy instead of mastectomy) and the greater the chance of survival. To insure early detection, you must:

1. Do a monthly breast self-exam (BSE).
2. Have an annual breast exam by your health care provider.
3. Have a mammogram as appropriate.

As a first step, we have to learn how to look at and touch our breasts.

Looking At and Touching Our Breasts

Your breasts are a part of your body. As women, we are used to looking at our breasts in terms of size and droop but have ignored looking at our breasts in terms of health. By looking at our breasts on a regular basis, we learn to recognize changes in them.

Touching our breasts makes us aware of what our breasts feel like, keeping in mind that during any month, normal shifts in hormones will change how our breasts feel. Some women have more sensitivity in their breasts a few days before they menstruate, while others may feel tender during the middle of their cycle.

When we look at and touch our breasts on

a regular basis, we learn to recognize what our breasts feel like most of the time. Once we feel comfortable looking at and touching our breasts, the next step is to learn how to systematically touch our breasts and the surrounding areas.

As she began to breast-feed her new son, Iris knew that there was something wrong. Something in her breast felt round and hard. She didn't know what it was, but she knew it should not be there. She had to go for a checkup and decided to let her doctor know about her concern.

She was scared when she softly told him that she had felt something in her breast. He looked at her and gently tapped her breast. No need to worry, he said. That type of thickening was common with mothers who were breast-feeding. She felt relieved that the lump was nothing to worry about.

But months passed and the lump was still there. And she knew that something was wrong. She decided to go for a second opinion.

Monthly Breast Self-Exam (BSE)

All women over age twenty should do a breast self-exam (BSE), which takes less than fifteen minutes, once a month. The BSE has three parts: shower or bath, looking at a mirror, and lying down. The order in which you do these does not matter. What is essential is that you do all three on the same day because each aspect gives you information about a different part of your breast and connected areas. Remember that 50 percent of all lumps are found in the upper area near the underarm.

Some women teach their partners how to conduct the lying down portion of the monthly breast exam.

If you still get your period, you should do your BSE a few days after your period ends. Women who no longer have periods should do their BSE the same day each month.

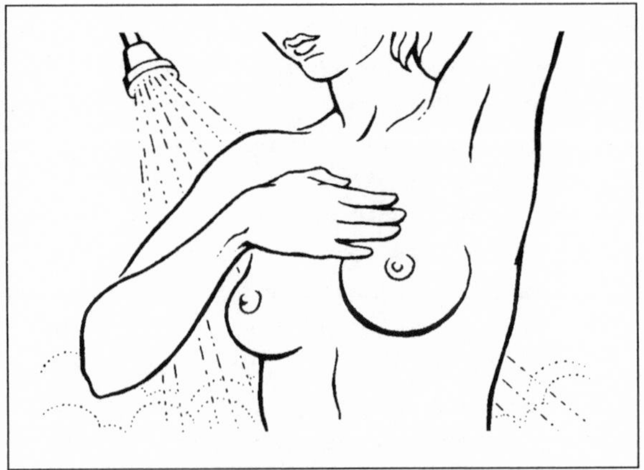

Breast Self-Exam—Shower

1: Shower or bath. This part of the BSE focuses on your nipples and your breast. The water and soap make your skin slipperier and thus make it easier to examine your breasts.

- Right breast exam. Begin by raising your right hand high over your head and using your left hand to examine your right breast. Using the fingertips of your left hand, apply light and deep pressure in either a clockwise spiral or an up-and-down grid pattern to your right breast. You may find that if you close your eyes you can focus better on what you feel. Be sure to cover the entire breast and the underarm.
- Left breast exam. Raise your left hand high over your head and use your right hand to examine your left breast in the same way. Using the fingertips of your right hand, apply light and then deep pressure in either a spiral or grid pattern to your left breast.

You may want to obtain a shower card by contacting the American Cancer Society.

If you feel a lump in your breast, you should see your health care provider. Keep in mind that some women's breasts have more non-

Average-size lump found by getting regular mammograms

Average-size lump found by first mammogram

Average-size lump found by women practicing regular breast self-examination

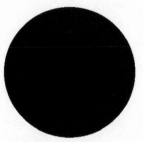

Average-size lump found by women practicing occasional breast self-examination

Average-size lump found by women untrained in breast self-examination

Size of Lump and How Found

cancerous lumps than others. Moreover, at different times of the month your breasts may feel more lumpy. Once you are in the regular habit of doing a BSE, you will know better how your breasts feel normally and be able to recognize when you feel something abnormal.

2: Looking at a mirror. This part of the BSE looks at overall differences between your breasts. You must look at your breasts from three different positions: (1) hands at your side, (2) hands clasped behind your head, and (3) hands on your hips, while flexing your chest muscles. In each of these positions you are looking for:

- Any change in the size of the breast
- Whether one breast is a lot lower than the other
- Any changes on the skin of the breast
- Any changes in the shape or skin of the nipple
- Any changes in the color of the skin (redness, discoloration)
- Nipple discharge

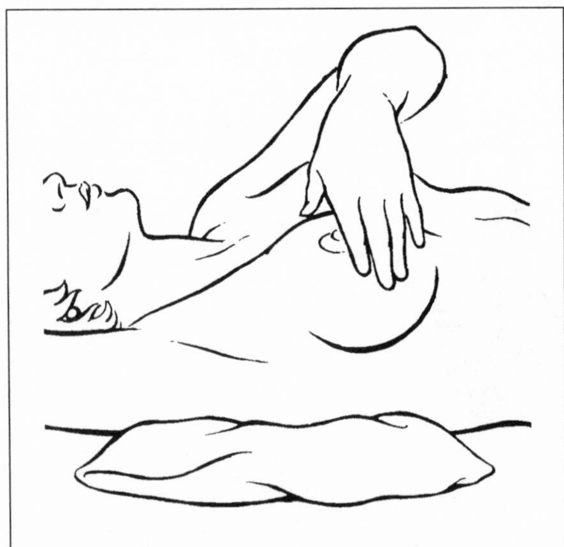

Breast Self-Exam—Lying Down

3: Lying down. The American Cancer Society recommends that you examine the breast and underarm while lying down. This part of the BSE helps you to better feel the area from your breast to your underarm to your collarbone.

To do this part of the exam, lie down and place a pillow under your left shoulder. Place your right hand under your left armpit, and with your fingertips make small spirals the size of your fingertips all the way to your left breast. You can either make the small spirals in a downward motion toward the nipple or in a circular motion around the breast and in toward the nipple.

Then move your right hand to your left collarbone, and again make small spirals with your fingertips all the way down to your left breast. Once you have done this for the area from your collarbone and left armpit to your left breast, repeat the same steps on your right breast.

Now place the pillow under your right shoulder, and use your left hand to examine the area from your collarbone and right armpit to your right breast.

You should be pressing firmly enough to move the skin. Notice how your skin moves and how it feels when you make the spirals with your fingertips.

Make sure that you see your health care provider if you notice:

- A swelling in the upper arm
- An increase in the size of the small, oval-shaped lymph nodes near your armpit

Not All Lumps in Your Breast Mean Cancer

For 4 out of 5 women, the lumps in their breasts may be unrelated to cancer. The American Cancer Society emphasizes that the woman's responsibility is *only* to find a change and *not* to make a diagnosis. Your health care provider may later diagnose some of the lumps you find as:

> **Warning: Possible Signs of Breast Cancer**
>
> 1. A lump in the breast
> 2. Any change in the size of the breast
> 3. One breast a lot lower than the other
> 4. Changes on the skin of the breast
> 5. Any changes in the shape or skin of the nipple
> 6. An increase in the size of the small, oval-shaped lymph nodes near your armpit
> 7. Cloudy or bloody fluid coming out of your nipple

- Cysts: liquid-filled sacs that are found usually in both breasts. They range from firm to soft and are tender to the touch right before your period (most typical in women ages thirty-five to fifty).
- Fibroadenomas: made up of different kinds of tissue. They feel solid, round, and rubbery. Sometimes they are easy to move. They are usually painless and are more prevalent in young women.
- Fibrocystic lumps: change size as a function of the menstrual cycle. They are found in nearly half of all women. They are difficult to distinguish from malignant lumps. They decrease in size with onset of menopause (ages thirty-five to fifty).
- Intraductal papillomas: small nodes underneath the nipple area. They can cause the nipple to bleed. They appear in women in their forties. Any bleeding from your nipple is reason for you to see your health care provider.
- Lipomas: made up of fatty tissue. These small lumps range in size from ¼ to ½ inch in diameter. They move around freely and grow slowly. Diagnosis is based on biopsy. They affect mainly older women.

Annual Breast Exam by Your Health Care Provider

Every woman should have a clinical breast exam at least every three years from the ages of twenty to forty and annually after age forty.

A breast exam is an important part of your annual screening visit to your health care provider. The breast exam done by your provider will be similar to your BSE, the difference being that your provider is more skilled in detecting lumps. During the exam if your health care provider feels a lump he or she will try to determine its size and will determine how easily it is moved around. All this is valuable information in determining what kind of a lump it is.

Although you may feel uncomfortable and vulnerable when your health care provider looks at your breasts, remember that this is part of the exam. Some women have indicated that if they are feeling embarrassed, it is easier to look at the top of the health care provider's head or away from the area being examined.

Despite your provider's skill in detecting lumps, he or she will not immediately know if a lump or thickness is normal or abnormal for you. You should know your breasts better than anyone else after conducting regular BSEs and will be able to report what is usual for your breasts and what is unusual.

Mammogram

Women age forty and over should have a mammogram every year. In 1987 Latinas were found to be the group least likely to have had a mammogram. As a result of good outreach to our community by the American Cancer Society and the National Alliance for Hispanic Health, however, by 1992 Latinas were the group most likely to have had a mammogram.

A mammogram is an x-ray of the breast. A high-quality mammogram can identify a lump before it can be felt by breast exam. Still, it is important to remember that a mammogram cannot detect all tumors because some tumors do not show up well on the x-ray. Your local health department can tell you where you can obtain a low-cost mammogram.

It is critically important that mammography be conducted in a manner that is safe and reliable. This means that the mammogram must be taken by trained technicians using equipment in good working order with the results read by a specialist. Although many people assumed that this was the norm, by 1992 it had become clear that although many women were getting mammograms, the mammogram was not always as safe or reliable as expected. At that point, Congress gave the Food and Drug Administration (FDA), which has responsibility for overseeing the safety and effectiveness of medical devices, the lead responsibility for carrying out the Mammography Quality Standards Act (MQSA).

Obtaining a quality mammogram. The purpose of MQSA is to insure the prevalence of high-quality mammograms through the development of standards and annual monitoring of the 11,000 mammography centers throughout the country. In 1994 the FDA published a set of standards that providers and centers had to meet in order to be certified by FDA-approved accreditation bodies. In order to be a legally operating center for mammography, a facility must have a prominently displayed certificate issued by the FDA. When your doctor sends you for a mammogram, be sure to call and find out whether the center has such a certificate.

Who should have a mammogram. There has been much debate with respect to the age at which women should obtain their first mammogram and the frequency with which follow-up mammograms should be scheduled. According to the Centers for Disease Control (CDC), a mammogram is not as informative for women under thirty as for older women. The American Cancer Society has indicated that at age forty, every women should begin

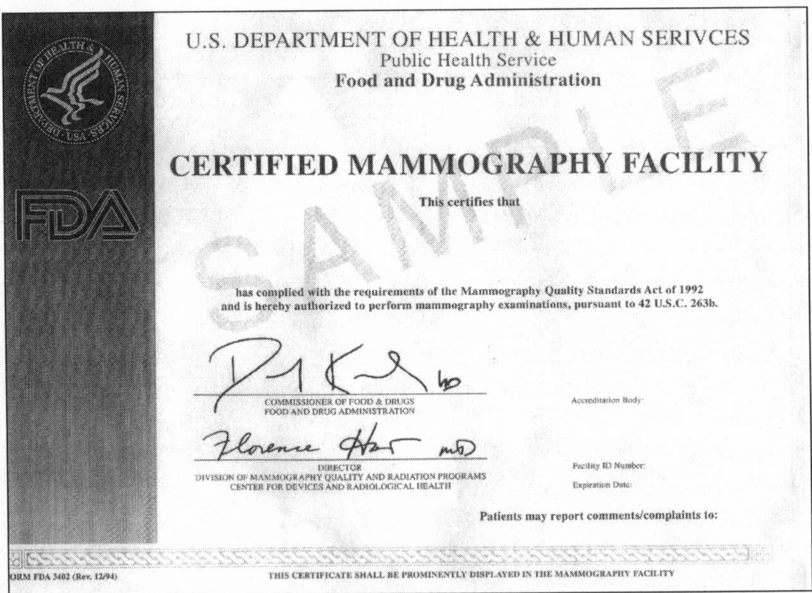
U.S. DEPARTMENT OF HEALTH & HUMAN SERIVCES
Public Health Service
Food and Drug Administration

CERTIFIED MAMMOGRAPHY FACILITY

This certifies that

has complied with the requirements of the Mammography Quality Standards Act of 1992 and is hereby authorized to perform mammography examinations, pursuant to 42 U.S.C. 263b.

COMMISSIONER OF FOOD & DRUGS
FOOD AND DRUG ADMINISTRATION

Accreditation Body:

DIRECTOR
DIVISION OF MAMMOGRAPHY QUALITY AND RADIATION PROGRAMS
CENTER FOR DEVICES AND RADIOLOGICAL HEALTH

Facility ID Number:
Expiration Date:

Patients may report comments/complaints to:

ORM FDA 3402 (Rev. 12/94)

THIS CERTIFICATE SHALL BE PROMINENTLY DISPLAYED IN THE MAMMOGRAPHY FACILITY

Sample Mammography Certificate

getting annual mammograms (women with a family history of breast cancer may be encouraged to begin mammography at an earlier age). The recommendations for women ages forty to fifty are currently the subject of much debate. Guidelines for this age group are under review. For women over sixty-five, Medicare pays for mammograms but only every other year. Additional references are provided in the resources section of this chapter.

What happens when you go for a mammogram. In the mammography dressing room, you will be asked to remove all your jewelry and clothing from the waist up. A garment that opens in the front will be given to you to keep you warm and covered.

You will then go to a room where a technician will ask you to open the garment and place one of your breasts on a plastic plate. The technician will move your breast gently to position it properly on the plate. A second plate is then placed on top of your breast to flatten it out as much as possible. All this positioning and pressing is done to get good pictures of your breast. One image is taken from the top and one from the side. After the images of one breast have been taken, the technician will repeat the same procedure with your other breast.

In most instances, you will be asked to wait while the technician develops the film. If the picture is not clear, the technician may take a second set of images.

Remember that the position for taking a mammogram may feel unnatural and even uncomfortable but *that it can save your life*. So make sure that you get your mammograms as often as is indicated for your age.

Results from your mammogram. The images of your breast will be reviewed by a physician trained to read what to the untrained eye seem to be just shadows. The physician who reads your x-ray will send a report on the findings to the health care provider that referred you.

Some lumps turn out to be liquid-filled cysts; other lumps contain coarse calcium deposits (resulting from old injuries, inflammation, or changes in the breast arteries due to aging). Some lumps contain tiny specks of calcium (microcalcification). These small calcifications can suggest the presence of a cancer.

If your health care provider has identified a lump and cannot be sure that it is noncancerous, the next step is to ascertain exactly what it is. According to the National Cancer Institute, the only way to diagnose cancer accurately is through biopsy.

Other Methods

The use of ultrasound to image the breast has led to more information about tumors. Ultrasound is often able to distinguish between a mass that is solid and one that is liquid. While a liquid mass is probably a benign cyst filled with liquid, a solid mass may be a cancer. Unfortunately, ultrasound cannot detect small calcium deposits or small tumors.

Increasingly, new technologies are being approved as improvements or adjuncts to mammography. Nevertheless, at this time the most commonly available diagnostic procedure for the breast is mammography.

Biopsy

In the past, women were routinely asked to give permission for the surgeon to do a mastectomy if cancer was found during a biopsy. Today, in most cases, diagnosis and treatment are two different parts of the process, although in some instances the surgeon will perform a lumpectomy during a biopsy. Usually there is a diagnostic biopsy first, and then, after a few days to a week, treatment begins. In most cases, the time between the biopsy and the beginning of treatment is used to carefully consider the treatment options and to prepare you for the consequences of treatment. Research shows that this delay has had no detrimental effect.

There are two major ways to obtain material from a lump: aspiration/needle biopsy and surgical biopsy.

1. Aspiration/needle biopsy

• Fine needle aspiration (FNA). The breast is anesthetized, and a long thin needle is inserted into the lump to remove part of it. It will be obvious whether the lump is filled with liquid or solid material. If the lump is filled with liquid, it is a cyst. This means that cancerous cells are not present, and your physician will remove the unwanted liquid. If the lump is solid, some of the material is taken out for further examination. This procedure is usually done on an outpatient basis.

Aspiration is a very effective technique as long as it is done properly. If a woman has large breasts and a small lump near the chest wall, this procedure is not recommended because it may not be possible to reach the lump. Neither is aspiration recommended if the lump cannot be seen on a mammogram, because the surgeon has to be able to direct the needle to the lump.

• Needle core biopsy (stereotactic breast biopsy/mammo-test). The breast is anesthetized, and a needle is inserted into the lump to extract some tissue. The needle is guided using a computerized x-ray technique. This procedure is increasingly used because it is highly accurate and, unlike surgical biopsy, leaves no scar.

2. Surgical biopsy. This requires removal of part of the lump (incisional biopsy). If the lump seems suspicious, the surgeon will remove 1 centimeter (about ½ inch) of healthy tissue in the area immediately surrounding the lump (excisional biopsy) to see if it contains cancerous cells. If the lump appears benign, the surgeon will remove less of the surrounding healthy tissue.

Stages of Breast Cancer

Carcinoma in situ	The cancer is isolated in one place and is found only in a few layers of cells. The cure rate for this type of breast cancer is over 90 percent.
Stage I	Cancer cells are found only in the breast, and the tumor is smaller than 1 inch (2.5 cm) at any point.
Stage II	Cancer cells are found in the breast area and under the arm in the lymph nodes. The size of the tumor is between 1 and 2 inches (2.5–5.0 cm).
Stage III	Sometimes referred to as locally advanced cancer, in this stage the tumor is more than 2 inches (5.0 cm) in size, and cancer cells are present in most lymph nodes and other areas near the breast.
Stage IV	In this stage the cancer has spread to other parts of the body (metastasized).
Recurrent cancer	If you have had cancer and were treated, sometimes the cancer will still return. This is considered recurrent cancer.

Surgery

This is always difficult to face, yet in the area of breast cancer, surgery provides the best chances of cure. Recent studies have

> *Consejos*
>
> Most women qualify for a lumpectomy. Be sure this option is discussed.

shown that when a woman qualifies for a lumpectomy, there is no difference in her survival rate and that of women who have a mastectomy. The different kinds of surgery are described below.

Lumpectomy

The tumor is removed together with some of the surrounding area. There is only a small change in how the breasts look. Some of the lymph nodes in the underarm will be removed.

Partial or Segmental Mastectomy

The tumor, up to one quarter of the breast tissue, and all or some of the lymph nodes are removed.

Total or Simple Mastectomy

The entire breast and sometimes a few lymph nodes are removed.

Modified Radical Mastectomy

The entire breast, all the lymph nodes under the arms, and the lining over the chest muscles are removed.

Radical Mastectomy (Halsted Radical)

The entire breast, all the lymph nodes under the arms, and the chest muscles are removed. Once the treatment of choice for breast cancer,

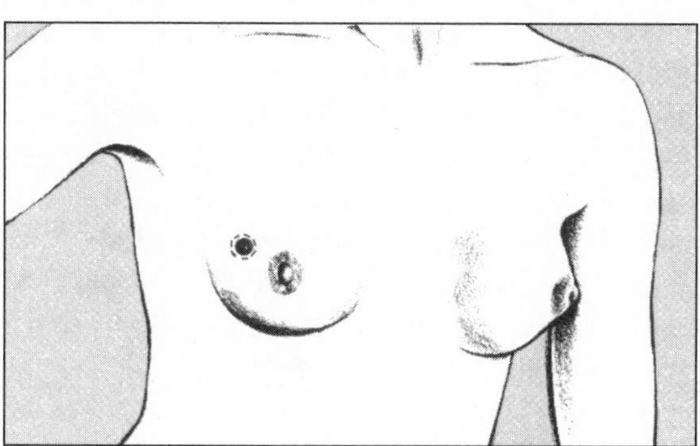

Lumpectomy

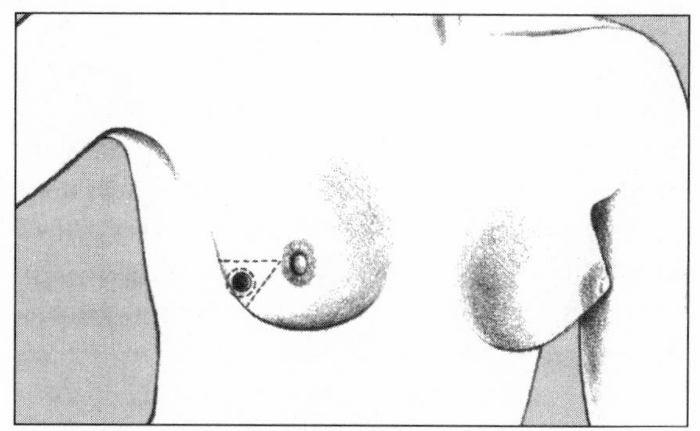

Partial Mastectomy

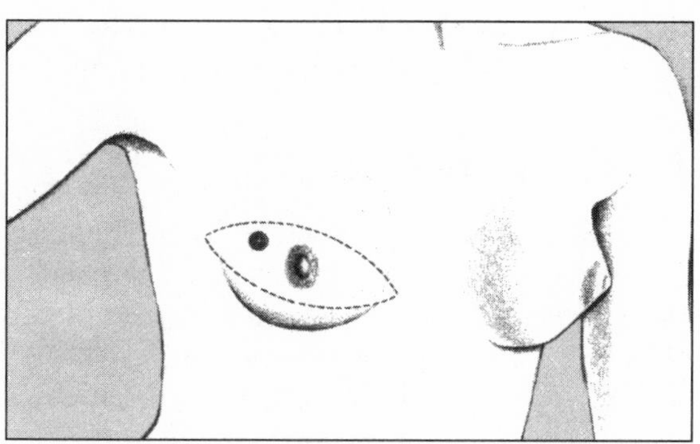

Total Mastectomy

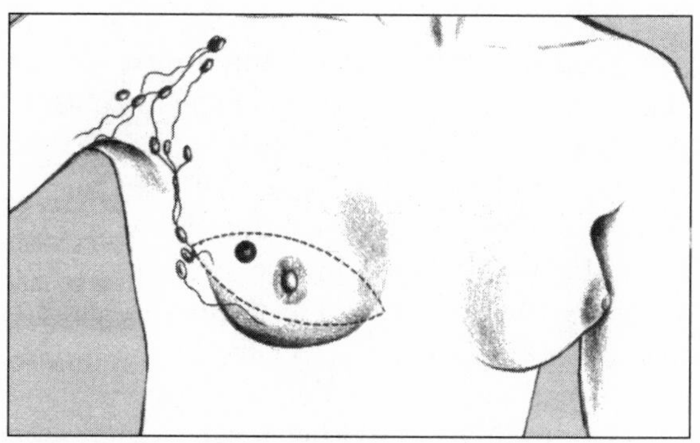

Modified Radical Mastectomy

it is now used only in those cases where the cancer is attached to the chest wall.

Follow-up and Re-screening

Of great concern is the large number of Latinas who do not come back for repeat mammograms that can detect abnormal breast changes over time. The initial mammogram establishes the baseline against which future mammograms can be compared. Monitoring changes over time can alert Latinas and their health care providers to abnormalities for which further screening or treatment may be required. Timely follow-up will help the health care provider reach a diagnostic resolution and make future recommendations that could potentially save a woman's life.

Although Latinas have one of the lowest rates of breast cancer, they have one of the highest mortality rates and are more likely to die from the disease than non-Hispanic white women. The higher mortality rates are due in part to late-stage diagnosis when treatment options are limited and less successful. Too often when a finding is suspicious, some women are lost to follow-up. This means they will not return to the clinic, even though a suspicious or abnormal finding may have been found.

Cervical, Uterine, and Ovarian Cancer

We need to listen very carefully to everything our health care providers say. Especially when it comes to our reproductive systems, we are often fearful of being told that we have a tumor. Some of us turn off our ears when we hear the word *tumor*, but we need to listen carefully because not all tumors are bad. Sometimes fibroids and functional cysts (see Chapter 6) are mistakenly called tumors, and in our minds we think that means cancer and that we are going to die. The quantum leaps our imagination takes may make it difficult for us to grasp what is going on with our body.

Warning

The more cigarettes a woman smokes in a day and the longer she has been smoking, the higher the risk for cancer of the cervix, stomach, esophagus, bladder, lung, throat, and larynx.

We know that we Latinas have more problems than other women with our ovaries, cervix, and uterus. Most of the time the problems we experience are part of the normal intricacies associated with the female reproductive system. Sometimes, however, there is something wrong that is much more serious. Cancer of the cervix, cancer of the uterus, and cancer of the ovaries are some of the things that can be very wrong. Often we mistakenly use the terms interchangeably, thinking that we can take care of our ovaries, cervix, and uterus with one simple test. One Latina stated, "I go for my annual Pap test, and if that is OK I do not worry about anything." The reality is that a Pap test only gives us information about the cervix, not about the ovaries or uterus.

We need to learn about cancer of the cervix, cancer of the uterus, and cancer of the ovaries. The only thing they have in common is that the earlier we know about a problem with them, the greater the success of treatment.

Cervical Cancer

Maria had known that she was working very hard. The high stress from her job had given her many sleepless nights. And now, to make matters worse, she was getting bad cramps, and sometimes she would bleed a lot. It was hard to know what was going on.

She was certain it was just some weird stuff

happening with her period and thought she had better just ignore it. After all these years of pain and discomfort, she knew it would just go away. She took some tea to calm herself down.

A few days later, Maria was having dinner with her friend Clarissa. Maria told Clarissa what had been going on with her period. With certainty, Maria gave Clarissa her own diagnosis, that this unusual bleeding was probably due to stress.

Clarissa listened to her friend's comments intently, but then she shook her head and said to Maria, "I know what stress looks like; I see it every day in the mirror when I look at myself. But when I look at your face—you do not look like someone with just stress. You look like there is something very wrong with you."

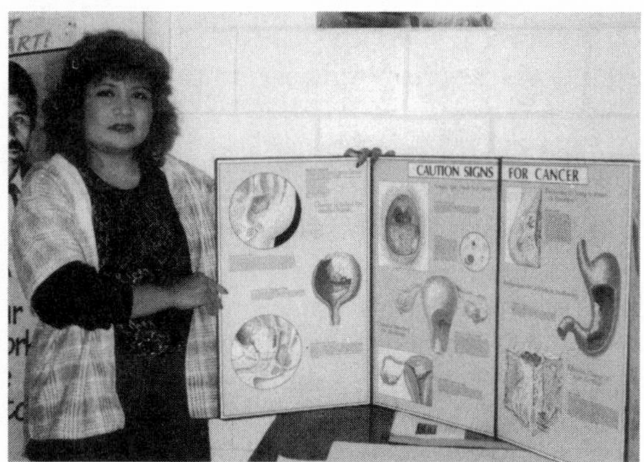

We need to have the best information available at all times.

Cervical cancer is typically without symptoms. Early detection helps determine when there are precancerous conditions. Because precancerous conditions may not cause pain, we should see our health care providers on a regular basis even if we do not feel sick or have pain.

Pain is not a symptom of cervical cancer until it has progressed to the invasive mode. The most common symptom in cervical cancer is abnormal bleeding—too much or too little bleeding at the wrong time of the month. The wrong time is any time when we are not having our regular period; for example, after sexual intercourse or douching or between periods. At the same time, every instance of abnormal bleeding is not a sign of a problem, since it is also found in women who are going through menopause.

A Pap test is the most effective method for early detection of cervical cancer. What little data there are about Latinas and cervical cancer indicate that Latinas are the group least likely to go for a Pap test (also known as a Pap smear) and most likely to get cervical cancer. The fact that we do not go for regular Pap tests explains our higher rates of cervical cancer. It is thus a matter of life and death for us to overcome our reluctance and our biases against Pap tests.

Some Latinas think that only if they are sexually active do they need to have a Pap test. The fact is that all Latinas over the age of eighteen, including those over sixty years of age, should have an annual Pap test. Latinas under eighteen who are sexually active should also have regular Pap tests. If your Pap test is normal three years in a row, your health care provider will be able to tell you when you should go for your next one. For the majority of women, an annual Pap test will be recommended.

Several studies indicate that women mistakenly believe that the need for Pap tests declines with age. In fact, cervical cancer deaths occur at a higher rate for women over 65 (9 out of 100,000) than for women ages 18 to 64 (2 out of 100,000). Medicare covers cervical cancer screening every two years for women and annual tests for those women who are at high risk.

Most recently research has focused on the role viruses play in cervical cancer. There is strong evidence of a relationship between human papilloma viruses (HPVs) and cervical cancer. HPV is considered a sexually transmitted disease (see Chapter 18). Women with HPV or whose partners have HPV have a higher risk of cervical cancer. The relationship between HPV and cervical cancer is not a one-to-one relationship; most woman exposed to HPV do not develop cervical cancer.

The data suggest that there is a greater risk of cervical cancer when the immune system is not working well. Thus Latinas who are HIV positive have higher rates of cervical cancer than other women. Similarly, women who are taking medications in order to suppress their immune systems (typically these are women who have received organ transplants) also seem to be at higher risk for precancerous lesions.

What we know suggests that various factors interact to cause cervical cancer. Sometimes it is difficult to understand the relationship between a specific factor and cervical cancer. For example, women who smoke have much higher rates of cervical cancer. The heavier the smoking habit, the higher the risk for cervical cancer.

Until recently Latinas smoked less than other women, but as mentioned above, that is changing, which in the future may increase our already high rates of cervical cancer. One thing is for certain—smoking is bad for us in many ways.

While we know that smoking is bad for us, there is some evidence that folic acid (found in dark green leafy vegetables, orange juice, dried peas, beans, and lentils) plays a role in protecting us from cervical cancer. Some women take it in the form of a daily dietary supplement or eat fortified cereals. The right amount to take is still to be determined. The nature of this protection is only now being seriously studied.

Diagnosis

The Pap test is used for diagnosing cancer of the cervix. It is not as reliable for diagnosing cancer of the uterus and cannot diagnose ovarian cancer. In the spring of 1996, the FDA indicated that a Pap test plus speculoscopy was more sensitive than the Pap smear alone in detecting cervical abnormalities.

What does it mean to have a positive Pap test? If your Pap test is positive, there are cell abnormalities. You will probably be asked to have a second test to confirm the initial findings (see Chapter 6 for information on preparing for your pelvic exam and Pap test).

A precancerous condition is an area in which abnormal cells exist but only in the top layer of cells. It is not known what causes these conditions. The technical name for these cell abnormalities is squamous intraepithelial lesions (SILs). There are two categories of SILs:

1: Low-grade SILs, also referred to as mild dysplasia or cervical intraepithelial neoplasm 1 (CIN 1), are typically found in women twenty-five to thirty-five years old. In some instances these abnormal cells go away on their own; in other instances they grow and become high-grade SILs. If these are found, your health care provider will probably want to monitor you closely and may recommend that you have a follow-up Pap test sooner than one year.

2: High-grade SILs are also called moderate or severe dysplasia, CIN 2, CIN 3, or carcinoma in situ. In high-grade SILs, the precancerous cells look very different from normal cells and there are many more of them. These abnormal cells are still found only in the cervix.

Test results are now based on the Bethesda System, which classifies the findings as low-grade to high-grade SILs. The previously used system classified cells using a 5-point scale, with 1 being normal and 5 being invasive cancer. Cervical cancer is considered invasive if the abnormal cells from the cervix have invaded other nearby tissues or organs. In order to determine whether you have invasive cervical cancer, it is important that cells from the other tissues and organs be examined under a microscope. Make sure to ask your doctor which system was used to grade the findings.

If a Pap test is not normal, your health care provider will probably want to obtain more information by using one or more of the following tests:

- Colposcopy. Health care providers should recommend a colposcopy if cells are abnormal or if your results from a series of several Pap tests are slightly abnormal. This procedure is similar to speculoscopy except that after the vinegar-like solution is used to coat the cervix, a colposcope (which is like a microscope) is used to look more closely at the cells on the cervix. Colposcopy is a means to grade the lesions more accurately and, if necessary, point to an area where there should be a biopsy.

- Schiller test. A Schiller test may be recommended as an adjunct to colposcopy. With the colposcope in place, the cervix is coated with an iodine solution. Abnormal cells turn white or yellow, while normal cells turn brown.

- Biopsy. In a biopsy, a very small piece of tissue is removed from the cervix. There are two major types of biopsy: surface biopsy and below-the-surface biopsy.

Surface biopsies are usually done in the office. There are several different methods. In one method, an instrument is used to pinch off little pieces of the cervix. Another method is the loop electrosurgical excision procedure (LEEP), in which a local anesthetic is administered and a very thin wire loop is inserted through the vagina to slice off a thin round piece of tissue. There is usually some bleeding or discharge after these procedures. Although they may hurt, the tissue heals quickly.

Biopsies below the surface usually require local or general anesthesia. In conization ("cone biopsy"), a cone-shaped sample of tissue is removed. For some precancerous conditions, conizations are used as a treatment if the entire precancerous area can be removed.

Additional Facts about Cervical Cancer

Precancerous Conditions

If your condition is precancerous, your health care provider may recommend treatment of the affected area by freezing (cryosurgery), cauterization (diathermy or burning), laser (which destroys abnormal tissue but leaves normal tissue intact), LEEP, or conization to remove unhealthy tissue. While you may experience some discomfort and light bleeding for one or two days, there are no side effects.

Surgery

A hysterectomy (removal of uterus and cervix) is done if abnormal cells are found inside the opening of the cervix and the woman does not want to have children in the future. When only the uterus and cervix are removed, there are no symptoms of menopause, since hormones are still being produced by the ovaries. If the fallopian tubes and ovaries are removed (salpingo-oophorectomy), menopause occurs. It is important to remember that sexual desire and the ability to enjoy sex physiologically are not changed by hysterectomy (see Chapter 6).

Radiation

More advanced cervical cancers are often treated with radiation. Some women report that they feel their vagina becomes narrower and less flexible as a result of radiation treatment. If this happens to you, your health care provider can instruct you on how to use vaginal dilators and water-based lubricants to increase the flexibility and size of your vagina.

Myths and Facts

Myth: Only women who are sexually active need to have a Pap test every year.

Fact: All women over eighteen need to have a Pap test every year. This is especially true for older women.

Myth: Having a hysterectomy will reduce my ability to have an orgasm.

Fact: A hysterectomy does not change your clitoris, and thus there is no physiological reason not to have an orgasm. You may need to address issues of your emotions and self-esteem.

Myth: If I have a hysterectomy, I will immediately start menopause.

Fact: You will start menopause only if your ovaries have been removed.

Uterine Cancer

There are two major types of uterine cancer: (1) endometrial cancer and (2) sarcoma. Endometrial cancer accounts for the large majority of all uterine cancer and is found most commonly in women who are postmenopausal. It begins with abnormal cell growth in the endometrium (lining of the uterus). There may be very few signs to indicate that there is a problem. Over time the growth in the endometrium can extend to other parts of the uterus and nearby areas.

It is unclear what causes the cells to grow abnormally or to spread beyond the uterus. On a preliminary basis, the roles of estrogen and progesterone are being closely watched. The research does not say for certain what the impact of these hormones is but rather suggests that prolonged exposure to estrogen alone, as in estrogen replacement therapy (ERT) instead of hormone replacement therapy (HRT), may be a factor in the development of endometrial cancer and that progestins act to protect you from it. Research on endometrial cancer is at a very early stage, with scientists just beginning to look at possible causal factors in its development.

Since most women who have endometrial cancer are over sixty, researchers have assumed that it is a slow-growing cancer. Given the historical dearth of research on women over sixty, new definitive studies are expected to answer some of the basic questions related to this disease by 2010.

Sarcoma, found in only 5 percent of cases of uterine cancer, begins in the walls of the uterus, in the smooth muscles. Over time a sarcoma may spread and reach the endometrial layer of the uterus. Very little is known about sarcomas.

Diagnosis

There is no test for early detection of uterine cancer. Ultrasound and biopsy of the uterus are used for early detection of uterine cancer. Uterine cancer occurs most frequently in women between the ages of fifty-five and seventy.

The pattern for at-risk women is inconsistent. What is known is that there is greater risk for women who are obese, have few or no children, began menstruation at an early age, and/or begin menopause late. The higher-risk group also includes women of higher income and education. The amount of risk that each of these factors contributes cannot be accurately predicted.

Additional Facts about Uterine Cancer

In endometrial cancer, treatment or combinations of treatment will be determined by your health care provider depending on the stage of the cancer.

Stage I	Tumor limited to the endometrium; five-year survival rate between 64 and 95 percent.
Stage II	Tumor involves cervix.
Stage III	Tumor spread throughout pelvic area.
Stage IV	Tumor spread to bladder or rectum or more distant organs such as the lungs or liver.

Surgery usually involves a hysterectomy (see Chapter 6).

Ovarian Cancer

What makes ovarian cancer a particularly difficult disease is that the symptoms are vague or even nonexistent in the early stages. Therefore, ovarian cancer is usually detected in the more advanced stages when it is more difficult to treat. For this reason, ovarian cancer is the leading cause of gynecological cancer death for women in the United States. Each year an estimated 23,000 new cases of ovarian cancer are diagnosed. In 1996 nearly 15,000 women died from this disease. This means that 1 in 58 women will get ovarian cancer in their lifetime. Although the cases we read about in the popular press involve younger women, ovarian cancer is usually found in postmenopausal women in their sixties.

While there are risk factors associated with ovarian cancer, it is important to remember that the majority of women who get ovarian cancer do not have the risk factors. Women at higher risk for ovarian cancer include those who have not borne any children and those who gave birth after age thirty. There is increased risk when there is a family history of ovarian cancer, breast-ovarian cancer syndrome, or hereditary nonpolyposis colorectal cancer. A personal history of cancer or a diagnosis of breast cancer is also considered a risk factor.

On the other hand, it seems that women who have been pregnant, those who breastfeed, and those who use birth control pills are less likely to get the disease. Unfortunately, the links between these factors and the disease are hard to decipher.

Diagnosis

The symptoms of the early stages of ovarian cancer are difficult to recognize and are thus often ignored. These symptoms include digestive complaints and some discomfort in the lower abdomen. Moreover, there is no accurate way of diagnosing ovarian cancer in the early stages.

Much has been written about a blood test known as CA-125. This is a test for a tumor marker (CA-125) that is found where there are ovarian cancer cells. Unfortunately, CA-125 lacks reliability as a marker and so is not that good as a screening test. Not only has CA-125 been found in women who have benign ovarian conditions, it has also not been found in cases of ovarian cancer.

Needless to say, screening techniques for ovarian cancer must be greatly improved. The lack of accurate screening procedures results in most diagnoses occurring after cancer cells have spread to the abdomen, colon, diaphragm, and stomach.

Although there are several types of ovarian cancer, the most common kinds occur in the lining of the ovary and are called epithelial carcinomas. Other types of ovarian cancer are very rare.

If ovarian cancer is suspected, a more exacting screening technique is transvaginal ultrasound. The use of ultrasound (in which high-frequency sound waves bounce off internal organs, creating images) can tell you if there is a mass present in the ovary. Understanding exactly what this mass is can only be accomplished through laparotomy or abdominal surgery.

During the laparotomy, a small piece of tissue is taken from the ovary. If cancer is found, the entire ovary is removed. During the laparotomy, some lymph nodes may also be removed, as well as some fluid from the abdomen. All these samples of tissue and fluid are essential to determining the stage of the cancer. Determining the stage is key to appropriate treatment.

Additional Facts about Ovarian Cancer

There are four stages of tumor progression:

Stage I — Disease is located inside one or both ovaries. The five-year survival rate (i.e., are alive five years after treatment) is 95 percent.

Stage II — Disease is located in ovaries and

	nearby pelvic structures. The five-year survival rate is 79 percent.
Stage III	Disease is located in ovaries, pelvic structures, and in mid- or upper abdomen. The five-year survival rate is 28 percent.
Stage IV	Disease is located in ovaries, pelvic structures, abdomen, and other parts of the body. About 10 percent of women have a five-year survival rate.

Because of the lack of early diagnostic screening techniques, 60 percent of women diagnosed with ovarian cancer are already in stage III or IV. Approximately 70 percent of women who are diagnosed with stage III or IV disease will relapse with tumors after apparently complete removal of their presenting tumor. To try to improve survival rates, women with stage III or IV disease are usually given chemotherapy after surgical removal of as much disease as possible.

Pancreatic Cancer

Very little is known about this type of cancer. The pancreas, which has two major components, the exocrine and endocrine glands, is about 6 inches long and is located behind the stomach. The exocrine area is responsible for helping you digest food, and the endocrine area produces hormones (like insulin) that help the body store and use food. About 95 percent of pancreatic cancers start in the exocrine area.

Diagnosis

Early detection of pancreatic cancer is nearly impossible because by the time it begins to cause symptoms like pain or signs like jaundice, it has usually spread way beyond the borders of the pancreas into the neighboring tissues and organs. You should see your health care provider when you have any of the following symptoms: nausea, loss of appetite, unintentional weight loss, pain in your upper or middle abdomen, or yellowing of your skin (jaundice).

Definitive diagnosis may involve a variety of procedures, including imaging techniques (CT or MRI) and endoscopic retrograde cholangiopancreatography (ERCP). In ERCP you are sedated as a flexible tube is inserted down your throat, through your stomach, and into your small intestine. As your physician looks through the tube, a dye is injected to see where it travels. Using the same tube, the physician can insert a fine needle into the pancreas to remove cells for biopsy.

Additional Facts about Pancreatic Cancer

Stage I	Cancer is found only in the pancreas or has started to spread just to the tissues next to the pancreas, such as the small intestine, or the bile duct.
Stage II	Cancer extends directly into the stomach, spleen, colon or surrounding large blood vessels.
Stage III	Cancer has spread to the regional lymph nodes.
Stage IV	Cancer has spread to areas farther from the pancreas such as the liver or lungs.
Recurrent	After surgery, the cancer has reappeared in the pancreatic area or another part of the body.

Different surgical procedures are available to remove the tumor and most of the areas surrounding the pancreas, but they often fail because the tumor has spread beyond the reach of the surgery.

According to the National Cancer Institute, "Most patients with cancer of the pancreas are not cured with standard therapy and some standard treatments may have more side effects than are desired. . . . Clinical trials are going on in most parts of the country for all stages of pancreatic cancer." There is new research into the possibility of biological therapy as a treatment for pancreatic cancer.

To get more information about clinical trials, call (800) 4-CANCER.

Mind

Sonia knew that she felt something in there. Her left breast was unusually tender, and something felt like the edge of a table. Maybe it would go away on its own.

She began to think about what it would mean if that lump were really something. How could she go on? She wasn't a particularly attractive woman, and she knew that she would be disfigured if it did turn out to be something. She couldn't bring herself to think the thought of what it might be.

How would Alfonso see her? How would she be able to go to the dressing rooms in the stores?—some of them did not have curtains. In the summer she never particularly liked getting into a bathing suit. But now if this were really something . . . No, it was better to hope that it would just go away.

As Latinas, perhaps the hardest thing is the belief that cancer is a death sentence. We need to focus on all the evidence that in many instances there is treatment and possible cure.

Because our self-esteem may be challenged by the changes brought about by the surgery or treatment we undergo, the support system we establish will be vital to our recovery. Partners who truly love us will continue to be supportive and affectionate during and after our treatment. These partners will experience our stress as we go through this difficult part of our lives. Those of us without partners will continue to have the support of our family and friends.

Some Latinas may find that a support group is a critical part of their support network. Many of the organizations listed in the resource section have organized groups of women to share each others' experiences and support each other throughout the process of treatment and recovery. These types of groups have a positive effect on survival as the members share with each other all that they have learned.

Your mind-set about treatment is very important. Researchers do not understand why, but there is clear evidence that a positive attitude is beneficial to all involved.

Most of us struggle throughout our lives trying to balance our feelings with realities. It is important to remember that we are more than our physical bodies—we are the totality of our experiences and relationships.

Susanna had known that she could not have children. She had told all her friends because, in her mind, she knew it was OK not to have children, that there were other things in her life. She had nieces and nephews and lots of cousins that she cared for.

And yet Susanna knew that for many years she had hoped and prayed that at the right moment something magical would happen. If God willed it, well, perhaps she would become pregnant.

But now she had to have this hysterectomy. She knew that any hope she had nurtured about bearing her own child would soon be gone. Whatever fantasies she had sustained that perhaps a miracle would happen were to be put aside forever. It was one thing to be infertile because her reproductive organs were not working—but it was another to have her organs removed.

Her secret hope of having a child could never become a reality now.

Spirit

Cancer scares us and makes us feel vulnerable. We feel violated, as if something has reached in and destroyed our very core. We may try to understand why we have been singled out. We may be forced to face our beliefs about death and dying.

At these times, even with the support of our friends and our health care providers we need to go deep inside ourselves and respond to our souls crying out. We may be afraid of what is in store for us in this life. We must allow ourselves to mourn our losses. We must let ourselves cry and also rejoice for the inner strength and resources of being a Latina—that is what keeps us going forward with *life*.

As Latinas, we know only too well that faith and prayer can sustain us in our loneliest moments. Sometimes, when the decisions we have to make are overwhelming and we are scared, we must turn to our innermost voices and listen.

If we have cancer, we may have a tendency to blame ourselves for some past failing. We may think that perhaps this is a cross that God has given us to carry. Yet, if you believe in a loving God, you know that cancer is just another part of the human condition. Within the concept of redemption is the belief in treatment and cure. So be hopeful and positive.

You must focus on the idea that God gave us brains so that we could solve our problems. Treatment, care, and aftercare are all part of the gifts we can give to each other. Empower yourself through prayer and knowledge. As Latinas, we know that they will take us a long way.

Summary

To most Latinas, just the mention of cancer is enough to scare them away from the conversation. Yet talking about the realities of cancer informs us of the facts. Although Latinas used to have low rates of cancer, we now have increasing rates of various types of cancer. Breast, colon, lung, cervical, uterine, ovarian, and pancreatic cancers are of major concern to Latinas.

The important message is that if we do not smoke, carefully monitor our own health, and have our health care provider conduct the appropriate annual exams, we will position ourselves well in the struggle against cancer. All the evidence makes it clear that the earlier the diagnosis, the better results we get from treatment.

Remember—with early detection and treatment, the chance for extended survival and even a cure is excellent.

RESOURCES

General

Organizations

American Association of Retired Persons
601 E Street NW
Washington, DC 20049
(800) 424-3410 or (202) 434-2277
www.aarp.org

American Cancer Society
1599 Clifton Road NE
Atlanta, GA 30329
(800) ACS-2345 (800-227-2345)
www.cancer.org

Make Today Count, Inc.
MACC (Mid America Cancer Center)
1235 E. Cherokee
Springfield, MO 65804
(417) 885-2588
(national support and self-help network)

National Cancer Institute
Cancer Information Service
Building 31, Room 10A-03
31 Center Dr. MSC 2580
Bethesda, MD 20892-2580
(800) 4CANCER (800-422-6237)
CancerFax: (301) 402-5874; (800) 624-2511
(for assistance in using CancerFax)
CancerNet: cancernet.nci.nih.gov

National Coalition for Cancer Survivorship
1010 Wayne Avenue, Suite 770
Silver Spring, MD 20910
(877) 622-7937
www.cansearch.org

National Institutes of Health Clinical Center
Recruitment and Referral Center
Warren Grant Magnusen Center
NIH
Bethesda, MD 20892-2655
(800) 411-1222
www.cc.nih.gov

National Women's Health Network and Women's Health Network Clearinghouse
514 10th Street NW, Suite 400
Washington, DC 20004
(202) 347-1140
www.womenshealthnetwork.org

Hotlines

American Cancer Society
(800) 227-2345

National Cancer Institute
(800) 4-CANCER (800-422-6237)

Books

Cook, Alan R., and Peter D. Dresser, eds. *Cancer Sourcebook for Women.* Detroit: Omnigraphics, 1996.

BREAST CANCER

Organizations

(Also see American Cancer Society and National Cancer Institute listed above.)

Breast Cancer Resource Committee
2005 Belmont St. NW
Washington, DC 20009
(202) 463-8040
www.afamerica.com/bcrc

LatinaSHARE
1501 Broadway, Suite 1720
New York, NY 10036
(212) 719-4454 (Spanish)
(212) 382-2111
www.sharecancersupport.org/latina.html

Look Good . . . Feel Better Cancer Program
1101 17th Street NW, Suite 300
Washington, DC 20036
(800) 395-LOOK (800-395-5665) or (202) 331-1770

My Image After Breast Cancer
6000 Stevenson Avenue, Suite 203
Alexandria, VA 22304
(703) 461-9595

National Alliance of Breast Cancer Organizations
9 E. 37th Street, 10th Floor
New York, NY 10016
(212) 719-0754 or (888) 80-NABCO (806-2226)
www.nabco.org

National Breast Cancer Coalition
1707 L Street NW, Suite 1060
Washington, DC 20036
(202) 296-7477
www.natlbcc.org

National Alliance for Hispanic Health
1501 16th Street NW
Washington, DC 20036-1401
(202) 387-5000
www.hispanichealth.org

Susan G. Komen Breast Cancer Foundation
5005 LBJ Freeway, Suite 370
Dallas, TX 75244
(972) 855-1600
www.komen.org

Y-ME National Breast Cancer Organization
212 West Van Buren
Chicago, IL 60607
(312) 986-8228 or (800) 221-2141
www.yme.org

YWCA Encore Plus Program
Office of Women's Health Initiatives
624 9th Street NW, 3rd floor
Washington, DC 20001-5305
(202) 628-3636 or (800) 95-EPLUS
www.ywcaencore.org

Hotlines

My Image After Breast Cancer 24-Hour HOPEline
(800) 970-4411 or (703) 461-9616

Su-Familia Family Health Helpline
National Alliance for Hispanic Health
866-SuFamilia (783-2645)

Y-ME National Breast Cancer Organization 24-Hour Hotline
(800) 986-2505 (Spanish) or
(800) 221-2141 (English)

Books

American Cancer Society. "A Breast Cancer Journey: Your Personal Guidebook," 2001. Atlanta, GA. American Cancer Society.

Kahane, Deborah Hobler. *No Less a Woman: Femininity, Sexuality, and Breast Cancer.* 2d rev. ed. Alameda, CA: Hunter House, 1995.

Komarnicky, Lydia, and Anne Rosenberg, with Martin Betancourt. *What to Do If You Get Breast Cancer: Two Breast Cancer Specialists Help You Take Charge and Make Informed Choices*. Boston: Little, Brown, 1995.

LaTour, Kathy. *The Breast Cancer Companion*. New York: Avon, 1994.

Love, Susan M., and Karen Lindsey. *Dr. Susan Love's Breast Book*. 2d ed. New York: Addison-Wesley, 1995.

Pressman, Peter, and Yashar Hirshaut. *Breast Cancer: The Complete Guide*. New York: Bantam Doubleday Dell, 1993.

Robinson, Rebecca Y., and Jeanne A. Petrek. *A Step-by-Step Guide to Dealing with Your Breast Cancer*. Secaucus, NJ: Carol Publishing, 1994.

Swirsky, Joan, and Barbara Balaban. *The Breast Cancer Handbook*. New York: HarperCollins, 1994.

Publications and Pamphlets

"Breast and Cervical Cancer Resource Kit." Guide for early detection of breast and cervical cancer among Hispanic women. 1997 National Alliance for Hispanic Health, 1501 16th Street NW, Washington, DC 20036; (202) 387-5000.

"Breast Cancer: Information and Support." General information on breast cancer treatment for women. Y-Me National Breast Cancer Organization, 212 West Van Buren, Chicago, IL 60607; (800) 221-2141 (English) or (800) 986-9505 (Spanish). Other titles include:

"Cuando la Mujer Que Tu Amas Tiene Cáncer Del Seno." Spanish language information on how to obtain treatment for breast cancer.

"For Single Women with Breast Cancer," 2000. Information on breast cancer treatment for single women. Available in Spanish.

"Just for Teens! The Teen Guide for Breast Care." Teen Guide on how to monitor breast cancer.

"When the Woman You Love Has Breast Cancer." Guide for those who know someone suffering from breast cancer.

"A Woman's Guide for Breast Care." General information on breast cancer treatment for women. Available in Spanish.

"Breast Cancer Fact Sheet." U.S. Public Health Service Office on Women's Health,

Dept. of Health and Human Services, 200 Independence Avenue SW, Room 730-B, Washington, DC 20201; (202) 690-7650.

"Preguntas y respuestas sobre el cáncer del seno." Pamphlet No. 4595-PS. American Cancer Society, 1599 Clifton Road NE, Atlanta, GA 30329; (800) ACS-2345 (800-227-2345) or 404-320-3333; www.cancer.org. Other publications (all available in Spanish) include:

"How to do Breast Self-Examination" (Pamphlet No. 2674)

"Mammography: What Every Woman Needs to Know" (Pamphlet No. 5024)

"Cancer Facts for Women" (Pamphlet No. 2623).

"Preguntas Para Hacerle a Su Médico Sobre el Cáncer del Seno," May 1993. Spanish language information on breast cancer. National Cancer Institute Cancer Information Service; (800) 422-6237. Other titles include "What You Need to Know about Breast Cancer," July 1993.

Cervical and Uterine Cancer

Organizations

(Also see American Cancer Society and National Cancer Institute listed above.)

LatinaSHARE
1501 Broadway, Suite 1720
New York, NY 10036
(212) 719-4454 (Spanish)
www.sharecancersupport.org/latina

National Alliance for Hispanic Health
1501 16th Street NW
Washington, DC 20036
(202) 387-5000
www.hispanichealth.org

YWCA Encore Program
Office of Women's Health Initiatives
624 9th Street NW
Washington, DC 20001
(202) 626-0700 or (800) 953-7587
www.ywca.org

Publications and Pamphlets

"Preventing Cancer," Sept. 2000. American College of Obstetricians and Gynecologists; (800) 762-2264. Other titles include:

"Disorders of the Cervix," Sept. 2000.

"Uterine Fibroids," Mar. 2000.

"Pap Smears," 1999. Pamphlet No. 1539. AAFP Family Health Facts series. American Academy of Family Physicians; 11400 Tomahawk Creek Pkwy, Leawood, KS 66211-2672; (800) 944-0000.

"Cancer Facts for Women." (Pamphlet No. 2623), 1998. American Cancer Society, 1599 Clifton Road NE, Atlanta, GA 30329; (800) ACS-2345 (800-227-2345) or (404) 320-3333.

"La Prueba Pap: Un Método para Diagnosticar el Cáncer del Cuello del Utero," January 1993. National Cancer Institute Cancer Information Service, Building 31, Room 10A-21, 9000 Rockville Pike, Bethesda, MD 20892-3100; (800) 4CANCER (800-422-6237). Other titles include:

"What You Need to Know about Cervical Cancer." Pamphlet No. 95-2047.

"What You Need to Know about Cancer of the Uterus," 1997. Pamphlet No. 93-1562.

Colorectal Cancer

Organizations

(Also see American Cancer Society and National Cancer Institute listed above.)

United Ostomy Association
199772 McArthur Blvd., Suite 200
Irvine, CA 92612
(800) 826-6826
www.uoa.org

Lung Cancer

Organizations

(Also see American Cancer Society and National Cancer Institute listed above.)

American Lung Association
1740 Broadway
New York, NY 10019
(212) 315-8700
www.lungusa.org

Ovarian Cancer

Publications and Pamphlets

"Cancer of the Ovary," January 1992. American College of Obstetricians and Gynecologists; (800) 762-2264. www.acog.org. Other titles include "Ovarian Cysts," June 1993.

"Cancer Facts for Women." (Pamphlet No. 2623), 1998. American Cancer Society, 1599 Clifton Road NE, Atlanta, GA 30329; (800) ACS-2345 (800-227-2345).

"What You Need to Know about Ovarian Cancer," 2000. Pamphlet No. 94-1561. National Cancer Institute Cancer Information Service, Building 31, Room 10A-21, 9000 Rockville Pike, Bethesda, MD 20892; (800) 4-CANCER (800-422-6237).

13

Depression

More Than Being Blue

Sonia and Anita had been close friends for years. They talked to each other about every aspect of their lives. They enjoyed giving each other support through all the happy and tragic events that marked their days.

During the last few months, however, Sonia had sensed that something was different. Now each time she called, she felt that Anita was finding it hard to talk to her.

Before there had always been the comfort of long talks in which they shared the dreams they had and recognized the dreams they knew would never come true. For years Sonia had listened to Anita comment on the ups and downs of her relationship with Alfredo. It seemed that Alfredo never had time for Anita. He was always working. What passion once punctuated their lives had become little more than a passing footnote.

Sonia had heard all this for years, but now it sounded different. Now when she spoke with Anita she would hear Anita cry. Anita would tell her how worthless she felt. Here she was with most of her life behind her and very little to show. It was getting too much to bear.

When Sonia saw Anita, she was stunned at what she saw. Anita did not look like herself. Sonia asked Anita if she had been trying to lose weight. Anita said no, she just did not want to eat. To make matters worse, she had found lately that she could not even get a good night's sleep. Anita confided that she had been waking up in the early morning hours. She would lie next to Alfredo and quietly weep.

Anita had not wanted to bother Sonia with all of this because she knew that this sadness would pass. But Sonia knew this was more than their usual exchange of lamentations. She was afraid that there was something very wrong with Anita. And she did not know what to do.

Depression is an illness. It is not something that is "all in our mind" or something that we "get over." And for those Latinas who are clinically depressed, the stigmatization that too often accompanies the diagnosis makes it difficult to acknowledge the condition or seek treatment.

What we know from every existing data system is that Latinas are more likely than other women to suffer from depression. Thus it was not surprising that when the Commonwealth Fund conducted its nationwide survey on women's health, over one-half of the Latinas reported that they suffered from severe depression. Tragically, and for unknown reasons, Latinas are also the group least likely to use mental health services.

The situation is worse for young Latinas. Latina teenagers have higher rates of attempted suicide than any other group of teenagers—19.7 percent have made at least one suicide attempt, compared to 11.2 percent for African-Americans and 11.3 percent for non-Hispanic white female teenagers. These numbers support what we find when each of us looks within our hearts and spirits. Depression is not new for us. It is a natural by-product of *aguantar*. For some of us, *aguantando* is how we stay in relationships or marriages that are considerably less than satisfactory.

In 1999 UCLA researchers documented that men and women have different responses to stress. The tendency towards "fight or flight" that had been assumed to describe everyone seemed to apply mostly to men. Women experiencing stress were more likely to "tend or befriend," i.e, focus on children or seek the company of other supportive females.

In recent focus groups, Latinas were asked if, given a million dollars, would they stay with their spouses. The overwhelming majority of women said no. One Latina qualified her response by saying that she would leave her husband but would give him half the money because he had been a good father.

What is compelling is that these women had made the choice to stay with their spouses because they felt that they had limited options. They stated it very clearly—they were *aguantando*. As the primary caretakers in their families, they knew that they had to be strong and endure for the sake of everyone but themselves. From childhood, we all learn to put everyone in the family ahead of whatever needs *we* may have. Many women report that even when they know there are other options, they feel incapable of changing the circumstances that are contributing to their depression. These fears that keep us frozen in a bad situation are too often fueled by our low self-esteem, which suffocates whatever desire we have to make a change.

As Latinas, our depression can look different from that of other women because we have developed coping skills encouraged by our cultural values, which mask the depth of our despair. Moreover, the relationships that define us are very often at the core of our inability to take control of our lives. Afraid of the risks involved in changing our lives, and not acknowledging how our most important and intimate relationships contribute to our feelings of despair, we close our minds, silence our hearts, and pray that our obedience to God or our sense of spirit will sustain us. But faith demands more than obedience—it requires that we honestly confront our feelings and fears. Until we are able to do this, our despair only worsens. As time passes and we can no longer cope with the cries of our innermost voices, we begin sleepwalking through our daily activities in a last desperate attempt to ignore what we feel.

What were once pleasurable activities become no more stimulating than anesthesia traveling through our veins. We allow ourselves to feel nothing because to feel would be too painful. Sex becomes not the lovemaking that is a source of joy and pleasure but something we do out of obligation. The result is depression, which is fed by our inability to see that no matter how hopeless we might feel, the reality is that we can create new opportunities for ourselves and our loved ones. It is our depression that keeps us where we are and makes us feel that we have nowhere to go.

We can overcome this hopelessness. There is hope, and we are not helpless. Fortunately, of all the mental illnesses, depression has the highest rate of successful treatment. The first hurdle in our recovery is to recognize when we are depressed and to begin to take the steps necessary to overcome it.

How Do We Know When We Are Depressed?

Sadness is one color in the palette of life. Sometimes we feel sad or blue, or we feel as though nobody loves us. We may not like the way it feels to be sad, but it is part of being human. It is important to understand that it is OK and even normal to feel sad—for a little while. But sometimes we feel sad for more than a little while, with the result that we are unable to perform our day-to-day activities. At those times we may be depressed.

Remember that depression is different from just being unhappy or sad. We suffer from depression when the color of sadness takes over the canvas of our lives with its darkness and leaves room for no color or light to enter. Depression permeates every part of our life and leaves no thought or feeling untouched. It affects how well our bodies function, how we feel about ourselves, our relationships, and our work. Depression touches our spirit and makes us feel that there is no hope of life getting better.

For some of us, depression may occur only once, during a particularly difficult period in our lives. For others it may recur several times.

As Latinas, we need to fully understand how the symptoms of depression affect our body, mind, and spirit. The symptoms need to be meaningful for us within the boundaries of the lives we lead. The following are the basic symptoms of depression.

Consejos

Symptoms of Depression

BODY

- Sleeping too much or too little or waking excessively early in the morning
- Appetite and/or weight loss or excessive overeating and weight gain
- Decreased energy over an extended period of time, including complaints of fatigue, feeling "slowed down"
- Persistent physical symptoms that do not respond to treatment, such as headaches, digestive disorders, and chronic pain

MIND

- Persistent sad, anxious, or "empty" moods
- Loss of interest or pleasure in activities, including sex
- Thoughts of death or suicide or suicide attempts
- Restlessness, irritability
- Difficulty concentrating, remembering, or making decisions

SPIRIT

- Feelings of hopelessness, pessimism
- Feelings of guilt, worthlessness, helplessness

Body

• **Sleeping too much or too little or waking excessively early.** We know how much we need to sleep in order to feel good. Some of us feel rested with six hours of sleep, but others need eight solid hours. When we are depressed, our sleep pattern changes. Some of us use sleep as an escape and sleep more than usual in a way that interferes with our lives. Others may experience recurrent insomnia and find that sleep is the escape that eludes us. For some Latinas, one of the clear signs of depression is that they start waking up early in the morning.

• **Appetite and/or weight loss or excessive overeating and weight gain.** A change in how much we eat and the respective change in our weight is another way our bodies signal to us when we are depressed. One Latina was so depressed that she did not notice she had eaten an entire box of chocolate truffles—and she did not particularly like chocolate. Another Latina who had always tried to maintain her weight knew that something was wrong when in addition to some of the other symptoms she noticed that she had lost 13 pounds without even trying. When you see yourself or your friends experiencing unintended weight loss or gain, it is important to consider depression as a possible factor.

• **Decreased energy, fatigue, feeling "slowed down."** When such statements as "*Me siento sin ánimo*" (I feel dispirited), "*Tengo fatiga*" (I am fatigued), and "*Estoy muy cansada*" (I am very tired) become a customary part of our conversation with a friend or loved one, it may indicate a problem that needs more serious attention. It is natural to feel tired some of the time, but when this reduction in energy is constant and debilitating, we need to look deeper for the root of the problem.

• **Persistent physical symptoms that do not respond to treatment, such as headaches, digestive disorders, and chronic pain.** Sometimes we do not allow ourselves to experience emotional or spiritual pain, and thus our bodies become the host for all of our concerns. The mental turmoil we try to ignore demands attention by bubbling out in other ways.

Mind

• **Persistent sad, anxious, or "empty" moods.** A depressed Latina is not necessarily sad all the time. More commonly the depressed person finds that her mood has undergone a change and that she suddenly feels overcome with recurrent feelings of anxiety or the tendency to worry excessively over things she cannot control. Often Latinas who are depressed describe a loss of feelings as one of the symptoms they experience. It is important to notice any radical changes in mood and outlook when determining whether you or a loved one is depressed. We do not have to be sad every day of our lives to be depressed. What we have to recognize is the change in our mood, so that we know when there is a change or we find that we are always sad. For some of us, the change may be one of feeling anxious. For others, while we may have usually felt happy or sad, we feel nothing now. Sometimes it is the absence of feeling which we can recognize as one of the symptoms of depression.

• **Loss of interest or pleasure in activities, including sex.** Sometimes the activities that once gave us pleasure no longer make us smile. At these times we might feel inconsolable because even the activities and people we once treasured now seem meaningless. We may find ourselves merely going through the motions of working, playing with our children, even having sex with our partner.

• **Thoughts of death or suicide or suicide attempts.** If you or a friend have thoughts of suicide, you should talk to a mental health professional. Although only 15 percent of persons who are depressed commit suicide, thoughts of suicide are one of the most common symptoms associated with depression. Some researchers have suggested that Latinas with a strong Catholic background are less likely to consider suicide because of the religious taboo. When you have a depressive disorder, however, you are less likely to make rational judgments. As a result, over half of suicides are committed by persons who have a depressive disorder.

• **Restlessness, irritability.** Even women who are typically calm and easygoing may find themselves becoming restless as their negative feelings increase. Small irritations or annoyances that we might have overlooked or even laughed at before suddenly seem unbearably frustrating and another indication of our displeasure with our lives.

• **Difficulty concentrating, remembering, or making decisions.** Depression can lessen our ability to remember or make choices, and thus the depressed person can find it difficult to focus on routine tasks. A depressed person may once have been very decisive, but as the depression deepens she can become incapable of acting or even recalling what she intended to do.

Spirit

• **Feelings of hopelessness, pessimism.** There are moments when each one of us feels that there is no way a difficult aspect of our life will get better. What sets clinical depression apart from the daily ups and downs of life is that these moments begin to occur more frequently and become a constant part of our lives. This constant sense of hopelessness is reinforced by the inability to do what were previously routine tasks.

• **Feelings of guilt, worthlessness, helplessness.** As Latinas, we often define ourselves by our relationships with others. Thus at times we may have difficulty realizing that we are valuable in our own right. Our feelings of worthlessness and helplessness may be exacerbated by the reality that we have not allowed ourselves to be individuals.

Types of Clinical Depression

We have all had some of these symptoms at some time in our lives, yet we may not have considered ourselves to be depressed. Most persons who are diagnosed with depression have at least five of these symptoms for an extended period of time. Indeed, as explained above, clinical depression is not a matter of temporary sadness or malaise. Rather, it is a condition in which the symptoms last so long that they interfere with our lives. Moreover, the types of clinical depression (described below) are not necessarily mutually exclusive. For example, a woman may be diagnosed with dysthymia and also experience episodes of major depression at different points in her life. Consequently it is difficult to state in absolute terms how common each type of depression is. What we do know is that major depression is relatively the most common and that manic-depressive illness is the least common.

Major Depression

I am so tired of everything. I do not want to live anymore. I am getting my life in order because I do not want to leave my things a mess. I know I have a friend who can take care of my cat.

I go to work and do my job. Nobody knows what I am going through. It is easy for me to do my job because I have been doing it for so long I do not have to think about it. I go in. I push papers around my desk and make a few phone calls.

These days I am not even hungry. This is the first time in my life I have lost weight without even trying. My clothes seem to be getting bigger, and I am getting smaller. It really doesn't matter. Nothing matters.

I go home and weep. No one listens and no one cares. I just want to die.

—*Evelyn, 45*

Major depression (also called unipolar disorder) is defined as having at least five of the symptoms listed above for at least two weeks and as a result being unable to be productive in daily life. Sometimes, such as when you are in mourning, you may show all the signs of major depression, but you will not be initially treated for it. If after several months your mood does not change, however, it may indicate that you are now having a major depressive episode.

Recently we have recognized that some women suffer from a special type of major depression—seasonal affective disorder (SAD). SAD occurs in fall and winter, with symptoms being alleviated in the spring. The typical symptoms of SAD are an increase in hours of sleeping and eating, as well as withdrawal from social activities. To be diagnosed with SAD, a woman usually has to experience this shift in two out of three consecutive years. SAD is believed to be related to the seasonal decrease in sunlight. Exposure to a fluorescent light without ultraviolet rays (i.e., light therapy) has been shown to be effective in the treatment of many cases of SAD.

Additionally, some women experience a change in mood after giving birth (postpartum depression). Postpartum depression is due to a combination of changes that occur after childbirth, which include alterations in hormonal levels, the need to adapt to new responsibilities, and reduced sleep as a result of caring for the infant.

Dysthymia

I cannot remember any truly happy moments of my life. There were nice things, I am sure, but in fact I cannot remember them. I actually do not remember most of my childhood. But those are just memories—or the lack of them. Whatever.

Sure there are times when I sleep too much. And sometimes I eat too much. But all this passes. I am just not a happy person. I do not even know what that would be like.

—*Millie, 28*

Dysthymia has the same symptoms as major depression. The difference is that the symptoms are milder but last longer. For example, while you may be able to work, you may be unable to perform at your optimal level. Usually dysthymia lasts at least two years.

Manic-Depressive Illness

When I would become manic it always seemed that there was so much to do and that I had this surge of drive that came out of nowhere. I felt I could do anything and everything. I ran around the office telling people what to do. Sometimes I would go on a shopping spree even though I knew my credit cards were at their limit. My energy seemed boundless.

Now I realize that all I ended up doing was alienating my coworkers and getting myself further in debt. I wish that when I was in a manic phase I could have been more constructive. I have learned that while I felt as if I was moving mountains, in fact all I usually did was make a mess.

—*Elena, 31*

In manic-depressive illness (also called bipolar disorder), the symptoms of depression alternate with the agitation and energy surges (mania) of manic episodes. It is important to note that major depression and dysthymia occur more commonly in women, while manic-depressive illness occurs equally in men and women. Persons in a manic phase are not very productive. They do a lot of things fast but do not accomplish any of their goals.

MYTHS AND FACTS

Myth: If I am depressed I can just shake it off.

Fact: Clinical depression is a serious illness that cannot just be shaken off, but with the proper combination of psychotherapy and medication, depression can be overcome.

Myth: There are pills that can cure depression.

Fact: While there have been great advances in the development of effective medication, the complexity of factors that create and maintain depression make it unlikely that any single medication alone will result in a long-term cure.

Myth: It is OK to feel sad all of the time.

Fact: Even though your life may be difficult, feeling sad all the time should not be acceptable. If you do, you should seek treatment.

Myth: This is not depression. I just went through a difficult divorce.

Fact: For each individual, depression is due to a combination of genetic, biochemical, social, and environmental factors. The causal factors are not what determine whether you are depressed. Depression is defined functionally (by how well you can perform your day-to-day tasks), physically (by changes in your eating and sleeping habits), and emotionally (by feelings of sadness or worthlessness). The length of time that you have a combination of these symptoms determines whether you are depressed.

Myth: All persons who are suicidal are depressed.

Fact: Not all persons who are suicidal are depressed.

Causes of Depression

It would be much easier to treat depression if there were just one factor that determined whether people became depressed. However, there are at least three major factors. Additionally, the combination of factors and the contribution made by each factor to the depressive episode vary with each individual. Thus for each depressed person, the cause and consequently the treatment will be different. The three major factors are genetics, biochemistry, and environment.

Genetics

Genetic research tries to identify two major things: whether depression can be inherited and whether there are genetic defects that are linked to depression.

With respect to heredity the evidence is not that strong. The research indicates that identical twins (who share all the same genes) are slightly more likely to suffer from bipolar disorder than are fraternal twins (who share only some of the same genes). With respect to the transmission of dysthymia or major depression, the evidence for a genetic factor is weak. This means that in most cases, even when there is a family history of depression, only some members of the family will develop the illness.

Research continues in the attempt to determine whether there are factors in the genes you are born with or factors that make genes mutate over time to change the brain or body chemistry and result in depression.

Biochemistry

Early research into the biochemical basis of psychiatric disorders stemmed from finding that the chemical treatment of certain physical conditions produced changes in the moods of patients. For example, some patients treated for tuberculosis with isoniazid became euphoric. Over time scientists began to understand the relationship between a variety of drugs and the brain.

The National Institutes of Health named

the 1990s the Decade of the Brain. With that mandate, much was done to increase our understanding of how the brain functions. What we have confirmed is that there are different chemicals in our brains that affect our behavior.

Some of these chemicals, called neurotransmitters, are responsible for sending messages from one part of the brain to other parts of the brain. Serotonin and norepinephrine are two key chemicals present in this system. Persons who are depressed, no matter what the causes, have an imbalance of these chemicals in their brains. Some people may become depressed when they have too much serotonin, while others become depressed when they have too little. Depression also seems to go hand in hand with other changes in the body. For example, levels of the hormone cortisol tend to be higher at night for those who are depressed. As a result, the depressed person is unable to experience the most restful stages of sleep. This explains why depressed people report that they are tired even though they may actually sleep more hours than usual.

As of this writing, we do not yet know whether these chemical imbalances are the cause or the result of the depression. What is certain is that when we lack the right balance of these chemicals, which varies by individual, symptoms occur that we define as depression.

Consejos

Just because you have a real reason to be depressed does not mean that you are not clinically depressed.

Too many of us believe that clinical depression is not a real illness, that it is only in your head, and that if you can pinpoint what caused the signs of depression—for example, loss of a relationship, a major unexpected shift in your life—you are not truly depressed. This is not true. While there may be an event that triggers the symptoms of depression, it is the duration of your symptoms that determines whether you are clinically depressed.

Environment

Birth, marriage, divorce, and death are the markers of our lives. These events, as well as violence, financial struggle, and abuse, all produce anxiety. And when the anxiety inherent in any of these events is left unresolved, the result can be depression.

Depression is too common in women. Up to the age of sixty-five, women suffer from depression at twice the rate of men. The picture is worse for Latinas, who report twice as many depressive symptoms as non-Hispanic women. To explain the various environmental factors that might be at work when an individual feels depressed, a host of theories have developed. Some of these are described below.

Everyone knew that Elena was a good daughter, a good wife, and a good worker. All through her life she had done everything for everyone. She often felt pulled in different directions, but all she did was try to meet each of the new demands placed on her days. She knew that there was no way out and no one to help her—her brother could barely manage his own life, and her husband, although a decent man, was not particularly helpful. She did it all herself because she knew that there was no way of escaping her ever-increasing responsibilities. She just accepted it all as part of what life had given her.

By aguantando she had been able to accept all the responsibilities that had landed on her lap.

She was just so tired. She felt so exhausted that even the energy for a smile seemed beyond her, but at the same time she found herself too restless to sleep. She chalked it up to all the things she was worried about. But lately it seemed to Elena that she was having trouble concentrating too. And when she found herself weeping, she felt it was just her frustrations coming out. This was her life, and she just accepted it.

Learned Helplessness

Martin Seligman's research on learned helplessness is often given as the best example of how experiential factors result in depression. In these studies, dogs were put into boxes with two compartments (shuttleboxes) and trained to jump from one compartment to the other when a light came on to avoid receiving an electrical shock. After several trials, the dogs learned to jump as soon as the light went on and thus avoid the shock.

In the next part of the experiment, a barrier, which the dogs could see, was placed to prevent them from jumping out of the compartment when the light went on. At first the dogs tried to jump over the barrier, but after a while, when the light went on, they would not even try to jump out. They would just lie in the boxes and take the pain. Later, when the barrier was once again removed and the dogs could see that it was no longer there, they still would not attempt to jump to escape the shock.

Seligman used the term *learned helplessness* to explain the behavior of the dogs. It was clear that in the beginning, when the barrier was first put up, the dogs had tried all sorts of actions to escape the unpleasant situation, but when it was obvious that no escape was possible, they learned to accept that the shock would come. The bulk of Seligman's career was committed to documenting the evidence of this theory and relating it to human issues of personal control.

For Seligman and many of his colleagues, the extrapolation to humans was straightforward—when there are barriers that we believe are insurmountable, we may learn to believe that we have no alternative but to tolerate unacceptable conditions. Thus people in these situations learn that the only way to survive is to become docile and accept the many barriers that society sets up. And for most people, the helplessness leads to depression.

For women, and especially Latinas, there are obstacles in the workplace, education, and all too often within our relationships, which we feel incapable of changing. Elena's experiences show how learned helplessness may lead to clinical depression.

Psychodynamic Factors

Depression has been defined by some theorists as anger turned inward. The cause of this anger is typically some unresolved conflict from childhood. These conflicts are usually related to difficulties in the parent-child relationship.

A psychodynamic interpretation of Elena's situation would focus on her unresolved, unconscious anger at her family for making her the child who took care of everyone. Rather than confronting the anger, she internalizes it and becomes depressed. Identifying the source of the anger and resolving it in a healthy way are important components of the treatment.

Cognitive-Behavioral Factors

In this view, depression is viewed as a result of a person's unreasonable and often irrational beliefs; for example, "I have to make everybody happy" or "I should always be a good daughter." These thoughts, or cognitions, then produce behaviors, which become self-defeating because we are trying to embody a set of beliefs that can never be fulfilled. Over time we become depressed because we are unable to live the kind of life we have unreasonably constructed.

Thus Elena defines her days as carrying out

> ### *Consejos*
>
> Psychotherapy is more than just talking.
>
> In psychotherapy, patients are asked to discuss various aspects of their lives. As the patient speaks, the psychotherapist listens and takes notes while thinking about the implications of what is being said, analyzing the words used by the patient, restructuring the thoughts in healthy ways, and developing potential intervention strategies. With all this going on in the therapist's head, it is no wonder that a therapist's response to a patient's statements is often, "Hmmm . . ."

those tasks that are required for everyone else but completely forgetting about herself.

Treatment

While it is always helpful to empathize with a loved one who is clearly suffering, your encouragement alone won't cure the depressed individual. Similarly, if you suspect that you are clinically depressed, confiding in a friend or relative is only a temporary salve and ultimately does not address the problem. If you think you are depressed or if you have a friend that you think is depressed, it is important to seek professional treatment. The risk of depression in pregnancy and in the postpartum period is higher than in the non-pregnant state.

Professional treatment typically involves both medication and psychotherapy. Medication may be required to alleviate the biochemical changes that occur with depression, and the psychotherapy helps the patient understand and change the self-defeating behaviors that often occur with depression.

Medication

Very often we wish there were a pill we could take that would make us feel all right. Although there are new, successful treatments for depression, they all take time to be effective, and sometimes you have to change medications several times before finding the one that works best for you. To complicate matters, we do not know all we need to know about women and medications.

What we know about women and medication is limited for two reasons. First, most of the research done to determine whether a drug works excludes women of childbearing age; that is, women between the ages of fifteen and forty-four. Second, most women who suffer from depression are in their childbearing years. What the available research does indicate, however, is that women, and especially Latinas, respond to drugs differently from the general population. For example, Latinas have more side effects from antidepressants and may actually require lower doses.

If medication is prescribed for your depression, it is important that your providers closely monitor how you are reacting to it. In general, the medications and treatments used in pregnancy to treat depression are safe in pregnancy and in the breastfeeding period. It is recommended that you work closely with

> ### *Consejos*
>
> How long will I be on medication?
>
> Most persons who are depressed will be on medication for less than a year; persons with a bipolar disorder will continue to take medication for the rest of their lives. You and your health care provider need to determine how long you will take medication.

your health care provider and undergo medical treatment of depression during this period since the consequences of untreated depression may increase the risk for you and your baby. Keep in mind that there is no single test to determine the exact nature of the biochemical imbalance that accompanies your depression. You should expect to try several different kinds of medication before you find one that works for you, and you may have to wait a few weeks to see whether a medication helps you feel better. If your health care provider decides to change your medication, you may have to go without medication for a few weeks before you are given a new one.

Make sure to enter all the information about how you feel in your health journal (see Appendix B). Much of the decision about whether a particular medication is effective for you is based on what you tell your provider.

Medications are usually sold as generic or nongeneric/brand (see Chapter 22 for a discussion of brand versus generic medicines). As with any medication, it is important to be aware of possible adverse interactions with other medicines you are taking. This is especially true when you are taking monoamine oxidase (MAO) inhibitors (see item 3 below).

The medication prescribed for you will be selected based on what your health care provider believes may be most beneficial for you. Following are the four main types of medications given for depression and bipolar disorders.

1: Selective serotonin reuptake inhibitors (SSRIs) are the latest addition to the chemical treatment of depression. These drugs make more serotonin available by preventing its destruction (reuptake). Prozac (fluoxetine) is the most well-known drug in this class. There are several others that are newer and are claimed to have more positive effects while reducing adverse reactions. These include paroxetine (Paxil), sertaline (Zoloft), venlafaxine (Effexor), and fluvoxamine (Luvox). Additionally, Venlafaxine (Effexor) and nefazodone (Serzone) have an effect on serotonin and norepinephrine.

2: Tricyclic antidepressants increase the availability of neurotransmitters, such as norepinephrine. They include amitriptyline (Elavil, Endep), amoxapine (Asendin), desipramine (Norpramin, Pertofrane), imipramine (Tofranil), and nortriptyline (Aventyl, Pamelor).

3: Monoamine oxidase (MAO) inhibitors also increase the availability of neurotransmitters, but they must be closely monitored because they may cause serious interactions with other drugs (prescription as well as over-the-counter substances) and require dietary restrictions. These medications are often successful with persons whose symptoms of depression are an increase in eating and hours of sleeping. These medications include isocarboxazid (Marplan), phenelzine (Nardil), and tranylcypromine (Parnate).

4: Lithium inhibits the release of certain neurotransmitters. This medication is most likely to be given to persons with bipolar disorder. For manic-depressives, the need for ongoing treatment with lithium is lifelong.

Finally, when other medications are not successful, medicines such as buproprion (Wellbutrin), maprotiline (Ludiomil), and trazodone (Desyrel) are also used to treat depression because of how they impact on specific substances. For example, buproprion (Wellbutrin) has more of an effect on norepinephrine and dopamine than on serotonin. You and your provider will determine which medicine works best for you.

> ### *Consejos*
>
> Treatment success is best achieved by a combination of medication and psychotherapy.

Psychotherapy

What we see in the movies about psychotherapy is often a caricature of what actually happens. Unfortunately, the stereotypes that are depicted often produce unrealistic expectations. As a result, we may begin therapy with the idea that we will be forgiven for our mistakes or be given the solutions for our turmoil—all after one visit. We often seek instant cure and to feel "all better" immediately.

If only it were that easy. Keep in mind that we did not become depressed instantly. Therefore it should not surprise us that the cure takes time. The benefits of psychotherapy are not the result of one visit, and there is no magical solution. Psychotherapy requires emotional work by both the patient and the therapist. It also requires a commitment to insight and change that extends beyond the therapeutic session. Therapy may last a few weeks or a few years.

To structure the process of psychotherapy, there are a variety of approaches, each with its own conceptual framework for explaining and impacting on the patient's behavior. Most therapists fall into one of the three categories described below.

Psychodynamic Therapy

Classical psychoanalysis is based on the teachings of Sigmund Freud and his followers. For Latinas, this type of therapy, which is based on the treatment of middle- and upper-class European women, may seem removed from their own experiences. In fact, some women believe that many core Freudian concepts (penis envy, castration anxiety) are detrimental to women.

Psychoanalysis involves a long-term commitment of time and money. Typically patients see their analyst at least twice a week for several years. This approach usually involves creating an environment where the patient can talk about whatever is on her mind. Often the analyst sits behind the patient and makes no eye contact, to make it easier for the patient to speak freely. This is a way of tapping into the patient's unconscious. Analysis of dreams also plays an important part in this therapy, as another means of glimpsing the patient's unconscious thoughts.

The principles underlying classic psychoanalysis have led to the development of many derivative treatment modalities; for example, Jungian therapy. In many of these, the role of the psychoanalyst is more active, and therapy may require fewer sessions.

Clarisa Pinkola Estés, in her landmark book, *Women Who Run With the Wolves,* shows how psychodynamic theories can be interwoven with the experiences of Latinas to create a successful type of therapy. Estés uses the stories and songs that are part of the Hispanic culture as a gateway into the Latina psyche. This provides a means for gaining understanding of one's own behavior.

Cognitive Behavioral Therapy

This therapy is based on the research evidence that there is a direct link between what we think and how we behave. Changing what we think so that our behavior changes too is the outcome of this therapy. The work in these sessions progresses through a series of steps: (1) identification of behaviors that you want to change, (2) assessment of the beliefs and thoughts that support the behavior, (3) establishment of the relationship between what you think and how you behave, (4) evaluation of the positive and negative consequences of thoughts and beliefs, and (5) development of a treatment strategy, which involves thinking of the situation in new ways in order to change future behavior.

Behavioral therapy may last a relatively short time (twenty weeks), although in the process of therapy other issues may emerge that must be addressed. As part of the therapy, patients are often required to do homework, keep a journal, or complete other activities that support the discussions in the sessions.

Eclectic Therapy

The reality is that most therapists have been trained in more than one modality and develop their own framework for therapy by combining the best elements of the interventions above. Eclectic therapy is not focused on one technique or procedure but rather on the knowledge, experience, and personal characteristics of the therapist.

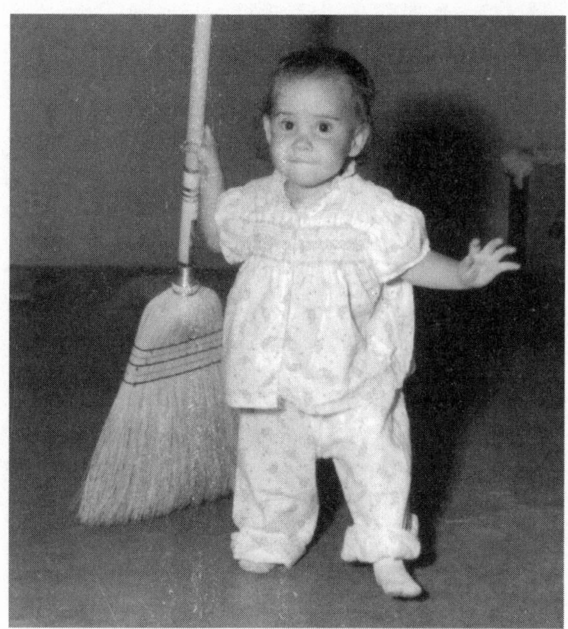

This baby girl grew up to become a psychologist.

Types of Mental Health Professionals

There are various kinds of mental health professionals, each with different areas of expertise, levels of experience, and techniques. The list below summarizes the educational and licensing requirements for some of the professions. There is great variability by state as to what mental health professionals may call themselves, as well as who can prescribe medication. In the majority of cases, only a physician or physician assistant can prescribe medication. Whether or not your mental health professional can prescribe medication herself, she should have extensive experience in working with internists and other medical professionals to insure that patients receive the best combination of medication and psychotherapy.

- **Clinical psychologist.** These professionals have earned a Ph.D. in clinical psychology. The course work involves a B.A. plus four years of courses, research, and direct clinical work, plus an additional one-year clinical internship. Licensing requirements vary by state.

- **Counselor.** The qualifications for counselors vary by state. A license may be required in some states.

- **Pastoral counselor.** There is great variability in training among pastoral counselors and minimal regulation.

- **Psychiatrist.** Training involves four years of medical school followed by a three- to four-year residency in psychiatry. There are strict licensing requirements. Recently some psychiatrists have focused less on psychotherapeutic methods and more on the use of medication to control depression and other mental illnesses. These specialists are called psychopharmacologists or neuropsychiatrists.

• **Psychoanalyst.** Previously the majority of psychoanalysts were psychiatrists. In recent years, in order to expand the numbers of formally trained psychoanalysts, other mental health practitioners have also been encouraged to participate in the training offered by psychoanalytic institutes. As part of the training, these professionals must undergo their own psychoanalysis to help them resolve their own issues.

• **Psychologist.** There is great variability among states in the qualifications required for using the title of psychologist. In some states, only a master's degree is needed, while other states require more advanced training.

• **Psychotherapist (therapist).** In many states this title is not protected, and persons may practice without meeting any formal educational or training requirements. Thus this term may encompass a wide variety of practitioners who are not licensed.

• **Social worker.** A licensed social worker has usually completed at least a master's degree in social work (M.S.W.). The degree of direct clinical experience varies greatly.

Steps for Selecting Your Mental Health Professional

In the treatment of depression, your cultural background and the language you feel most comfortable speaking play an integral part. More so than with a physical illness, where a provider can read an x-ray and see a broken bone, the ability to communicate with you and understand you is the only way a mental health professional can be helpful in your

Consejos

How to Select a Therapist

1. Develop a list of names.
   - Ask friends for recommendations.
   - Ask your health care provider for recommendations.
   - Ask for suggestions from your local chapter of the Mental Health Association and other professional societies and from your local community mental health center.
   - Ask your priest, pastor, or rabbi for suggestions.
2. Schedule an introductory visit. Keep in mind that most mental health professionals will not charge you for this first visit. The purpose of the visit is to determine whether this is someone you can work with.
3. Develop a list of questions to ask during the visit, such as:
   - Do you speak Spanish?
   - How long have you been seeing patients?
   - What type of therapeutic approach do you take?
   - What experience do you have working with Latinas?
   - What is the average length of time for treatment?
   - How will the need for medication be determined?
   - How will the impact of my medication be measured?
   - What fees will be charged?
4. After the first visit, ask yourself:
   - Do I feel comfortable with this person?
   - Do I trust this person?
   - Does this person show an understanding and appreciation of my culture?

treatment. Make sure that your therapist is not only someone you like but someone who can understand what you say and the cultural dynamics that make you who you are. Selecting a mental health professional must be done thoughtfully because the establishment of a therapeutic alliance between you and the therapist requires that you feel comfortable with respect to your body, mind, and spirit.

The first step in selecting a mental health professional is to develop a list of names of potential providers. Follow the suggestions given in *Consejos* to obtain references.

Once you have a list of names, you should call and find out some basic information. Ask about insurance coverage and languages spoken. Given the importance of the ability to establish a relationship, many mental health professionals encourage an initial low-cost or no-fee visit. The purpose of the visit is to determine whether this is someone you can work with. During the visit you may want to ask some of the more specific questions suggested in *Consejos*.

After the initial visit, you need to think about whether you can feel comfortable talking to this person. The most important factors are that you be able to talk freely, feel confidence in their ability, feel that you can develop trust in them, and feel that they demonstrate an understanding and appreciation of your being a Latina. Keep in mind that a mental health professional is neither a friend nor a family member but rather a respected, skilled professional who will work with you to alleviate your depression.

Once you have chosen a mental health professional, you must also make a commitment to treatment. This means that you have to be honest and truthful. Very often patients have to reveal aspects of their lives or relationships that they have tried to ignore.

In a mutually honest and respectful partnership with your mental health professional, you will be on your way to recovery from depression.

Spirit

Alicia could not confide to anyone how she felt. She was sad—but it was more than that. Every moment and every day she felt completely overwhelmed. She was sleeping more than usual and was not surprised to find that she had been gaining weight.

With every passing day, life was getting more and more hopeless. The hollowness of her spirit, which at first had been like a dull ache, now seemed to encompass her every movement.

She started to go to church every day and prayed that God would give her the strength to endure. She wept as she wondered how God could have abandoned her during these difficult days.

Too often we ask our faith to intervene when science and reason have provided us with an understanding of what we are experiencing. For many of us, the denial that depression is an illness is rooted in our belief that if the illness does not result in clear-cut physical symptoms, it is only in our head. And we believe that the things in our head are the result of our moral weakness or a test by God of our obedience.

The reality is that sometimes we seek refuge in our faith because we want to shield ourselves from the possibility that we have a mental illness. A mental illness is treatable, and our responsibility to have a healthy spirit requires that we seek appropriate care for our condition.

While prayer is an important source of strength, and for many of us serves as the guiding framework by which we accept the way life unfolds for us, we must understand that sometimes the answer to a prayer lies in our ability to use the resources that are available. Prayer combined with psychotherapy and medication may be the powerful combination necessary to alleviate or overcome clinical depression.

Summary

Depression is a treatable illness that is caused by a combination of factors: genetic, biochemical, and environmental. Each person's depression is the result of a unique combination of these factors.

The specific symptoms of depression, the intensity of the symptoms, and the length of time we experience the symptoms provide the basic information for diagnosis. Once a diagnosis has been made, a combination of psychotherapy and medication are usually required for successful treatment.

Although there are various schools of psychotherapy, the critical elements for success in therapy are identifying a mental health professional with whom you can work and being committed to the therapeutic intervention.

RESOURCES

Organizations

American Psychiatric Association
Division of Public Affairs Department SG
1400 K Street NW
Washington, DC 20005
(202) 682-6000 or (888) 357-7924
www.psych.org

Depressive Awareness, Recognition and Treatment Program
National Institute of Mental Health
6001 Executive Blvd., Rm 8184 MSC 9663
Bethesda, MD 20892
(800) 421-4211 or (301) 443-4513
www.nimh.nih.gov

Knowledge Exchange Network Center for Mental Health Services
PO Box 42490
Washington, DC 20015
(800) 789-2647
www.mentalhealth.org

National Alliance for the Mentally Ill
Colonial Place 3
2107 Wilson Blvd., Suite 300
Arlington, VA 22201-3042
(800) 950-NAMI (800) 950-6264 or (703) 524-7600
www.nami.org

National Depressive and Manic-Depressive Association
730 N. Franklin, Suite 501
Chicago, IL 60601
(800) 826-3632 or (312) 642-0049
www.ndmda.org

National Foundation for Depressive Illnesses, Inc.
P.O. Box 2257
New York, NY 10016
(800) 239-1265
www.depression.org

National Mental Health Association
1021 Prince Street
Alexandria, VA 22314-2971
(800) 969-6642 or (703) 684-7722
www.nmha.org

National Mental Health Consumers' Self-Help Clearinghouse
1211 Chestnut Street, Ste. 1207
Philadelphia, PA 19107
(800) 553-4539 (English); (800) 553-4539, ext. 290 (Spanish); or (215) 751-1810

National Women's Health Network
514 10th Street NW, Suite 400
Washington, DC 20004
(202) 347-1140
www.womenshealthnetwork.org

Books

Carter, Rosalynn. *Helping Someone with Mental Illness.* New York: Times Books, 1999.

Formanek, R. *Women and Depression.* New York: Springer, 1987.

Gilligan, Carol. *In a Different Voice: Psychological Theory and Women's Development.* Cambridge: Harvard University Press, 1993.

Jack, Dana Crowley. *Silencing the Self: Women and Depression.* Cambridge: Harvard University Press, 1993.

Wells, K. B., R. Strum, C. D. Sherbourne, and L. S. Meredith. *Caring for Depression.* Cambridge: Harvard University Press, 1996.

Publications and Pamphlets

"Clinical Depression in Women." National Mental Health Association Information Center, 1021 Prince Street, Alexandria, VA 22314-2971; (800) 969-6642 (Spanish language materials also available). Other titles include Depression Fact Sheets and "Depression in the Latino Community."

"Depression: What Every Woman Should Know." (Also available in Spanish.) National Institutes of Health, National Institute of Mental Health; (800) 421-4211. www.nimh.nih.gov

"Depression: You Don't Have to Feel this Way," 1999. AAFP Family Health Facts series. Pamphlet No. 1547. American Academy of Family Physicians, 11400 Tomahawk Creek Pkwy, Leawood, KS 66211-2672; (800) 944-0000.

"Depression Is a Treatable Illness." Pamphlet No. 93-05. U.S. Department of Health and Human Services, Public Health Service, Agency for Health Research and Quality, Executive Office Center, 2101 East Jefferson Street, Suite 501, Rockville, MD 20852; (800) 358-9295 or www.ahrq.gov

"Desórdenes del Estado de Animo ó de Talento: Depresión y Psicosis Maniaco-Depresiva." To request a copy of this pamphlet, contact National Alliance for the Mentally Ill, Colonial Place 3, 2107 Wilson Blvd. Suite 300, Arlington, VA 22201-3042. www.nami.org; NAMI Helpline: (800) 950-6264 or (703) 524-7600. Other titles include "Understanding Major Depression: What You Need to Know about This Medical Illness."

"Let's Talk Facts about Depression," 1994. American Psychiatric Association, Division of Public Affairs, 1400 K Street NW, Washington, DC 20005; (888) 357-7924 or (202) 682-6220 (Spanish language materials also available).

"What You Should Know about Women and Depression." American Psychological Association, 750 First Street NE, Washington, DC 20002-4242; (800) 374-2721 or (202) 336-5500 or www.apa.org/pubinfo

"Women and Mental Health: Issues for Health Reform," June 1995. The Commonwealth Fund. To order call 888-777-2744.

14

Diabetes

My uncle had diabetes, my mother had diabetes, and I guess I will get it too. It just seems to run in my family. My uncle lost his foot, but my mother was more careful. I guess there is nothing I can do but just accept that it will happen to me.

—RINA, 28

Latinas are twice as likely as the general population to have diabetes. According to the National Institute of Diabetes and Digestive and Kidney Diseases (NIDDK), 1.2 million Hispanics have been diagnosed with diabetes and about 675,000 more Hispanics have diabetes but do not know they have it. Ask any Latina, and she will be able to name several of her relatives who have diabetes. And then the stories will begin about how one family member nearly lost his or her vision, how someone else had to have a foot or a leg amputated. It was all to be blamed—or so the stories went—on all those sweets the person had indulged in. The discussion will seem practically matter-of-fact as we resign ourselves to the inevitable—that we too will get diabetes.

Some Latinas recall reading or being told that the diabetes was due to their Indian ancestry and that it is literally carried in their genes. However, Latinas who trace their origin to Cuba or Puerto Rico also have high rates of diabetes, and in the Caribbean region the Spanish *conquistadores* (conquerors) virtually exterminated the Native Indian populations before any intermixing of blood could occur.

While we do not know what causes the higher rates of diabetes among Latinas, we do know that diabetes is a very manageable chronic disease. So, the task ahead of us is to learn how we can prevent this disease, which when left untreated can be devastating, and how we can manage diabetes if we get it. The first step is to get some of the facts about it.

What Is Sugar?

Catalina knew that her craving for sweets was to be blamed on all that sugar she had when she was a baby. Someone had told her mother that babies who were no longer breast-fed needed to be given sweet milk. Consequently, while she was still an infant her mother had given her bottles filled with sweetened condensed milk.

That is how Catalina explained her love for sweets. She loved candies and she loved chocolate, and because she had had sweets all her life, she knew that she would end up with diabetes. So she popped another chocolate into her mouth, knowing that diabetes was caused by having too much sugar as a child.

Carbohydrates are chemical compounds that contain carbon, hydrogen, and oxygen, with a typical ratio of two atoms of hydrogen to each atom of oxygen. Sugar is a sweet carbohydrate in crystalline form.

Simple carbohydrates are common white sugar, fructose, glucose, and other natural sugars. They are easily absorbed by the body because they are made up of only one or two molecules of sugar. Complex carbohydrates (found in rice, beans, potatoes, and bread) take longer to be absorbed because they are made up of many molecules of sugar strung together.

In order to function efficiently, we have to eat the different types of compounds the body needs. The body needs simple and complex carbohydrates, proteins (complex nitrogen compounds that contain amino acids), and fats (a complex compound). We need all three, but each to a different degree—mostly carbohydrates, some protein, and relatively small amounts of fat.

Consejos

Sugar or Artificial Sweetener?

Sugar has only 16 calories per teaspoon. Gram for gram, it is relatively low in calories for all the energy it provides. Most important of all, it is a natural product.

If you are not diabetic, there is no real reason to use artificial sweeteners. The long-term side effects (known and unknown) of the chemicals in artificial sweeteners should be a greater source of concern to you than the number of calories you take in.

To keep your weight under control, you may have become accustomed to drinking soda with artificial sweetener, but if you are truly concerned about your health and appearance, drink bottled water. Water is good for your skin and for your body.

Think about it.

What Is Diabetes?

Our bodies all need sugar to function properly. Diabetes is the group of medical conditions that occurs when your body cannot use sugar properly. It is not that you have too much sugar, but rather that the body cannot use the sugar that you take in. Therefore, instead of being used by the cells in the body, the sugar remains in your bloodstream.

A hormone called insulin, which is naturally produced by the pancreas in a healthy body, plays a critical role in the body's ability to use sugar. The pancreas releases insulin into the bloodstream, which carries it throughout the body. Once insulin arrives at its designated site, it acts as a gatekeeper, allowing sugar to enter the cells and provide the fuel the cells need to function. When a person has diabetes, there are problems with this process.

Diabetes must be carefully treated and monitored. When diabetes is undiagnosed or untreated, many long-term complications may ensue: cardiovascular disease, stroke, hypertension, blindness, kidney disorders (end-stage renal disease), loss of sensations in feet and legs, and amputations. The onset of these conditions may not be gradual but instead abrupt and severe. Diabetes is the leading cause of blindness in adults over age thirty and the leading cause of end-stage renal disease. It is also a major contributing factor to amputations of the feet and legs.

Diabetes occurs in three major forms.

Type 1 diabetes (previously called insulin-dependent diabetes mellitus [IDDM] or juvenile diabetes) accounts for 5% to 10% of diagnosed cases. Autoimmune, genetic, and environmental factors are hypothesized to cause this type of diabetes. It is unclear what are the specific risk factors.

Type 2 diabetes (previously called non-insulin-dependent diabetes mellitus [NIDDM] or adult-onset diabetes) accounts for 90% to 95% of diagnosed cases.

Gestational diabetes (GDM) may develop during pregnancy and occurs in 2% to 5% of pregnancies.

Type 1 Diabetes (Insulin-Dependent Diabetes or IDDM)

Type 1 occurs when the pancreas is unable to produce the necessary amount of insulin. In the late 1980s, researchers began to hypothesize that type 1 was an autoimmune disease. This changed the definition of diabetes from a malfunctioning of part of the body (i.e., the pancreas) to a more systemic malfunction.

The immune system is the mechanism by which the body fights illness. When the system malfunctions, it may attack itself instead of foreign bodies. In type 1 the immune system destroys the insulin-producing cells of the pancreas. The exact reason for this has not yet been determined, but the current theory is that it is due to a combination of genetic factors and viruses. Type 1 occurs equally in males and females.

Type 2 Diabetes (Non-Insulin-Dependent Diabetes or NIDDM)

In type 2 the pancreas is producing insulin in normal quantities, but the body is not recognizing the messages transmitted by the insulin. In other words, type 2 is likely to be the result of cells not accepting insulin as the gatekeeper.

Type 2 is usually found in adults over forty. It is more common in women than in men, and it is almost always found in individuals who are overweight. Definitive studies of the role of weight in the onset of type 2 are yet to be done. What we know is sometimes confusing. For example, while Latinas tend to be overweight, African-American women tend to be more overweight than Latinas but have lower rates of type 2. What is certain is that being overweight is a complicating factor in type 2 and may accelerate the progression of the disease.

Gestational Diabetes

We do not know what causes healthy pregnant women to become diabetic, but we do know that this can occur nearly twice as often in Latinas (see Chapter 8).

How Is Diabetes Diagnosed?

Because Latinas are at high risk for diabetes, you should be familiar with the symptoms of the disease. Make sure to tell your health care provider if you have such symptoms. Also, try to find out which members of your family have had diabetes because there is believed to be some degree of genetic predisposition to diabetes. Sharing information about health conditions among family members is a good way to help one another. Although your health care provider should have a detailed history of your family as a matter of good clinical practice, remember the realities of health care in today's environment. The infor-

Signs of Diabetes

- being very thirsty
- urinating often
- feeling very hungry or tired
- losing weight without trying
- having sores that are slow to heal
- having dry, itchy skin
- losing feeling in your feet or having a tingling feeling in your feet
- having blurry eyesight

Source: What is Diabetes, NIDDK, 2000.

mation may not be at the top of your file, and with a limited amount of time it is unlikely that your health care provider will be able to read through your entire file.

Good health today requires that you work in partnership with your health care provider and alert the professional to symptoms that concern you. Since in the early stages of diabetes the symptoms may go unnoticed or be similar to those found in other conditions, you should be sure your provider knows about the history of diabetes in your family.

Only your health care provider can diagnose whether or not you have diabetes. In order to confirm the diagnosis of diabetes, you will have to have a test to assess how much sugar is contained in your blood.

Sandra was feeling fine. She was losing weight, and her exercise program was going well. But she felt tired. "Too much exercise," she thought to herself.

She knew what would also make her feel better—no more soda. She would just drink a lot of water. And that was a really good idea because it seemed she was always thirsty. Sandra laughed because all the water she had been drinking just seemed to wash right through her. She knew that must mean that all the toxins in her body were being cleared out.

So when at work she participated in one of the free screening tests, she could not believe the results. Her blood sugar levels were higher than normal—she was diabetic.

Different Types of Tests

To confirm a diagnosis of diabetes, your health care provider will request a test to assess how much sugar is in your blood. Information about your blood sugar level may be obtained by urine tests or blood tests. Many of us prefer urine tests because although they may be messy they do not hurt. Unfortunately, urine tests are not the best way to measure glucose levels, since there is great variability among people with diabetes as to how much glucose they spill into their urine. A more accurate diabetes test requires that your blood be analyzed. It may only be necessary to prick your finger (finger stick), but your health care provider may decide to obtain a larger sample by drawing blood from a vein.

Screening Tests

A screening test is a test given regardless of whether a person is displaying any symptoms of a disorder. Health professionals are increasingly aware of the problem of diabetes in Hispanic communities. As a result, many community fairs and other local activities include free screening for diabetes. These tests help to quickly determine whether you have more glucose in your blood than your body can process.

In the typical screening test, you will be asked when you ate your last meal and a series of other questions. One of your fingers will be pricked so that a drop of blood can be collected and placed on chemically treated paper. The paper is placed in a machine for analysis, and in a few minutes the results are available for you.

If the results are negative, you do not have too much glucose in your blood. If the test is positive, your health care provider should administer diagnostic tests.

Diagnostic Tests

A diagnostic test is given when your health care provider is reasonably certain that you may have diabetes. The three best-known tests for diabetes are the fasting plasma glucose test (the preferred test for diagnosing type 1 or type 2 diabetes), the random plasma glucose test, and the oral glucose tolerance test (only for gestational diabetes.) Diabetes is diagnosed when one of these tests is positive and there is a second positive test on a different day.

Fasting plasma glucose test. Before this test is administered, you are asked to eat or drink nothing but water for at least 10 hours but no more than 16 hours. If the test is scheduled for the morning, this usually just means eating nothing after dinner and not eating anything in the morning. Blood is drawn and sent to a laboratory for analysis. In some offices, these services are located near each other and you will be able to wait in the office for your test results. If your blood level is above 126 mg/dl (milligrams per deciliter) you will be asked to take a second test. If both of your tests are over 126 you will be diagnosed with diabetes. Your health care provider will not have to request additional tests to confirm the diagnosis.

Random plasma glucose test. For persons who have some of the signs and symptoms of diabetes, it may be easier and faster to take a blood sample at random without having them fast. When blood is obtained after you have eaten a meal, it may be acceptable to have a glucose blood level of 140 to 200 mg/dl. If the numbers are much higher, your health care provider may diagnose diabetes.

Oral glucose tolerance test. At one time this was considered the best way to get information about the body's ability to use glucose. It has been replaced by the fasting plasma glucose test. Today the oral glucose tolerance test is used mostly during and after pregnancy.

What the Future Holds

Scientists are coming closer to developing less invasive ways to measure blood glucose levels. Most of these technologies do not require a blood sample. Instead a beam of light is aimed into your eye or your finger to detect your blood glucose levels. In the near future, some of these less intrusive diagnostic devices will be in use by health care providers.

How Diabetes Affects the Health of Latinas

The reason diabetes is such a devastating disease is that we are often able to ignore its symptoms until it affects some major part of our body. Since all of our cells need sugar to function properly, not getting the right amount creates problems. Some of these are listed below.

Eye Problems

Nearly half the people with diabetes will develop some degree of diabetic eye disease. Diabetic eye disease is the leading cause of blindness in persons over thirty years of age. Take the test on the next page and see how much you can learn about diabetes and eye disease from the answers below.

Answers

1: True. Diabetic eye disease includes diabetic retinopathy—a leading cause of blindness in adults—cataracts, and glaucoma. The

How Much Do You Know About Diabetic Eye Disease?

1. People with diabetes are more likely than people without diabetes to develop certain eye diseases.
   True False Not Sure
2. Diabetic eye disease usually has early warning signs.
   True False Not Sure
3. People with diabetes should have yearly eye examinations.
   True False Not Sure
4. Diabetic retinopathy is caused by changes in the blood vessels in the eye.
   True False Not Sure
5. People with diabetes are at low risk for developing glaucoma.
   True False Not Sure
6. Laser surgery can be used to halt the progression of diabetic retinopathy.
   True False Not Sure
7. People with diabetes should have regular eye examinations through dilated pupils.
   True False Not Sure
8. Cataracts are common among people with diabetes.
   True False Not Sure
9. People who have good control of their diabetes are not at high risk for diabetic eye disease.
   True False Not Sure
10. The risk of blindness from diabetic eye disease can be reduced.
    True False Not Sure

Source: National Eye Health Education Program, National Eye Institute, National Institutes of Health, 2020 Vision Place, Bethesda, MD 20892-3655.

longer someone has diabetes, the more likely he or she is to develop diabetic eye disease.

2: False. Often there are no early warning signs of diabetic eye disease. Vision may not change until the disease becomes severe.

3: True. Every person with diabetes should have an eye examination at least once a year. Because diabetic eye disease usually has no symptoms, regular eye exams are important for early detection and timely treatment.

4: True. In some people, blood vessels in the retina may swell and leak fluid. In other people, abnormal new blood vessels grow on the surface of the retina.

5: False. People with diabetes are at higher risk of developing glaucoma than those without diabetes.

6: True. In laser surgery, an intense beam of light is used to shrink the abnormal blood vessels or seal leaking blood vessels. Laser surgery has been shown to reduce the risk of severe vision loss from advanced diabetic retinopathy by 90 percent.

7: True. An eye examination in which drops are used to dilate the pupils is the best way to detect diabetic eye disease. This allows the eye care professional to see more of the inside of the eye and check for signs of disease.

8: True. People with diabetes are at higher risk of developing cataracts at an earlier age than are those without diabetes.

9: False. Although good control of blood glucose can reduce the risk of diabetic eye disease significantly, it cannot prevent it in everyone. All people with diabetes should have an eye examination through dilated pupils at least once a year.

10: True. With early detection and timely treatment, the risk of blindness from diabetic eye disease can be reduced.

Infections

Latinas who have diabetes are more likely to develop yeast infections than those who do not have diabetes. Microorganisms that exist in the vaginas of all healthy women reproduce more rapidly when there is an elevated level of glucose in the bloodstream. Fortunately, a variety of medicines can be bought without a prescription (over-the-counter, or OTC, medicines) to treat these infections (see Chapter 6 for more information about the treatment of yeast infections).

Women who have diabetes also have two to three times the usual number of urinary tract infections, and the complications of these infections are more serious. As a result, when Latinas with diabetes develop a kidney infection, they may be given more aggressive treatment with antibiotics, including larger doses taken over a longer period of time.

Ironically, the antibiotics used for the treatment of a urinary tract infection may also kill the natural and necessary bacteria found in the vagina, thus increasing the likelihood of vaginal infections. These vaginal infections are typically treated with nonprescription topical ointments or suppositories in a cream formula.

Since infections change the composition of the blood, making it difficult to control blood glucose levels, it is important to treat them promptly.

Heart Disease

Diabetes has a negative impact on the cardiovascular system. Latinas who have diabetes and are premenopausal are at greater risk for heart disease than men of the same age with diabetes. Diabetic women are encouraged to follow the dietary recommendations given for heart disease (see Chapter 15).

Kidney Disease

Diabetes is the most frequent cause of end stage renal disease (ESRD). ESRD is managed by dialysis.

Neuropathy

Uncontrolled diabetes alters the way the nerves work that supply sensation to our arms and legs. The lack of sensation in our feet especially combined with the higher rate of blockage in the small blood vessels of persons with diabetes can lead to non-healing sores. These non-healing sores can often only be treated by amputating the foot or lower leg.

Hormonal Use

The interplay between hormones and diabetes is unclear, but the little research that has been done suggests that women with diabetes should avoid taking synthetic hormones. This means that they are advised not to use hormonal contraception methods. Research on hormone replacement therapy (HRT) is still inconclusive in this area.

High-Risk Pregnancies

Latinas with type 1 diabetes are encouraged to talk to their health care providers before they conceive. Counseling is essential to understanding how to reduce the high risks involved in pregnancy.

While some Latinas who have diabetes become pregnant, other Latinas acquire diabetes (GDM) during pregnancy. Many health care providers test women for diabetes between the twenty-fourth and twenty-eighth week of pregnancy. However, given the high rate of GDM in Latinas, it may be advisable to test Latinas earlier.

If you are pregnant and have either type 1 diabetes, type 2 diabetes, or GDM, it is essential to keep your blood glucose levels under control throughout the pregnancy through medication, proper nutrition, and exercise. When glucose levels are not acceptable, the baby may be born too big.

Uncontrolled diabetes in early pregnancy may lead to development of congenitally abnormal fetus. There is a higher risk of a baby developing a neural tube defect, a heart defect and many other types of genetic defects. Uncontrolled diabetes in pregnancy also places the mother at risk for development of other complications such as thyroid disease, hypertension, cardiovascular problems and a greater risk for complications at delivery. To protect the health of both mother and child, pregnant women with diabetes are often advised to monitor their glucose levels four to five times a day using an at-home test kit that can be purchased at a pharmacy. This is necessary because of the hormonal fluctuations that occur during pregnancy. In some cases insulin shots may be prescribed for women with type 2 diabetes during pregnancy.

Developing gestational diabetes or diabetes in pregnancy is a strong predictor that the patient may develop diabetes within the next five years. If a patient develops gestational diabetes this should be seen as a sign to alter diet and physical activity as a life long change to delay the progression of diabetes.

Consejos

For diabetics the extremes are bad. Know the signs.

Hyperglycemia—Very **high** levels of blood glucose

1. Excessive thirst
2. Frequent urination
3. Weakness, confusion
4. Dry lips and tongue
5. Cool hands and feet

Hypoglycemia—Very **low** levels of blood glucose

1. Feeling nervous, shaky, and weak
2. Sweating
3. Feeling hungry
4. Having headaches

Steps to Staying Healthy

As Latinas we are all aware that diabetes is a very common problem in our community. The best way to deal with diabetes is to try to prevent its appearance in the first place. This is most easily done with type 2 diabetes. Although its causes are not all well understood, insufficient exercise and being overweight are the greatest risk factors for all of us.

To the extent that we exercise regularly and maintain a healthy weight we can do a great deal to block the appearance of this disease. If diabetes develops despite these efforts, we need to understand that many of the complications of diabetes can be prevented by paying careful attention to how we take care of ourselves and by working closely with our health care providers. With diabetes, almost more than any other disease, our attitude day by day will determine how the disease will affect the quality of our lives.

Our focus as Latinas with diabetes is to take control of the situation by monitoring our blood levels on a daily basis using a glucometer, being well informed about how diabetes affects our health, and keeping ourselves healthy through proper diet and exercise. By knowing what to expect and what we can do, we will be prepared to meet any challenges.

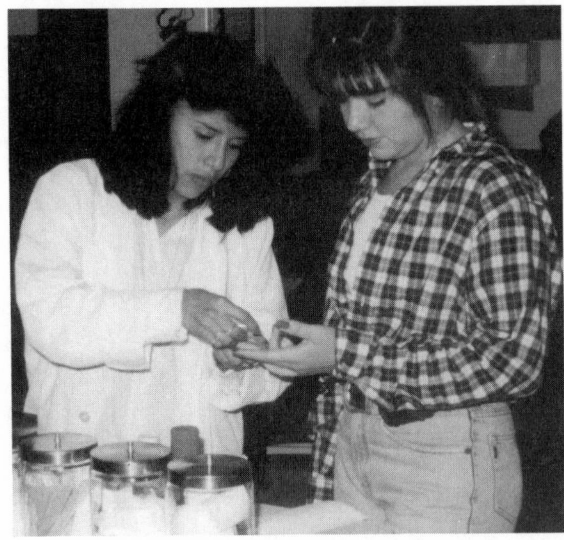

It is important to monitor our glucose levels.

Continuous Monitoring

When you have diabetes, it is essential to monitor your glucose level on a daily basis. Your health care provider may ask you to monitor yourself several times a day to help determine how different foods, activities, emotions, and thoughts make your blood glucose levels fluctuate.

The most effective method is to use a portable meter monitoring kit (i.e., a glucometer). The machines are easy to use. Simply prick a finger so that a drop of blood falls on a paper strip. The paper strip is inserted into the monitor, which analyzes the paper and gives you a readout of the blood level.

Based on your blood glucose level, you may decide to change your diet or change the amount of medication you take. If your blood sugar is too high, you may decide to take more insulin or more medication. If your blood sugar is too low, you may decide to drink some orange juice or eat a piece of candy.

Once you know you have diabetes, you must monitor and control your blood sugar every day of your life. You are the only one who can make sure you stay in line and control your intake of glucose. Some of us try to skip days and get by, but the truth will come out. A glycosylated hemoglobin or Hemoglobin A1-C (HgA1-C) test of your blood sample will let you and your health care provider know how well you have actually controlled your levels of glucose in the preceding eight to twelve weeks.

With diabetes, the reason it is so important to control your blood glucose level is that the damage to nerves and blood vessels caused by high glucose levels is cumulative and usually irreversible. On days when your diabetes is out of control, the cells in your body are being damaged. It is this damage that leads to all the complications of diabetes—i.e., blindness, heart disease, and kidney failure.

Taking Your Medication

Oral hypoglycemics are pills we can take to reduce the amount of glucose in our blood by increasing the production of insulin. Currently several pills are available that can reduce blood glucose levels. Each is different in how it works on the body. Your health care provider will prescribe the pills that are best for you.

These pills are not prescribed for women who are pregnant or for nursing mothers. They are recommended for those who have type 2 diabetes.

Pills are only effective if taken as prescribed, in combination with healthy eating habits (see Chapter 19) and light to moderate exercise.

Some people with type 2 diabetes may be told that they are better candidates for controlling their blood glucose through injections of insulin. In this case, your health care provider will give you the necessary instructions.

Controlling Hypertension

While controlling hypertension is important for all of us, it is especially important if you have diabetes. Numerous studies have shown that careful control of blood pressure combined with control of blood glucose can prevent the onset of kidney disease in diabetics.

No Smoking

As Latinas, we used to be the group least likely to smoke, and that was good. Today things are changing for the worse. Our collective health chant should be "If you smoke, stop, and if you don't smoke, don't start."

It is not clear how smoking impacts on diabetes, but it is clear that persons with diabetes who smoke are more likely to get heart disease than persons with diabetes who do not smoke. Since diabetics are already at increased risk for heart disease and the link between smoking and heart disease is well documented, clearly smoking is quite dangerous for the person with diabetes.

Careful Eating

If you have diabetes, what you eat affects how much glucose is in your blood. If you do not have diabetes, what you eat has little impact on the glucose in your blood. Having diabetes changes your eating in two main ways, making it necessary to (1) maintain a comfortable weight and (2) reduce the amount of sugar you eat.

Maintaining a Comfortable Weight

You need to talk to your health care provider to determine what would be a good weight for you to try to maintain. Sometimes it is not good to set up these goals on our own because we may be focusing on the appearance aspect rather than the health aspect of weight. This is particularly true for young girls with type 1 diabetes, who may become anorexic or bulimic in order to control their weight. Chapter 20 provides some commonsense approaches to addressing this issue.

Myths and Facts

Myth: Fructose, found in honey and fruit, is better than sucrose, from sugar cane, sugar beet, and maple sugar.

Fact: There is no advantage to eating fructose instead of sucrose.

Myth: If you are diabetic, you must restrict your salt intake.

Fact: Persons who have diabetes should follow the same guidelines for salt intake as nondiabetics.

Myth: I can eat all the bread I want, but I can't have sugar.

Fact: Sugar and bread are both carbohydrates, which will turn to glucose in the bloodstream, and you must limit the amount you eat of them both.

Myth: Cooked foods are better for you than uncooked foods.

Fact: Food that is raw and unpeeled raises your blood glucose less than cooked foods.

Myth: All you need is two well-spaced meals a day.

Fact: It is best to have several small meals spaced throughout the day.

Myth: If you are beginning to feel hypoglycemic, you should drink water.

Fact: If you are feeling weak, you should drink something with sugar in it, such as orange juice.

Myth: You can never do too much exercise.

Fact: If you exercise too much and you are taking pills to reduce your blood glucose levels, you can become hypoglycemic.

Myth: If I take my pills to control my diabetes, I can eat when and what I want.

Fact: When taking pills to control diabetes, you must continue to be thoughtful about what and when you eat.

Eating the Right Foods at the Right Time

As Latinas, we like tasty food. With a little bit of innovation we can eat the right food and still enjoy it. Most persons with diabetes will be encouraged to eat a diet that is 50 to 60 percent carbohydrates, 12 to 20 percent protein, and less than 30 percent fat.

Preprinted diets are very difficult for most of us to follow because we usually have to prepare meals for the entire family. A good way to think of meals is that you are trying to prepare healthy meals for your entire family while adapting some of your favorite foods to keep in line with the percentages above. Chapter 19 provides lots of tips for this. The person with diabetes has to be especially vigilant to reduce intake of all carbohydrates and to have a mixture of complex and simple carbohydrates.

Eating at the right time means having several (four to five) small meals spaced throughout the day so that blood glucose levels will not become extremely high (as when you binge eat) or extremely low (as when you skip meals).

More Activity

Activity and exercise are good for all of us. This is especially true when we have diabetes because activity and exercise improve the way our bodies use insulin and food.

There are many things we can do to be more active than most of us are. Activity does not mean that you have to join a class or take time from your schedule. In many instances it means that we rethink how we are doing our every-day activities. Some of the things we can keep in mind are:

1: Doing things a little faster. This means that whether we are going to the store, up a flight of steps, or cleaning, we try to move a little faster and in the process use a little more energy. And that is good.

2: Adding incidental exercises. Incidental exercise is also a result of making slight changes in our normal day-to-day activities rather than doing planned exercises. Taking the stairs instead of using the escalator and walking instead of driving are ways to increase our incidental exercise.

Once you have increased your level of activity, you may want to do some more formal exercises. The best way to do this is to (1) do something you enjoy, (2) start out slowly, and (3) increase the speed and quantity of the exercises over time.

As Latinas, although we tend to be "other-oriented," some things we prefer to do on our own. Exercising is definitely one of these activities. Doing exercises at home is a good way to begin since we can have a degree of privacy. You can try dancing to music or doing floor exercises (see Chapter 21).

Those of us who prefer the encouragement and support that a group activity provides can investigate what is available free or at a reasonable cost in our local community centers, churches, or health clubs and join up.

As part of our daily life, we can be more active with children and young people. If there are children around, it would probably be better for everyone to play an active game rather than sitting around watching television.

While activity and exercise are important, keep in mind that they will reduce your glucose blood level. So make sure not to take too much medication before you exercise and to exercise in moderation and not to the point where you make yourself hypoglycemic.

Mind and Spirit

As Latinas, we are even more prone to stress than other women because we have to negotiate the pressures of living in two cultures that do not seem to mesh. For Latinas who have diabetes, managing stress levels is not just important but essential. Stress increases the level of glucose in the blood, so we must learn to monitor the effect of the fluctuations in our lives so that we can keep these levels under control.

We must learn what things upset us. If we monitor ourselves carefully and honestly, we may be able to identify some of the triggers in our lives that make our blood glucose levels rise. We may also learn to fully appreciate how much it helps us to fulfill our spirits.

As we monitor ourselves, we can become attuned to the intermingling of our body, mind, and spirit. Our blood glucose levels, which fluctuate with our emotions, may reveal how those closest to us affect our lives. The results may surprise us. We might decide to see a mental health professional for help in learning how to handle the more challenging aspects of relationships we endure.

Summary

Diabetes is a major health concern for Latinas and we need to know the best information about how to prevent diabetes, recognize the early symptoms, and how to live with diabetes once we know we have it. By carefully monitoring ourselves, including during pregnancy, we can control diabetes and live full and complete lives.

RESOURCES

Organizations

American Association of Diabetes Educators
100 West Monroe Street, Ste 400
Chicago, IL 60603-1901
(800) 832-6874 or (312) 424-2426
www.adanet.org

American Diabetes Association
ADA National Service Center
1660 Duke Street
Alexandria, VA 22314
(800) 232-3472 or (703) 549-1500
www.diabetes.org

Juvenile Diabetes Foundation International
120 Wall Street, 14th Floor
New York, NY 10005-4001
(800) JDF-CURE (800-533-2873)
(212) 785-9500
www.jdf.org

National Diabetes Information Clearinghouse
1 Information Way
Bethesda, MD 20892-3560
(301) 654-3327
www.niddk.nih.gov/health/diabetes/ndic.htm

Hotlines

Diabetes Information and Action Line
American Diabetes Association
(800) 232-3472 (bilingual staff available)

Su-Familia Family Health Helpline
National Alliance for Hispanic Health
866-SuFamilia (783-2645)

Books

Jovanovic-Peterson, Lois. *The Diabetic Woman: All Your Questions Answered.* New York: Tarcher, 1996.

Publications and Pamphlets

"Diabetes and Your Body: How to Take Care of Your Eyes and Feet," 1999. Pamphlet No. 1553. AAFP Family Health Facts series. American Academy of Family Physicians, 11400 Tomahawk Creek Pkwy, Leawood, KS 66211-2672; (800) 944-0000. Other pamphlets on diabetes are also available.

"Diccionario de la Diabetes." NIH Publication No. 91-3016S (also available in English as NIH Publication No. 94-3016). National Diabetes Information Clearinghouse, 1 Information Way, Bethesda, MD 20892-3560; (301) 654-3327. Numerous publications; many in Spanish. Other titles include:

"Insulin-Dependent Diabetes," September 1994. NIH Publication No. 95-2098.

"Noninsulin-Dependent Diabetes," September 1992. NIH Publication No. 95-241.

"Gestational Diabetes: A Practical Guide to a Healthy Pregnancy," February 1993. NIH Publication No. 93-2788.

"Facts about Hispanics and Diabetic Eye Disease." National Eye Health Education Program, 2020 Vision Place, Bethesda, MD 20892-3655; 301-496-5248. Other titles include "¡Ojo Con su Vision!" NIH Publication No. 96-4032.

"Living with Diabetes." Juvenile Diabetes Foundation International, Diabetes Research Foundation, 432 Park Avenue South, New York, NY 10016-8013; (212) 889-7575. Other pamphlets on diabetes, including Spanish language publications, are available.

"La Diabetes Entre Latinos," 1992. American Diabetes Association, 1660 Duke Street, Alexandria, VA 22314; (800) 232-3472. www.diabetes.org

15

Heart Disease

"Me Duele el Corazón" . . .

"My Heart Hurts"

Mi corazón . . . Just the words in Spanish seem to imply so much more than they do in English. *Corazón.* Saying it can practically make you sigh. No part of our body is closer to our soul than our heart. For Latinas, passion, deep feeling, and our spiritual center reside in our heart.

And because we know that the pain in our heart is often due to the turmoil of our mind and spirit, we are too often likely to disregard the early symptoms of heart problems. Because we can attribute what we feel to something nonphysical, we disregard it and continue *aguantando*, taking it all in stride, as part of the way life unfolds. Yet if we listen carefully, we may discover that our body is trying to tell us something else.

The good news about Latinas and heart disease is that we seem to have less heart disease than other women do. Despite that, heart disease is still the leading cause of deaths for Latinas over sixty years of age.

How does heart disease change our lives? It is typically a gradual process that occurs when we have finished menopause. Therefore, we often mistakenly think the symptoms are just part of growing older. So although we may feel tired or out of breath, we fail to point out these very important symptoms to our health care providers. Given the importance of prevention and early treatment to avoid damage to the heart, we must learn to recognize the gradual changes in our life.

While only your health care provider can diagnose a heart problem, it is up to you to know how your heart works, recognize when there are problems, and understand the treatment options if a problem is diagnosed. Unfortunately, much of what we know about heart disease among women is inferred from knowledge gained from earlier studies that used mostly male subjects. There is no question that some problems with heart disease affect women differently than men and a greater understanding of this will come from studies yet to be done. Marianne Legato's book *The Female Heart* describes in great detail what we do know now about women and cardiovascular disease (CVD).

There is even less information and scientific data concerning CVD among Latinas. Of the few major CVD studies that included women, none attempted to describe what happens to the Latina heart. Even in the mid-

1990s, when the National Institutes of Health (NIH) began an ambitious ten-year study of women's health, the inclusion of Latinas was only minimal. While the information from the Women's Health Initiative should be a big step forward in understanding what happens to women with heart disease, as Latinas we still need to press for further studies to understand what might be unique in the way heart disease affects us. Thus we must educate ourselves and learn from each other.

How the Heart Works

We have all heard that the heart is a pump. If we are honest, we also recognize that although most of us know what a pump is, few of us understand how a pump actually works, and even fewer of us know how to take care of one.

The heart is the center of a system that transports oxygen and nutrients to cells throughout our body and takes away the waste those cells produce while doing their routine work.

Blood is the medium that picks up new oxygen supplies from the lungs, delivers that oxygen to all the organs of the body, and in exchange takes the product of the utilized oxygen known as carbon dioxide (CO_2) back to the lungs for elimination. The blood also carries glucose from the foods we ingest to all parts of the body where it is used for energy and in return takes the waste products of metabolism back to the liver and kidneys for elimination. The heart is the machine that pumps the blood through the body so that it can carry out all these tasks.

The heart is made up of very strong muscle tissue (myocardium) divided into four sections

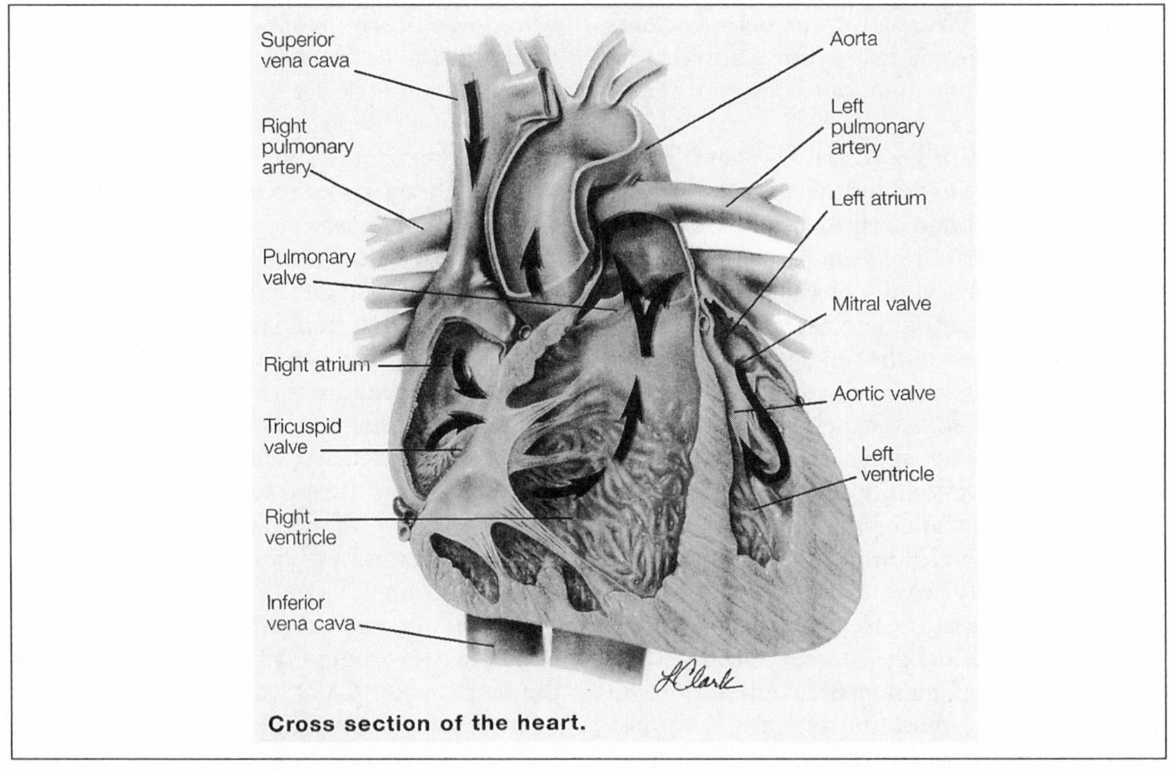

Cross section of the heart.

(chambers). The two top chambers are called *atria* (the plural of the word *atrium*)—one atrium on the right and another on the left. The two lower chambers are the ventricles, again, one on the right and another on the left. Between these chambers are valves that function to keep blood flowing in the proper direction. Blood travels through the four chambers as a result of the coordinated opening and closing of the valves that separate the chambers of the heart. The opening and closing of the valves is determined by the contractions of the heart.

The heart contracts in response to small electrical impulses generated by a group of cells located in the right atrium. The small electrical charge produced by these cells stimulates the heart to contract in a set pattern. Each heartbeat is a contraction, and as the heart contracts, it makes the blood flow. The upper chambers contract a fraction of a second before the lower chambers. This allows the lower chambers to fill up. Deep emotions as well as changes in our hormones can alter the rate at which the electrical impulses are released. The basic rhythm of the heart is determined by built-in programs, but these rhythms can be altered by chemical messages delivered to the heart by our nerves. That is why at times of stress caused by exertion, emotions, or fear our heart rate speeds up and at times when we are resting our heart rate is much slower.

Looking at the diagram of the heart, imagine the route that a drop of blood takes as it travels through the heart. Blood carrying carbon dioxide and other waste from the cells travels through the veins and is received by the heart's upper right chamber (atrium). As the atrium contracts, the valve between the upper and lower right chambers opens, allowing the lower right chamber (right ventricle) to fill.

When the heart beats, the blood is pumped from the right ventricle into the lungs where blood exchanges the carbon dioxide it carries for fresh oxygen. The blood then pulses through to the upper left chamber (left atrium) and across the mitral valve to the lower left chamber (left ventricle). Finally, the blood is then pumped from the left ventricle into the body's largest blood vessel, the aorta, which sends it to the entire body so that the blood can deliver its oxygen and nutrients.

When we measure blood pressure we are basically measuring the amount of work the heart is doing to push the blood through the arteries. The higher the blood pressure, which is determined by the relative size of our arteries, the more work the heart has to do. Arteries can dilate and contract according to a variety of factors such as our genetic makeup, the amount of salt in our diet, and the amount of exercise we get. When the blood pressure is too high we can end up with an exhausted heart muscle which is known as heart failure.

Each day the average heart beats 100,000 times, distributing 2,000 gallons of blood throughout the body. All this work is accomplished by an organ the size of a fist. Moreover, a woman's heart and coronary arteries are smaller than a man's.

Keeping the Heart Healthy

1: Don't smoke. Many Latinas know that smoking is not good for their lungs. Now that you know how the heart and lungs work together, it is easier to see the direct and strong relationship between them. If you smoke, stop, and if you do not smoke, please do not start.

2: Eat salt and fat in moderation. When the body retains water (which may be a result of excessive salt intake) or when the arteries are clogged (which may be a result of excessive saturated fat intake), the heart has to work harder. This means more wear and tear on the heart. Try not to add salt to your food, and follow the nutritional tips in Chapter 19.

3: Increase your activity. You do not have to run a marathon or swim 5 miles, but be honest about how much movement or exercise you engage in, and try to increase it gradually over the next few weeks until you reach your goal in terms of time. The increase in activity should be gradual, but the goal you reach must be maintained for the rest of your life. Chapter 21 suggests some good exercises with Latinas in mind.

4: Take your medicines as directed. If you are prescribed medications for your heart, even when you feel well, it is important to take them as directed. Some medicines have bad side effects if you stop taking them abruptly, and others (such as medicines to control hypertension) do not work unless a constant level is maintained in your body. If you think the medicines are making you sick discuss this with your health care provider.

5: Develop a more positive attitude toward life. Research shows that being happy encourages a healthy heart. So enjoy what you can, and let go of what you cannot control.

6: Learn to relax. Latinas work so hard at taking care of everyone that sometimes the hardest thing for them to do is to make time to relax. But relaxation is part of what your heart needs.

7: Focus on your faith. Whether you go to an organized church or feel that the world is God's house, you have your own faith. Your faith should give you peace—and peace keeps your heart healthy.

Consejos

How to Keep Your Heart Healthy

1. Don't smoke.
2. Eat salt and fat in moderation.
3. Increase your activity.
4. Take your medicines as directed (prescription and nonprescription).
5. Develop a more positive attitude toward life.
6. Learn to relax.
7. Focus on your faith.

When the Heart Does Not Work Well

Luisa knew she should be more energetic. She continued to work in the house and did all her chores, but for the past few months she had felt tired all the time. She just could not do the things she used to do, but she knew that this was just part of getting older.

What was worse than being tired was that lately she seemed to be developing asthma. She just couldn't breathe the way she used to. But she had learned how to take care of that. She found that if she rested a little, her sensation of being out of breath would pass.

Luisa continued doing all her work because she had so many things to get done. And yet she did not feel like her old self. Oh well, she thought, that must be what happens with time.

The majority of us recognize the images of a heart attack that the media has implanted in our minds. In one scene, a perfectly healthy person grips his chest, grimaces in pain, falls over, and is dead before the ambulance arrives.

The second scene you have seen countless times. The patient is in the hospital, and suddenly you know his heart has stopped beating because all you see is a monitor and a line that has gone flat. As that happens, a long beep signals to all the staff nearby what has happened. A nurse calls for a crash cart and lets everyone know that it is a "code blue" situation. The hospital staff all come running down the hall to where the patient is lying. One physician reaches over, gets the electrical charger, shouts "Clear!" and everyone jumps back while he applies the electrical pads to the patient's chest. Usually, for added drama, nothing happens.

Then the physician, looking worried, begins to sweat at the thought of losing a patient and again yells, "Clear!" as he shocks the patient a second time. At this point the monitor shows a blip as the heart begins to beat, and everyone looks relieved.

These scenes are meant to be dramatic. They are not factual, and they do not represent what actually happens in life. Contrary to popular perception, heart attacks are not always so dramatic and this makes their diagnosis sometimes difficult.

What a woman who is having a heart attack feels runs the gamut from heartburn or indigestion to severe chest pains. Over one-third (35 percent) of women who have heart attacks either do not notice them or the symptoms are so mild that they do not feel a need to report them.

The signs of a heart attack are difficult to list because data indicate that these symptoms may be different for women than for men, on whom most of the research has been done. The American Heart Association says the body likely will have one or more of these symptoms:

- Uncomfortable pressure, fullness, squeezing or pain in the center of the chest that lasts more than a few minutes, or goes away and comes back.
- Pain that spreads to the shoulders, neck, or arms.
- Chest discomfort with lightheadedness, fainting, sweating, nausea, or shortness of breath.

Less common warning signs of heart attack:

- Atypical chest pain, stomach or abdominal pain.
- Nausea or dizziness (without chest pain).
- Shortness of breath and difficulty breathing (without chest pain).
- Unexplained anxiety, weakness, or fatigue
- Palpitations, cold sweat, or paleness.

If you have these symptoms, you should call 911 or your emergency medical system or have someone take you to an emergency room and receive attention. Keep in mind that the faster you receive appropriate treatment, the smaller the amount of heart muscle that is damaged.

A heart attack is usually the result of an acute blockage of one of the arteries that supplies blood to the heart muscle. Most of the time this total blockage is superimposed on a process called atherosclerosis which has been slowly narrowing the diameter of the artery for years. These narrowed arteries are capable of delivering enough blood to the heart for it to do its work under normal circumstances. However, sometimes these narrowed arteries are not capable of delivering enough blood to the heart when the heart is being asked by the rest of the body to increase its pumping activity. Under these circumstances the heart sends off messages of pain telling us we need to slow down because the heart isn't getting enough blood flow. This pain is called angina. These exercise related pains are often the first sign of atherosclerotic disease in our coronary arteries.

If an acute blockage is superimposed on the narrowed arteries and the blood flow is 100% occluded, a heart attack results. A heart attack is more dangerous than angina because the heart muscle is in danger of being permanently damaged. A damaged heart muscle reduces the efficiency of the heart's pumping activity causing heart failure.

The acute blockage that causes the heart failure is the result of a blood clot forming on top of the atherosclerotic lesions in the heart's blood vessels. If we get to a hospital quickly enough when this is happening we can be given medicine that dissolves the blood clot and prevents the muscle from being permanently damaged. Preventing this damage is very important. Since aspirin can interfere with the formation of blood clots, if you think you might be having a heart attack call 911 or your emergency medical system and take one aspirin immediately.

Men at risk for heart attack develop atherosclerosis of their arteries in their 40's and 50's while in women it often doesn't appear until after menopause in their 60's. Since women begin to develop heart disease when they are older, it is more likely that they will also have other health problems, which may change the course of treatment. This is especially true for Latinas, who are more likely than other women to develop diabetes as they get older. Diabetes is known to contribute to the weakening of the walls of the arteries and reduce the usefulness of angiograms (diagnostic tests) and angioplasty (treatment).

Consejos

Angina Is Chest Pain

Everyone hears that a person with chest pain may have angina, which is a symptom of problems with the heart muscle. The question is, how does this kind of pain differ from other pains? How does it differ from indigestion? For many women, the symptoms are so similar that it is difficult to tell what is going on.

Health care providers cannot always tell the difference either. That is why they may run a series of diagnostic tests to see whether there is any other evidence to corroborate the presence of heart disease.

As Latinas, we need to listen to our bodies carefully and attend to the nuances that reveal what is going on. If you feel pain, and if you are concerned, make sure you get yourself to an emergency room. If you are having a heart attack, early medical intervention can help save more of your heart muscle.

• Arteriosclerosis and atherosclerosis. A good supply of blood requires that blood flow to the heart easily through unobstructed arteries. As we grow older, the arteries frequently "harden," or become less flexible, making it more difficult for the blood to flow through them. The disease process leading to hardening of the arteries is called arteriosclerosis.

Other problems arise when the arteries get clogged. This condition is called atherosclerosis. Arteries get clogged when their protective lining is damaged, allowing substances to build up inside the artery wall. This buildup is called plaque, and it is made up of cholesterol, waste materials from cells, fatty materials, and other substances.

Atherosclerotic plaque builds up in people at a higher risk for heart attack mostly because of genetic factors. However, there are at least five known factors that cause the buildup to proceed more rapidly: cigarette smoking, high blood pressure, high levels of cholesterol, diabetes, and lack of exercise.

• Smoking. When we think of smoking, we may focus on the effect smoking has on our lungs. But our lungs are not an isolated part of our body. Rather, they are an important partner of the heart because they are where the blood exchanges carbon dioxide for oxygen. Researchers are unable to explain all the reasons why smoking increases plaque in the arteries. However, it is clear that tobacco products injure the artery linings. If we stop smoking, our lungs clear in a few years, but the plaque that has built up in our arteries remains. The good news is that heart risk decreases in one to three years after a person stops smoking.

- High blood pressure. High blood pressure makes the heart work harder and adds strain to the entire system. The strain of high blood pressure makes it likely that an artery lining will be injured and in time be prone to blockage. High blood pressure is particularly damaging to the heart, brain, and kidneys. In 95 percent of cases, the cause of hypertension is unknown.

- Cholesterol. The body needs some cholesterol to function properly. In most instances, the liver produces all the cholesterol the body needs. Because of its structure, cholesterol does not dissolve in the blood. Consequently, the body attaches another substance (lipoprotein) to cholesterol so that the blood can carry it throughout the body. Blood carries cholesterol in two major forms: as low-density lipoprotein (LDL) and as high-density lipoprotein (HDL). When there is too much LDL, some of the cholesterol may settle into arteries. In contrast, HDL is believed to help keep the arteries clear of plaque.

In the best of situations, you have low levels of LDL and high levels of HDL. The risk of atherosclerosis is reflected by the ratio of LDL to HDL in your blood. Premenopausal women tend to have higher HDL levels than men, presumably as a result of estrogen production.

- Diabetes
- Lack of exercise

Since angina is a warning sign of severely narrowed arteries it should be evaluated promptly. Remember angina is best defined as chest pain that appears with exertion and disappears quickly with rest. If you develop angina it is often a red alert that a heart attack might be soon to follow. If you develop these symptoms see your health care provider immediately.

Some other heart problems are:

1: Valve problems. The four heart valves are critical to keeping the blood flowing in the right direction, and women tend to have more problems with these valves than men do. In more than 5 percent of all women (compared to 3 percent of men), the valve between the two left chambers does not close correctly, a condition called mitral valve prolapse (MVP). The cause of MVP is usually genetic, and usually there are no serious consequences. The condition is not clearly understood, and usually there are no symptoms. When there are symptoms, they may include lightheadedness, palpitations (rapid heartbeat), fatigue, or breathing difficulties. In rare instances, MVP may be associated with significant abnormal heart rhythms. Persons with MVP are at higher risk for infective endocarditis (an infection of the heart valves or inner lining of the heart) and slightly higher risk for a stroke. To reduce these risks you should take antibiotics before dental procedures.

2: Irregular heartbeats. The heart beats in a very systematic manner. Sometimes it beats faster (as when we are exerting ourselves), and sometimes it beats slower (as when we are resting). When the heart beats too fast, too slow, or very irregularly, it has what is called an arrhythmia. Many arrhythmias are harmless but if they are associated

Consejos

A stroke is not a heart attack. A stroke occurs when the brain does not get enough blood.

Your brain needs blood to function. Sometimes the blood cannot reach the brain because the pathway is blocked or because the path no longer exists (i.e., when an artery bursts or leaks). When this happens, the area of your brain that is unable to get blood dies, and the part of your body controlled by that area of your brain can no longer function. You may be unable to walk, move, speak, and/or comprehend spoken language. This condition is called a stroke.

Most strokes are due to a blockage—either a blood clot that forms in the brain (cerebral thrombosis) or a blood clot formed elsewhere in the body that travels to the brain (cerebral embolism). Some strokes occur when an artery in the brain bursts (cerebral hemorrhage). A few strokes occur when the surface of the brain bleeds into the space between the brain and the skull (subarachnoid hemorrhage).

In 1 out of 10 cases, the body gives us an early warning that we will be having a stroke. These early warning symptoms are referred to as transient ischemic attacks (TIAs). TIAs are best recognized as mild and temporary (usually less than 5-minute) versions of the symptoms that accompany a stroke. While a TIA lets you know that your likelihood of having a stroke has increased, it does not predict when the stroke will occur. If you have a TIA, you should immediately let your health care provider know.

Among the warning signs of a stroke are:

- Sudden numbness or weakness of the face, arm or leg, especially on one side of the body.
- Sudden confusion, trouble speaking, or understanding.
- Sudden trouble seeing in one or both eyes.
- Sudden trouble walking, dizziness, loss of balance or coordination.
- Sudden, severe headache with no known cause.

with symptoms of dizziness or shortness of breath contact your health provider.

Diagnostic Tests

As part of your annual checkup or if you complain of a problem, your health care provider may do some tests and measures to get a better sense of how your heart is functioning. Some tests are routine and simple; others are more sophisticated.

Latinas prefer to be informed about what a diagnostic test will entail so that they can prepare themselves. This is especially true when we have to explain the procedure to a parent or older relative we may be taking care of. We need to be able to prepare them and ourselves for the discomfort that some of these procedures produce.

The types of diagnostic tests used cover a broad range, from easy to do and relatively painless to more intrusive and uncomfortable. It is important to remember that the purpose of diagnostic tests is not to make you feel better but to find out if anything is wrong so that you can be properly treated. The following are part of a good heart exam.

Pulse

Your pulse rate is a basic measure of how hard your heart is working—that is, how many times it has to pump in order to supply the body with a sufficient quantity of blood.

Heart Sounds

In most instances, your health care provider will begin by listening to your heart with a stethoscope. You will be asked to breathe so that the sounds of your heart can be heard from the different points on the chest where the stethoscope is placed. A good clinician will be able to recognize the sounds of a healthy heart and be able to discern sounds that might indicate a damaged heart.

Blood Pressure

Your health care provider will use a special instrument (sphygmomanometer) to measure your blood pressure (i.e, how hard your heart has to work to pump blood). A cuff will be placed on your upper arm and inflated. Then your provider will place a stethoscope under the cuff and listen to the sound of the blood traveling through your artery. Some of us may find the pressure of the cuff uncomfortable, but that only lasts a short time.

Blood Test

When you have a heart attack, enzymes are released from the heart muscle into the blood. Your health care provider can measure these enzymes if you are having chest pain and they will help determine if the pain is because of a heart attack.

Electrocardiogram (EKG or ECG)

For this painless procedure, electrodes are attached to your body to measure the natural electrical impulses produced by your heart. These impulses usually follow a certain sequence. A change in the normal sequence is called an arrhythmia. When your heart beats

What the Numbers of Our Blood Pressure Mean

When we are told that our blood pressure is within the normal range, we usually sigh with relief and vaguely remember the two numbers involved. But what do they mean?

Most blood pressure readings are stated as one number over another number; for example, 120 over 72. The first number is the measure of systolic pressure, which is the pressure of the blood in the arteries when the heart beats and fills them with blood. The second number is the diastolic pressure, which is the pressure of the blood in the arteries between heart beats. The first number is always larger than the second.

There is great variability in the blood pressure of individuals, depending on age and other factors. That is why blood pressure is evaluated in terms of an acceptable range of numbers rather than one acceptable number.

What the numbers tell us is very important—the higher the number, the more difficult it is for the blood to flow through the body. Most adults are said to have high blood pressure, or hypertension, if the first number is 140 or greater or the second number is over 90 or greater. Within certain limits, the lower your blood pressure reading the better. Optimal blood pressure with respect to cardiovascular risk is less than 120/80. However, unusually low readings should be evaluated to rule out medical causes. If your blood pressure is less than 90/60 you should ask your health care provider to check it.

less than 60 beats per minute (bradycardia) or more than 100 beats per minute (tachychardia), you are experiencing an arrhythmia. The duration of such episodes and the speed of the heartbeat determine whether the condition is serious. Some episodes are so short that we may just feel a slight flutter. Longer episodes may cause more permanent damage. Sometimes the electrical signature will show signs of an old or new heart attack or excessive strain on the heart. An EKG will document the kind of electrical signature that your heart produces.

Echocardiogram (or Echo)

A wand producing sound waves is passed over the chest area. As the sound waves bounce off the heart, they produce a picture of the heart on a screen. The picture shows the structure and size of the heart, the movement of the valves, the beating of the heart, and other vital information.

The MUGA (Multigated Graft Acquisition) Scan Exercise Thallium Scintigraphy

In this category of diagnostics, the functioning of the heart is measured by tracking the movement of radionuclides injected into the bloodstream of the patient. The movement is tracked on a monitor showing computer-generated pictures. The images provide details about how the different chambers of the heart are working and how well blood is reaching the heart muscle. In women, breast tissues may create shadows that make the images harder to interpret, thereby lessening the test's accuracy.

Coronary Angiography (Cardiac Catheterization and Angiogram)

Undeniably this can be an unpleasant procedure. If you need this procedure, make sure that your health care provider has performed it on women many times before.

Cardiac catheterization is done in a hospital. A physician cleans and numbs an area where there is a major artery, usually the inner thigh or an arm, and then makes an opening in the skin. The next step involves slowly inserting a thin plastic tube into the opening and guiding it through the artery until it reaches the arteries that supply blood to the heart.

A dye, visible in x-rays, is injected through the catheter and released in the arteries of the heart. By watching on a monitor how the dye travels, it is possible to see where there is blockage. A picture called an angiogram can thus be obtained.

If an angiogram is being done to investigate the size of arteries in individuals with angina, the cardiologist will often decide to perform a therapeutic procedure called angioplasty with stent placement. In this procedure a balloon is used to dilate an area of narrowing and a plastic stent is inserted to prevent the narrowing from reappearing. Sometimes there is too much blockage for angioplasty to clear, and other therapies then must be considered, including surgery (see below).

The Heart's Collateral Circulation

Evidence suggests that in addition to the major arteries of the heart, some people can develop a secondary system of microscopic arteries around an area of blockage. It is unclear what causes these vessels to be generated or to open, thereby creating a natural bypass around the blockage.

This process may be a key factor in the development of new treatments for heart disease. Preliminary research suggests that the condition that causes chest pain (angina) may stimulate the growth of these vessels. Unfortunately, most current diagnostic tests do not yet have the capacity to measure this system.

Talk to your provider about whether you are a good candidate for angioplasty. Women with weak or brittle arteries, such as diabetics, are not good candidates. If your health care provider thinks you are a good candidate for catheterization, be sure that when the diagnostic procedure (angiogram) is done, the cardiologist is prepared to decide on the spot whether your condition can be treated by performing angioplasty at the same time. Unfortunately, sometimes the possibility of doing the two procedures simultaneously is not offered, for a variety of reasons that should be unacceptable to you (e.g., scheduling, the provider available does not know both procedures, reluctance to ask for a specialist to stand by).

Treatment

In and of itself, treatment does not necessarily mean that you will feel better or even be able to return to your old level of activity. You must carefully discuss with your health care provider what the consequence of each treatment will be for you.

For some people, medication combined with changes in diet and lifestyle improves the way the heart functions. For others, surgery has provided a new, more energetic lease on life. In some instances the result of a treatment may not provide the quality of life that a patient might have expected.

Especially when it comes to the surgical alternatives for treatment, you should know what the success rate of a given procedure is for women and preferably for Latinas of an age similar to yours. Health care providers are obligated to discuss this information with you in order to obtain your informed consent. Make sure they explain it to you in a way you can understand. You are the one who must decide if the quality of life you can expect after surgery is worth the risk involved in the treatment.

Coronary Heart Disease, Coronary Artery Disease, and High Blood Pressure

Coronary heart disease (CHD) and coronary artery disease (CAD) are the terms used to describe heart and blood vessel disease. The end result of these problems can be a heart attack (myocardial infarction, or MI). This occurs when part of the heart does not receive blood (ischemia). The longer the blood is blocked from getting to the heart, the greater the likelihood that the heart will suffer irreversible damage.

For those of us who have high blood pressure, the most important thing to remember is that high blood pressure can damage the arteries of the brain and heart. This damage occurs over the course of many years. It is also essential to remember that it is possible to have dangerously high blood pressure and not to have any physical awareness of it. That's why it is often called the "silent killer." This damage can be completely prevented by keeping the blood pressure in a normal range by exercise, maintaining a healthy weight, meditation, and if necessary medications.

Some Latinas have high blood pressure, and others have heart disease. Some have both. Because heart disease and high blood pressure are interrelated, you will be given a similar three-part strategy to improve your heart: medication, nutrition and exercise, and stress management. The specifics of each strategy are determined by the health care provider and the patient working together closely to determine which combination works best.

Nonsurgical Solutions

1: Medication. There are many medications that can be used to lower high blood pressure. Medications that reduce blood pressure are called antihypertensives.

Each of the medications has a specific goal, which will improve how the heart and circula-

Warning

While we may think we know how we feel when our blood pressure is high, there are times when blood pressure is high and there are no symptoms. Make sure to take medication to control your blood pressure regardless of how you may feel. It could save your life.

tory system functions: diuretics reduce the amount of excess water and salt in the body; beta blockers reduce the heart rate; sympathetic nerve inhibitors reduce the constriction of blood vessels; vasodilators relax the blood vessels; angiotensin-converting enzyme (ACE) inhibitors block the production of the chemical that causes the blood vessels to constrict; calcium antagonists reduce the heart rate and relax the blood vessels.

MYTHS AND FACTS

Myth: Latinas can feel when they have heart disease.

Fact: Sometimes the symptoms of heart disease are so mild that even a heart attack may go unnoticed.

Myth: If you have high blood pressure you will have a heart attack.

Fact: The relationship between high blood pressure and heart attack is unclear.

Myth: If you have a heart attack you cannot have sex for at least 6 months.

Fact: Your health care provider will tell you when you may have sex again. It may be as soon as a few weeks after your heart attack.

Myth: Drinking red wine will prevent heart disease.

Fact: Regular exercise and eating healthy meals are the best way to prevent heart disease.

If a person is having a heart attack, federal guidelines for care recommend that within 30 minutes of arrival in the emergency room, eligible patients receive one of the "clot-buster" drugs tissue plasminogen activator (TPA) or streptokinase (brand names Activase and Streptase). These drugs are called thrombolytics. When given promptly, they dissolve a blood clot and thus reduce damage to the heart. For these revolutionary drugs to work, you must get to the emergency room quickly. Certain underlying conditions, as well as delayed arrival in the emergency room, make some patients ineligible for thrombolytics.

After a heart attack, your health care provider will work with you to select the best medicine for your situation. The biggest mistake most of us make is to stop taking our medication when we feel better. It is critical that we take medication as directed for it to be fully effective.

2: Nutrition and Exercise. Many persons, especially those with hypertension or heart failure, are told to reduce the amount of sodium in their diet. The first step is not to add salt to any of the foods we cook or eat. The second is to practice good nutrition (see Chapter 19).

If we are overweight, weight loss will also help reduce the stress on our heart and may even reduce our blood pressure (see Chapter 20). Moderate physical activity is also considered an important part of a treatment plan to help strengthen the heart and control high blood pressure (see Chapter 21).

If your cholesterol level is high you will be advised on dietary ways to reduce it. If your cholesterol level remains too high despite dietary efforts, you may be advised to take medication to reduce the cholesterol level. The most commonly used medications for this today are called "statins."

I take bubble baths. Wherever I go, whomever I visit, I always make sure that I pack bubble bath

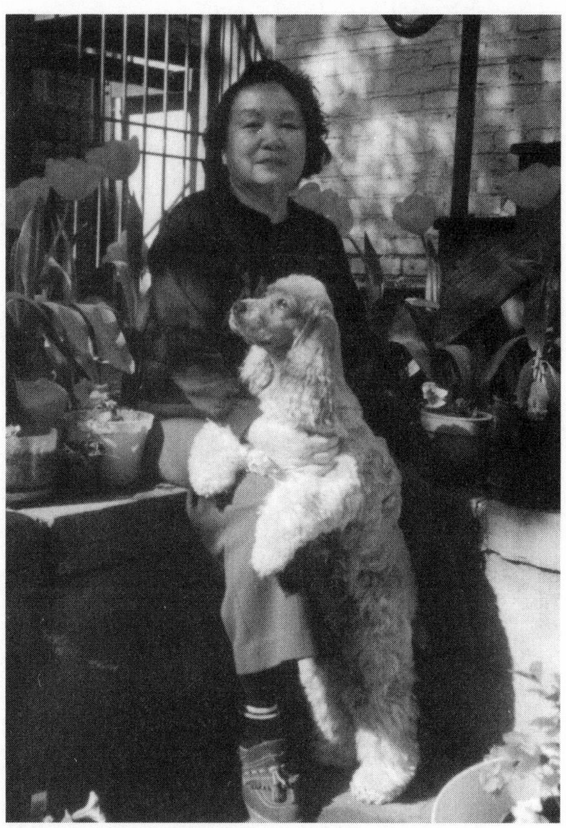

Keep active and exercise—just walking your dog is good for your heart.

and some reading. It makes me feel good to just soak and read a book.

I don't know when I started to do this. I do know that when I take my bubble bath, no matter what went on in the day, I just let it go.

—*Guadalupe, 54*

3: Stress Management. Latinas appear to cope well, but that does not mean we are actually doing well. Too often we bear the burden of all the concerns in our families, and we must learn to manage that. To find emotional and spiritual release, as well as ways to replenish ourselves, is an essential part of controlling our high blood pressure. Recent research indicates that mental stress is associated with higher rates of heart attacks. Thus the reduction of mental stress is essential.

Some women may join a church prayer group; others may just want to stay home and read. Whatever you do, it should be an activity that relaxes your mind and renews your spirit. One Latina said that knowing she had heart disease made her recognize her own vulnerability and redirect her efforts for the benefit of her community.

Each one of us has to define stress management in our own terms. After all, this is something that must resonate with our inner selves, and only we know what those needs are.

Interventional Solutions to Coronary Heart Disease and Coronary Artery Disease

Once you have been diagnosed with ischemic heart disease, the first choice may be to pursue the solutions described above. When these have not been successful, you may be referred to a surgeon, who may offer a surgical solution. These are discussed below.

1: Angioplasty. Angioplasty, commonly known as the balloon procedure, is usually done along with an angiogram. In this medical procedure, after the catheter has been guided into the coronary arteries, it serves as a tunnel that allows a second smaller catheter with a deflated balloon tip to be inserted through it. When the second catheter reaches the blocked area, it is inflated so that it can compress the material causing the blockage and thus widen the space. A plastic stent is then placed to prevent the artery from closing up again.

While angioplasty is less traumatic than coronary bypass surgery, there is always a concern that the procedure will have to be repeated again, because the buildup will sometimes recur even with a stent. If angioplasty does not work, you might be directed to having coronary bypass surgery. In contrast to surgery, most people go home on the same day after an angioplasty procedure.

When considering angioplasty, one of the most important factors is how often and how successfully your physician has performed this procedure.

> *Consejos*
>
> There are new, less invasive surgical ways to heal the heart. Recent research suggests that, using new instruments, heart surgery may be done with only a 3-inch opening in the chest. By April of 1997 nearly 1,500 patients had undergone this procedure.

2: Coronary bypass.

It was the day before her surgery. Estela's cardiologist had spent time talking to her about how she would recuperate after the surgery. He told her that she would have some discomfort when she came out of surgery, but in the end she would feel better.

Estela listened with great interest as her doctor explained how they would take a good vein from her leg and put it into her heart so that the blood would flow easily again. She knew that bypass surgery was a fairly common procedure. Some of her friends' husbands had had it, and they were all feeling better than they had before. She took in each word the doctor said and considered it carefully as she tried to understand what was going to happen the next day.

Later that night, Estela lay in bed thinking about what her surgery would be like. She gently placed her hands against her chest. She knew where her heart was—there, under her left breast—but when she pressed down, all she could feel was bone. She pushed down harder on her chest and poked it with her fingers. Yes, bone—that is what she could feel.

As she lay there, she tried to understand how her cardiologist would get down to where her heart was. All she knew was that her heart was under the bone.

There has been a lot of medical experience with coronary bypass surgery. The problem is that most (70 percent) of that experience is with men, and with men who are younger than most of the women who undergo the procedure. This is major surgery—it takes several hours and involves cutting through the chest bones, being on a mechanical heart-lung machine during surgery, and needing physical as well as emotional support afterward.

In this type of surgery, a healthy blood vessel is removed from one part of your body (leg or chest) and reattached (grafted) to your heart so as to reroute the blood around the blocked area. The number of times a rerouting or bypass is needed depends on the type and number of blockages you have. It may be a single, double, triple, or quadruple bypass.

Women are twice as likely as men are to die from bypass surgery. When women survive the surgery, their long-term survival is the same as men's, even though it is likely that they will have more complications. There has been no study focusing on the outcomes for Latinas.

This type of surgery is followed by a difficult recovery period, and women who undergo it should be prepared to need some assistance for several weeks.

3: Valve repair or replacement. Sometimes a heart valve does not close (insufficiency). This allows blood to flow in the wrong direction (regurgitation or leakage) and places strain on the heart. Other times, a valve cannot open all the way (stenosis). This also puts a strain on your heart. Your surgeon may recommend a valve repair or replacement. Artificial valves are made of plastic or metal or specially adapted from a pig's heart valve.

This procedure is much more than switching parts; it is major heart surgery. It is essential that you discuss the various options with your cardiologist and surgeon before deciding whether this is a course you want to pursue.

4: Pacemaker implants. If your heart is not producing the necessary electrical impulses to function properly, your health care provider may recommend that a pacemaker be implanted. For some patients it may be desirable to implant an automatic defibrillator, which generates an electrical shock when it detects a problem with the heartbeat (e.g., very rapid heartbeat). Your cardiologist and surgeon will help you determine what will make your heart work best.

5: Heart transplant. When neither medicine, lifestyle changes, nor other surgical options have been successful, your surgeon may recommend that you have a heart transplant. A heart transplant is therapy for end-stage heart failure, and it is effective in some cases. This may be a viable option for you to consider. This procedure is extremely difficult, and there is very little information on the success of the procedure with women. Outcomes vary with different centers and surgeons. Make sure to get information on the outcomes for Latinas.

Mind and Spirit

I know it sounds silly, but since my mom died I think I have gotten heart disease. At first I thought I was being a hypochondriac or overly dramatic. But the feelings are real, and I am too embarrassed to share them with anyone. Whenever I get very upset, I seem to have this ache in my chest. It is on the left side, beneath my breast.

When my mom had surgery, I know that is where they did one of her grafts. And now I find that I have pain in the same area when something happens that wounds me deeply. Somehow the spiritual or emotional pain that I tell myself I am handling is making this ache in my chest.

And after so many times, I know it is too real to be something I just imagine or that is only in my head. At the same time I have learned that closing my eyes and focusing on the good things in life helps the pain go away.

—*Juanita, 44*

We must learn to take care of our mind and our spirit. The electrical impulses that control the heartbeat are only one part of the heart. Our heart is controlled also by how we feel.

Death is a natural part of life. Our spiritual and religious life tells us that. Thus to be told that heart disease is the number one cause of death for Latinas should not so much alarm us as inform us. There are ways to make our heart and the system it supports work better and be healthier longer. We need to rethink how to live.

The heart is at the center of our being, and if we are to take care of our heart, we must take care of our mind and our spirit. Many of the strategies for getting beyond *aguantando* (see Chapter 1) need to be a part of any heart disease prevention program. Knowing how to set limits on the burdens we take on is also important to our mental health.

With respect to our spirit, we have to focus on our faith as a source of joy and understanding. Harboring anger, rancor, or other negative feelings will only have a detrimental effect on the health of our heart.

We must learn to do these things not only when we know we have heart disease but wherever possible, as a means of preventing heart disease. A healthy spirit (see Chapter 2) is essential to a heart that functions at its best.

Summary

To have a healthy heart, we know that it is good not to smoke, not to add salt to our food, to keep our weight at a moderate level, to exercise regularly, and to reduce our intake of fat. While there are specific guidelines for taking care of the physical aspect of our heart, we must also nourish our emotional and spiritual heart.

But sometimes there are signs that our heart is not doing so well. Several diagnostic tests are available to help identify the nature of the problem and to help point the patient and health care provider in the right direction for treatment. There are a variety of treatments available for hypertension and heart disease, all of which include some combination of medication, diet, exercise, and stress management tailored to the patient.

In more advanced cases of heart disease, surgery may be required. The choice of surgical intervention is made by the cardiologist, surgeon, and patient working together to develop a treatment plan that promises the most success.

RESOURCES

Organizations

Alliance for Aging Research
2021 K Street NW, Suite 305
Washington, DC 20006
(202) 293-2856
www.agingresearch.org

American Heart Association, National Center
7272 Greenville Avenue
Dallas, TX 75231-4596
(800) 242-8721
www.americanheart.org
www.women.americanheart.org

National Heart, Lung, and Blood Institute Information Center
P.O. Box 30105
Bethesda, MD 20824-0105
(301) 592-8573
www.nhlbi.nih.gov

National Institute on Aging Information Center
P.O. Box 8057
Gaithersburg, MD 20898-8057
(800) 222-2225 or (301) 496-1752
www.nih.gov/nia

National Women's Health Network
514 10th Street NW, Suite 400
Washington, DC 20004
(202) 347-1140
www.womenshealthnetwork.org

Hotline

(888) My Heart (694-3278)
Information for women regarding heart disease and stroke.

Su-Familia Family Health Helpline
National Alliance for Hispanic Health
866-SuFamilia (783-2645)

Books

Cambre, Suzanne. *Lady Killer: Heart Disease. Women at Risk*. Atlanta: Pritchet & Hull Associates, 1995.

Diethrich, Edward B., and Carol Cohan. *Women and Heart Disease: What You Can Do to Stop the Number-One Killer of American Women*. New York: Ballantine, 1994.

Legato, Marianne J. *The Female Heart: The Truth about Women and Coronary Artery Disease*. New York: Avon, 2000.

Pashkow, Frederic J., and Charlotte Libov. *The Women's Heart Book: The Complete Guide to Keeping Your Heart Healthy and What to Do If Things Go Wrong*. New York: Dutton, 1993.

Publications and Pamphlets

"Activity After a Heart Attack," 1997. Pamphlet No. 1528. AAFP Family Health Facts series. American Academy of Family Physicians, 11400 Tomahawk Creek Pkwy, Leawood, KS 66211-2672; (800) 994-0000. Other titles include "High Blood Pressure," 1993. Pamphlet No. 1541.

"La Angina de Pecho Inestable." Pamphlet No. 94-0605 (also available in English). Agency for Health Care Research and Quality; (800) 358-9295. Other titles include:

"What You Should Know about Stroke Prevention." Fact Sheet.

"Heart Failure Patient Guide."

"La Insuficiencia Cardíaca." Pamphlet No. 94-0615 (also available in English).

"Caring for Your Heart," 2000. National Alliance for Hispanic Health, 1501 16th Street NW, Washington, D.C. 20015; 202-387-5000 (also available in Spanish).

"The Healthy Heart Handbook for Women," 1992. NIH Publication No. 92-2720. National Heart, Lung and Blood Institute, P.O. Box 30105, Bethesda, MD 20824-0705; (301) 592-8573. Other titles include "Heart Disease and Women: So You Have Heart Disease," September 1995. NIH Publication No. 95-2645.

"Silent Epidemic: The Truth about Women and Heart Disease." American Heart Association National Center, 7972 Greenville Avenue, Dallas, TX 75231-4596; (800) 242-8721; www.women.americanheart.org. Materials in Spanish are also available.

16

HIV/AIDS

Margarita had known for a long time that her marriage was not the best, but she also felt she did not have the freedom to leave Patrick. After all, they had two children, whom they loved, and more important, she knew that the children would never understand. And if she were to leave Patrick, she knew her family would never accept it.

So she had stayed with Patrick. As the children grew up, she knew that with time she would eventually leave Patrick, and eventually she did. Still, she could not help but feel sad at the way things ended.

To make matters worse, everyone said how bad Patrick looked and how obvious it was that he needed her. He had always been thin, but now he was getting thinner. In addition, his drinking had gotten worse. But she was not living with him anymore. Of course, she was still his wife, but now she could have that little bit of solace that she had needed for so many years. She was finally at peace with herself. Her apartment was only one room with a kitchen in a closet, but it was hers and she could enjoy it.

Then one evening the phone rang. It was about Patrick. He was in the emergency room, and he had said that she was his wife. Margarita rushed to see him, answer questions, fill out what seemed like endless forms, and then she waited. All night long, while the hospital personnel tried to control his life signs, she wondered what had happened to him this time that he had gotten so sick.

She shook her head at the sadness—too many years of smoking cigarettes and drinking beer. She leaned back in the chair, sighed, and rested her head against the wall. Even sitting she needed support to get through this night.

In the morning, when the physician on duty came looking for her, he had only one question to ask: "Why didn't you tell us your husband was HIV positive?" As soon as the words left his lips, the doctor realized he had made a mistake. The expression on Margarita's face revealed that she had not known.

There is never a way to be prepared for what happens when HIV/AIDS strikes in our lives. Too often Latinas think of AIDS as something that happens to gay white men. Yet the numbers, the research, and the many Latina lives that have been touched by HIV/AIDS tell a very different story.

Warning

According to the Centers for Disease Control, most Latinas who are HIV positive have been infected by having sex with a man they did not know was HIV positive. Most Latinas who are HIV positive are married and monogamous.

We may want to bury our heads and think, not us, not me, not my friends. But if you look around you, it is obvious that HIV/AIDS is a concern for Latinas—not only as mothers, sisters, and friends of persons who are HIV positive, but also because we ourselves have become infected with HIV.

Since the early 1980s, when the Centers for Disease Control began to track what would later be known as HIV/AIDS, Hispanics have been overrepresented among the cases. Moreover, the proportion of Latinas who are HIV positive has increased steadily. Not only are the numbers growing, but the magnitude is dramatic. In 1993 *Women and the AIDS Epidemic: An impending Crisis for the Americas* was published by the Pan American Health Organization. In 2000 Latinas represented only 12 percent of the general population but fully 20 percent of women with AIDS, and the situation is getting worse.

High-Risk Behaviors

In the early days of HIV/AIDS, public health officials talked about groups at high risk for HIV/AIDS. It was easier to say that HIV/AIDS happened to those people in those communities. And we found it comforting to tell ourselves that those people were not our men, not our community, and certainly not Latinas.

We know better today. Everyone is at risk for HIV/AIDS. And it is not being a member of a certain group that puts one at high risk for HIV/AIDS but engaging in certain behaviors.

The HIV/AIDS prevention message is still very difficult to communicate for several reasons. First, most of the behaviors that increase the likelihood of being exposed to HIV are either private sexual behaviors or behaviors that are illegal (injecting illegal drugs and sharing needles) and are therefore not openly discussed.

Second, since we are dealing with private behaviors, the accuracy of what people say about their HIV status and their risks to you may be questionable. Many persons either don't know their status or deny that they engage in activities that put them at risk. In other words, people either do not know or they lie.

Finally, it is difficult to admit that we have HIV/AIDS concerns when we know that our

Preventing Exposure to HIV

1. Do not engage in activities through which your blood may come into contact with someone else's blood. This means that you should not engage in:
   - Unprotected vaginal-penile intercourse
   - Unprotected anal-penile intercourse
   - Unprotected oral-penile sex
   - The sharing of needles during ear piercing, body piercing, or injecting drugs (legal or illegal)
2. Use a condom and use it correctly. If you feel uncomfortable talking to your partner about using a condom, ask yourself why you feel comfortable having sex with him.
3. Share information about HIV/AIDS with your family and friends.

family and friends disapprove of our sexual practices or our intimacy with men and women who share needles when injecting drugs.

To make matters worse, early HIV/AIDS education sometimes took a negative moral tone and used the opportunity to judge people's behavior while ignoring the reality of how people live their lives. The messages were "Do not be promiscuous" and "Do not inject drugs." Another approach was to address the lives of real people: "Have only safe sex" and "Do not share needles." Remarkably, all the while, the messages that were being transmitted about HIV/AIDS still left out Latinas.

How were Latinas to talk about *safe* sex when many of us did not even talk about *sex*? We may do it, but we do not talk about it. And if we do talk about it, we talk to other Latinas but not to our male partners. Moreover, for many of us, using a condom evoked any number of taboos. Some of us felt that it conflicted with our religious beliefs, while others felt that a man only used a condom when he was with a "dirty" woman. The idea that perhaps the man she was sexually intimate with might be the carrier of HIV/AIDS would not be considered by a woman who was brought up to trust and obey the men in her life. To complicate matters, even if you could gather the courage to ask, how could you force a man to use a condom?

Many Latinas still sidestep the issue of sharing needles. How are we going to get our partners or ourselves to stop sharing needles? Of course, these are all relatively private events, and for us Latinas, what is private stays private.

We are still wrestling with these issues while the number of Latinas exposed to HIV continues to rise. In many ways, HIV/AIDS has forced us to have the discussions that *costumbre* (custom) and tradition may have silenced. However, when it comes to HIV/AIDS, it is important for us to know the facts. Our lives and the lives of our families may depend on it.

Consejos

Condom Sense Can Save Your Life

How many of these have you done?

1. Bought some condoms.
2. Taken condoms out of the wrapper and looked at them.
3. Unrolled a condom onto your finger and focused on what it felt like.
4. Long before you made the commitment to engage in sexual activity, talked to your partner about using a condom.
5. When you both decided to have sex, made sure that you had condoms within easy reach.
6. Said, "No, thank you" to someone who claimed to love you but wanted to have unprotected vaginal-penile sex or penile-anal sex.
7. Found ways to incorporate condom use into sexual foreplay.
8. Decided to wait before having sex with someone until you were more certain about the person's history.
9. Decided not to have sex with someone because neither of you had condoms.

If you are sexually active and answered "yes" to less than 5 of the actions above, you do not have condom sense and are probably engaging in high-risk behavior.

Diagnosis

Angela could trace it back to Steve.

She had first met Steve three years ago. He was a good-looking man. He had a good job, and as her mother would say, he looked muy limpio *(very clean). Angela felt she knew everything about him. He had been so honest, telling her about his troubled youth, his family, and even about the many sexual partners he had had. And he let her know how special she was to him. After a while they began to make love regularly. She really loved him and was looking forward to building a life with him.*

Sometimes, however, things do not seem to work out. Angela found him becoming distant, and one day he just disappeared. She was sad, but she kept hoping that he would come to terms with whatever was bothering him and return. Months went by, however, and eventually she stopped thinking about him.

Recently she had begun having trouble sleeping. And even though she was no longer having sex with anyone, she was getting more frequent yeast infections. After trying some of the medicines that usually helped with her yeast infections, she consulted her health care provider, who ran a series of tests.

Soon afterward she learned the truth. She had tested positive for HIV. Fear gripped her—would she get AIDS?—and with the fear, the realization: it had to have been Steve.

A woman has AIDS when she is HIV positive and has at least one of the following:

- One or more life-threatening opportunistic infections;
- A blood test that shows a CD4 count of less than 200 (see "What HIV Does," page 244);
- An AIDS-related cancer, severe wasting, or dementia, e.g., invasive cervical cancer;
- Severe ulcers in her genital area from herpes simplex.

Acquired immune deficiency syndrome (AIDS) is the name given to a cluster of illnesses that result from having been exposed to the human immunodeficiency virus (HIV). These illnesses develop because the immune system—our body's mechanism for fighting off infections and some types of cancer—can no longer do its job. As a result, the body becomes vulnerable to a variety of illnesses caused by viruses, bacteria, parasites, and fungi.

These illnesses are called opportunistic infections. For many years, the diagnosis of AIDS focused on the illnesses that were most common. Because most of the persons with AIDS were men, there was only slight interest in what was happening to women who were HIV positive. It was not until January 1993 that the Centers for Disease Control expanded the definition of opportunistic illnesses to include a disease process specific to women, which includes invasive cervical cancer.

When a person is first exposed to HIV, there are no symptoms. And this can go on for quite a while. Today the average is ten years without a major symptom. As time passes, the first symptoms for women are similar to those of men—aches and pains, fevers, sore throat from swollen glands. As the immune system becomes weaker, Latinas have Pap smears that are abnormal, yeast infections that are frequent and/or do not seem to respond to treatment, or cases of herpes that are very severe. Latinas also begin to acquire the other symptoms common in persons who have HIV in their system: night sweats; rapid weight loss; dry cough that does not go away; swelling of the lymph nodes by the neck, armpits, and groin; swollen joints; and unexplained fever.

In the most advanced stages of AIDS, it is likely that Latinas will also get pneumonia. The pneumonia that men get, pneumocystis carinii pneumonia (PCP), is rare among persons who do not have AIDS. Women who have AIDS get PCP and, more often than men, bacterial pneumonia. Bacterial pneumonias are more common in the general population. Three or more bacterial pneumonias within one year in a person with HIV is an AIDS-defining diagnosis. Over time, for both men and women, there is increasing deterioration as the disease progresses and the body cannot fight off opportunistic infections.

Transmission

In order to get AIDS, a person must come into direct, blood-to-blood contact with the human immunodeficiency virus (HIV). Technically, HIV is a difficult virus to transfer from one person to another. It is not airborne and cannot survive on its own. It is not passed by casual contact—shaking hands or sharing utensils. It is passed by blood, semen, and through an HIV-positive mother's milk to her baby. Although HIV is found in saliva, it is not passed in saliva.

What HIV Does

HIV is considered a retrovirus because it reproduces itself using the enzyme called reverse transcriptase. When HIV enters the body, it infects the CD4 cells, also called T cells or T lymphocytes, whose function is to fight off infection and certain kinds of cancer. When HIV moves into a CD4 cell, it begins to reproduce itself using parts of the CD4 cell. Over time HIV uses so much of the CD4 cell that it kills it. In the meantime, it has reproduced itself many times.

Once we are infected, our immune system kicks in and tries to fight off the invading HIV by making antibodies. Unlike most other viruses, however, HIV is able to hide from these antibodies by taking on different disguises. While most viruses are recognizable, HIV is a quick-change artist with the ability to change its outer protein shell.

Over time the immune system cannot keep up with HIV. As the immune system gets weaker, the body becomes vulnerable to opportunistic infections.

HIV Tests—Diagnosis and Treatment

Diagnosis of HIV is based on a blood test. You can be tested in the privacy of your home using a home test kit, by your health care provider, or without cost by some local health departments. Some sites offer anonymous testing (blood is taken and you are assigned a number) or confidential testing (information is kept confidential but in many instances may be reported to a medical records service). Each method provides some degree of confidential counseling for persons who test positive.

Following are the two principle tests used to diagnose HIV.

- The enzyme-linked immunoabsorbent assay (ELISA) test indicates whether your body has produced the antibody that signals the presence of HIV. The term *seroconversion* is used to describe the point at which the new antibody is produced. Because HIV is a very special virus, it can take up to a year for seroconversion to occur, but most people (95 percent) produce the antibody within the first six weeks after exposure. The results from this test are available within several hours.

- The Western Blot test is more sophisticated and is given after a positive result on an ELISA. It is considered a confirming test.

Viral load testing is used for monitoring response to treatment and is not approved by the FDA for diagnosis of HIV. Viral load testing calculates the amount of HIV present in the blood by measuring how much HIV genetic material (i.e., RNA) is present. It was not until the late 1990s that this test became available. Recent research indicates that it is essential to measure the change in viral load on an ongoing basis in an individual who has been diagnosed with HIV/AIDS. The goal of anti-HIV treatment is to keep the load as low as possible.

Consejos

The medication regimen for HIV/AIDS is not only complex but evolving. It is a good idea to make certain that your health care provider either specializes in HIV/AIDS or has access to others who do.

Treatment

Currently there is no cure for AIDS. What we have accumulated in a relatively short time is a pantry filled with medicines to (1) reduce the viral load and (2) treat the opportunistic infections that occur when someone is HIV positive. Some of these medicines are taken to prevent illness; others are taken to treat illness.

The treatment of HIV/AIDS has been improving over time. The medicines of the late 1980's brought us a family of reverse transcriptase inhibitors (so that HIV cannot reproduce) called nucleoside analogs. By the mid 1990's there were protease inhibitors (inhibits the production of protease—an enzyme that HIV needs to duplicate) and a new kind of reverse transcriptase inhibitors called non-nucleoside analogs. The combination of these powerful medicines resulted in the triple drug combination of highly active antiretroviral therapy (HAART) or "cocktail" therapy.

HAART has been the most effective therapy available even though it is a strict and complicated sequence of pills (as many as 21 in a day) that must be taken at specific times of the day. HAART usually requires a daily assortment of medicines that include one protease inhibitor and two other drugs that are reverse transcriptase inhibitors. The most commonly used medicines are listed below.

These are all very strong and relatively new medicines. AZT, which is the oldest medicine for the treatment of AIDS, seems to be associated with higher rates of liver disease in women who take it. At the same time, women who are HIV infected and pregnant and take a combination therapy reduce the risk of transmission to their baby to less than 5 percent. In more advanced stages of HIV the risk to the baby is greater. Moreover, even though the babies may have antibodies for HIV, they do not always develop the virus itself. It is not clear how this happens. It is suggested that these babies be seen by a health care provider at two weeks of life, monthly through six months, and every three months thereafter through the age of two years. Health care providers pay special attention to the early physical findings of pediatric HIV.

Suffice it to say, we are just learning how to monitor the effects of these medicines. There is only minimal information on the effect of these drugs on women.

Reverse transcriptase inhibitors nucleoside analogs (NRTIs)	non-nucleoside analogs (NNRTIs)	**Protease inhibitors** (PIs)
AZT, Retrovir® (zidovudine)	Rescriptor® (delavirdine)	Agenerase™ (amprenivir)
ddi, Videx® (didanosine)	Sustiva™ (efavirenz)	Crixivan® (indinavir)
ddc, Hivid® (zalcitabine)	Viramune® (nevirapine)	Fortovase™ (saquinavir)
d4T, Zerit® (stavudine)		Invirase™ (saquinavir)
3TC (lamivudine)		Norvir™ (ritonavir)
Ziagen™ (abacavir)		Viracept® (nelfinavir)

Until the late 1990s, the focus in the management of HIV/AIDS was on the number of CD4 cells. When the CD4 cell count fell below 300, the risk for opportunistic infections increased, and therefore more aggressive treatment was necessary. Now that there is viral load testing, treatment can be adjusted more accurately according to the viral load.

This is a critical part of monitoring the effect of the new drug cocktails, which combine protease inhibitors with the older medications. Your viral load will be monitored every three to four months. Since it is relatively new, it will take a few years to see how HAART impacts on the health of women, including Latinas, who are HIV positive.

We know very little about how most drugs work in women because it was not until April 1, 1993, that the Food and Drug Administration issued guidelines that all new drugs had to be evaluated in women as well as men.

Clinical Trials: Are They for You?

Clinical trials offer you an opportunity to have your health monitored free and to be part of advancing the science of HIV/AIDS management. These are facts about clinical trials that you should consider.

- Women, and especially Latinas, are less likely to be part of a clinical trial than men.
- If your health care provider is a public institution, you are even less likely to be part of a clinical trial.
- What happens in a clinical trial can vary greatly. You may be given a new drug, a placebo (sugar pill), or nothing. You may feel much better or much worse (see Chapter 22).
- Whether or not you take part in a clinical trial should always be up to you.

AIDS Clinical Trials Information Service (ACTIS)

(800) TRIALS-A (800-874-2572)

ACTIS is a collaborative project of the Public Health Service, the National Institute of Allergy and Infectious Diseases, the National Library of Medicine, the Food and Drug Administration, and the Centers for Disease Control and Prevention. It provides free, up-to-date information on clinical trials that evaluate experimental drugs and other therapies for adults and children with HIV infection and AIDS. Bilingual reference specialists are available.

It is not surprising that with each new drug added to a woman's regimen of medicine there is some likelihood of a reaction that is not intended. Some drugs may combine with other drugs and become stronger when taken at the same time; others may become weaker. Since we are still learning about the impact of drugs on women, Latinas who are HIV positive need to carefully monitor how they react to the medicines they take and to share that information with their health care provider. Keeping a health journal (see Appendix B) is a good way of documenting what happens.

If you are HIV positive, one thing is certain: you will be taking an assortment of medicines and treatments that will not only lengthen your life but help you to maintain the best quality of life possible. Compared with the reality just a few short years ago, this is a big step forward.

Myths and Facts

Myth: There are cases of people who were HIV positive and over time became HIV negative.

Fact: This has occurred only in children who were born HIV positive because their mothers were HIV positive.
Myth: If I am HIV positive, I cannot travel.
Fact: You can still travel, but you have to be careful not to expose yourself to new sources of infection, because your immune system is suppressed.
Myth: Now that I am HIV positive, I can never have sex again.
Fact: Latinas who are HIV positive need to use protection to have sex with their partners (e.g., condoms or dental dams). They and their partners may also develop other ways to show love and affection that are safe and satisfying, such as massage and mutual masturbation.
Myth: There is a vaccine for HIV.
Fact: There is no vaccine for HIV. Even if one were to be discovered tomorrow, it would be too late for the thousands of Latinas who are already HIV positive.
Myth: You can get HIV when someone with HIV/AIDS sneezes near you.
Fact: No, HIV is not an airborne virus.
Myth: Someone with HIV swimming near you in a lake or pool can transmit the virus to you.
Fact: No, HIV is not a waterborne virus.
Myth: You can tell when someone is HIV positive by looking at them.
Fact: You cannot.

As knowledge about HIV has grown, so has the number of new treatments and medicines. Two pieces of advice in this regard:

- Be careful of advertising on radio or television about natural products that claim to cure AIDS.
- Do not purchase new medicines or treatments that have not yet been approved by the Food and Drug Administration. These simply put money in the pockets of unscrupulous companies that are taking advantage of HIV-positive people's desire to be HIV-free.

How to Stay Healthy

Body

1: Do not smoke. We do not understand all of the mechanisms that come into play, but we do know that smoking seems to suppress our immune system. We also know that it has a negative effect on our lungs and heart. There is no good reason to smoke, and there are a lot of good reasons to stop.

2: Eat a healthy diet; eliminate alcohol and all illegal drugs. It is important to maintain your weight. This may be harder for

Consejos

Tips to Staying Healthy If You Are HIV Positive

BODY

1. Do not smoke.
2. Eat a healthy diet; eliminate alcohol and all illegal drugs.
3. Engage in moderate exercise, and make sure you get enough rest.
4. Drink bottled or filtered water.
5. Take your medicines.
6. See your health care provider on a regular basis or when you notice some change in your body.

MIND

7. Keep informed about progress in HIV/AIDS research.
8. Keep a positive mental attitude.

SPIRIT

9. Reach out to your family and friends.
10. Renew your faith.

some of us than it is for others. If you are HIV positive, being able to maintain your weight is a sign that you are doing well. Food is the fuel that provides the energy your body needs. Since your body is fighting to make you better, you need to have a good and consistent source of energy. Eat regularly and eat well. Alcohol and illegal drugs compromise your immune system.

3: Engage in moderate exercise, and get enough rest. When we exercise, our body uses energy more efficiently. Exercise is also good at producing endorphins, which are the body's natural agents in charge of making us feel good. When we feel good, all of our systems work better. It is also important to get enough rest.

4: Drink bottled or filtered water. Unfortunately, the water supply is not as pure as it should be. To reduce the likelihood of getting an opportunistic infection, you must drink bottled or filtered water. Remember that the water from a lake, river, well, or natural spring may look clean but in most cases is not.

5: Take your medicines. Much of the care designed to manage HIV requires that you take your medicines and follow your treatment in the way they are prescribed. Keep in mind that as HIV/AIDS becomes more of a chronic disease, you will be able to enjoy your life more if you take your medications rigorously as directed.

6: See your health care provider on a regular basis or when you notice a change in your body. There are a lot of things your health care provider can do to keep you healthy. Each visit will include a physical examination, a review of medicines and vaccines that can be given to protect you, and an examination of aspects of your life that you may want to change.

It is likely that your health care provider will want to give you a tuberculosis test and a Pap smear on an annual basis to detect opportunistic infections. At variable intervals your CD4 level and viral load level will be measured. The frequency of Pap tests will be based upon your T-cell count and previous Pap results. For women with CD4 counts under 200 a Pap test is recommended every six months. Your health care provider may also want to give you some vaccines against preventable illnesses (e.g., influenza or the hepatitis B vaccine if your blood is negative to the antibody for HBV).

Your health care provider must be your partner in securing your wellness, but this can only be done if you make regular visits and provide complete information about what you have been doing. Make sure to let them know of any changes, good and bad, that you have noticed in your body.

Mind

I could never look at the AIDS quilt. After all these years it was still too painful. It never got easier.

I knew that other people had made quilts to honor and cherish those they had loved and lost. I knew that if I looked at what had become a sea of lost lives punctuated by pieces of fabric sewn together, I would be too overwhelmed.

I wondered if there would be anyone left who would make a quilt for me.

7: Keep informed about progress in HIV/AIDS research. Since the first cases of HIV/AIDS were reported, there has been much progress in what we know. We now understand more about the immune system, how it works and what happens when it does not work. The rapid pace of progress in treating many of the opportunistic infections and slowing the deterioration from HIV to AIDS has made it possible for people to live with the disease for many more years.

The resource list at the end of this section should be used regularly by you and your family.

8: Keep a positive mental attitude. There is no doubt that being HIV positive changes our life and having AIDS makes our life more difficult. But we can lessen the negative by working through our feelings.

Coping with HIV/AIDS is not a time to be the *aguantando mujer*, but rather a point in our life where we have to learn to acknowledge our fears, sadness, and even our outrage. And after we acknowledge them, we must release them. It is a time when we have to think about the importance of each day of our lives.

Spirit

9: Reach out to your family and friends. For many Latinas this is very hard. We feel guilty and worry that somehow we will give HIV to those around us, so some of us hesitate to reach out to those we love. Others of us insulate ourselves or cocoon ourselves in our own fears so that no one can touch us.

To stay healthy, we need love and affection. The positive feelings that come from our family and friends are critical to maintaining our health.

My sister, Cristina, was one of the few people I had told in the family that I was HIV positive. We had always been close and now more than ever I needed to have someone who would be there for me and my children.

Cristina would come over and help me with my food shopping. I was getting tired and really appreciated that she would come over to make dinner for us. So many times I was able to enjoy her support. It made all the difference to me to have someone who understood what was happening with me.

10: Renew your faith. Think about what you see when you go to most places of worship. There seem to be many more older women on their knees praying than younger ones. When you look at their faces, there is often a look of peace. Prayer seems to comfort

Alert: Taking Care of Yourself and Your Pet

Pets are wonderful companions and have been proven to actually help us feel better. A word of caution, however: if you are HIV positive, you must be careful that you are not exposed to the bacteria that your pet may carry. Here are some things to do so that you can continue to enjoy your pet(s).

- If you touch or handle your pet, be sure to wash your hands before eating.
- If your pet has diarrhea, do not touch the feces.
- Pets that are less than six months old should be examined by your vet for *Cryptosporidium, Salmonella,* and *Campylobacter.*
- Use heavy rubber gloves to clean aquariums.
- Avoid contact with exotic pets and reptiles.

To reduce the risk of toxoplasmosis, Latinas who are HIV positive and have cats should:

- Have someone who is neither HIV positive nor pregnant change the litter box.
- Avoid contact with cat feces.
- Keep cats indoors.
- Not allow cats to hunt.
- Not feed cats raw or undercooked meat.

In addition, it is important to control fleas to prevent the transmission of *Bartonella* infection. The Centers for Disease Control does not recommend that you test your cat for bartonellosis or toxoplasmosis.

them as they carry on with the burdens of day-to-day life. To find some of that solace or strength, some Latinas may take this as an opportunity to renew or discover their spiritual self.

One day when we were coming home from food shopping, my sister Elsa and I decided to stop by her church. It had been a long time since we had gone to church together.

We went inside. And as I walked behind my sister, I relived the early years of my life. So much had happened since then . . . school, love, marriage, divorce, and still more things in between. I shook my head in amazement, trying to understand how I had gotten where I was.

With that, I blessed myself and knelt down beside her. What else could I do?

Having AIDS in your life or in the life of those you love forces you into moments of quiet reflection and despair. It is a time when you question everything. Why are babies getting sick? Why are young women dying when they should be living? How did things get so out of control? Why me? Why us?

There is no single answer to any of these questions. For many, prayer helps them along their way. It may be that looking within ourselves we will find the answers we need.

Summary

HIV/AIDS touches all of our lives. No longer can we look at others and say that *they* are at risk for HIV/AIDS. We know that each one of us is also at risk. It is the behaviors we engage in—and the behaviors of those with whom we are most physically intimate—that put us at risk for HIV/AIDS. Remember: when you have sexual intercourse with someone, you are not only with that person, you are also with every person they have been with before you.

Today, with new ways to measure the extent of HIV in the body, there are new treatments; some are better than others. How much of this will benefit women or Latinas is still to be determined.

In the meantime, we must stick to the facts about HIV/AIDS and do all we can to keep ourselves as healthy as possible for as long as possible. What we do must heal the body, attend to the mind, and nurture the spirit.

RESOURCES

Organizations

American Red Cross-National HQ
Hispanic HIV/AIDS Education Program
8111 Gatehouse Road
Falls Church, VA 22042
(703) 206-6000
www.redcross.org/services/hss/hivaids/hispanic.html

Hispanic AIDS Forum
184 Fifth Avenue, 7th floor
New York, NY 10010
(212) 741-9797
www.hispanicfederation.org

Kaiser Family Foundation AIDS Public Information Project
2400 Sand Hill Road
Menlo Park, CA 94025
(650) 854-9400 or (800) 656-4533
www.kff.org/sections.cgi?section-hivaids

National Prevention Information Network
Centers for Disease Control
P.O. Box 6003
Rockville, MD 20849-6003
(800) 458-5231
(Call for further information on hundreds of HIV/AIDS materials and resources.)
www.cdcnpin.org

National Association of People with AIDS
1413 K Street NW, 7th floor
Washington, DC 20005
(202) 898-0414
www.napwa.org

National Minority AIDS Council
1931 13th Street NW
Washington, DC 20009-4432
(202) 483-6622
www.nmac.org

National Alliance for Hispanic Health
1501 16th Street NW
Washington, DC 20036
(202) 387-5000
www.hispanichealth.org

National Resource Center on Women and AIDS Policy
Center for Women Policy Studies
1211 Connecticut Avenue NW, Suite 312
Washington, DC 20036
(202) 872-1770
www.centerwomenpolicy.org

National Women's Health Network
514 10th Street NW, Suite 400
Washington, DC 20004
(202) 342-1140
www.womenshealthnetwork.org

Office of Minority Health Resource Center
P.O. Box 37337
Washington, DC 20013-7337
(800) 444-6472
www.omhrc.gov

Hotlines

AIDS Clinical Trials Information Service (ACTIS)
(800) 874-2572
www.actis.org

Su-Familia Family Health Helpline
National Alliance for Hispanic Health
866-SuFamilia (783-2645)

CDC National AIDS Hotline
(800) 342-2437 (English) or (800) 344-7432 (Spanish)

HIV/AIDS Treatment Information Center
(800) HIV-0440

Publications and Pamphlets

"1-800-TRIALS-A (1-800-874-2572) for the Latest Information on Clinical Trials for HIV and AIDS," How to get the most up-to-date information on treatment for those infected with HIV and AIDS. AIDS Clinical Trials Information Service, U.S. Dept. of Health and Human Services, Washington, DC: B172; (800) TRIALS-A (800-874-2572).

"AIDS-Related CMV: How to Help Yourself," NIH Publication No. 94-3718. Information for those suffering from HIV/AIDS-related cytomegalovirus (CMV). National Prevention Information Network, Centers for Disease Control, P.O. Box 6003, Rockville, MD 20849-6003; call (800) 458-5231; www.niaid.nih.gov

Other titles include:

"AIDS-Related MAC: How to Help Yourself," NIH Publication No. 94-3719. Information for those with HIV/AIDS-related *Mycobacterium avium* (MAC).

"The Brain Infection; TOXO: How to Help Yourself," NIH Publication No. 93-3326. Information for those with HIV about their risk for toxoplasmosis, a serious brain infection.

"HIV-Related TB: How to Help Yourself," NIH Publication No. 93-3327. Information for those with HIV about their risk for tuberculosis (TB).

"Infections Linked to AIDS: How to Help Yourself," NIH Publication No. 93-3324. Information about HIV and the cause of AIDS.

"The Lung Infection PCP: How to Help Yourself," NIH Publication No. 93-3325. Information for those with HIV about their risk for pneumocystic carinii pneumonia (PCP), a lung infection.

"Taking the HIV (AIDS) Test: How to Help Yourself," NIH Publication No. 95-3322. Information about HIV and the cause of AIDS.

"Testing Positive for HIV: How to Help Yourself," NIH Publication No. 93-3323. Information about HIV and the cause of AIDS.

"Como Hablar con Sus Hijos Sobre el SIDA." Sexuality Information and Education Council of the United States (SIECUS), 130 West 42nd Street, Suite 350, New York, NY 10036; (212) 819-9770. Call or order online at www.siecus.org/pubs. Spanish language materials also available.

"Cómo protegerse contra el SIDA." Publication No. 99-12965. Spanish language information on how the use of condoms can reduce the transmission of HIV/AIDS. U.S. Dept. of Health and Human Services, Public Health Service, Food and Drug Administration, Center for Devices and Radiological Health, Washington, D.C.; (800) 463-6332; www.fda.gov/oashi/abls.

"Stories of Discovery," Feb. 1999. NIH Publication No. 88-2773. Information about immunology as it relates to AIDS, allergies, asthma, and sexually transmitted diseases. Division of Research Grants, NIH, Westwood Building, Room 449, Bethesda, MD 20892. Call (800) 458-5231 or order online www.niaid.nih.gov/publications

"Facts on HIV/AIDS." Kaiser Family Foundation AIDS Public Information Project. Fact sheets on both prevention and treatment topics are available in English and Spanish by calling the Request Line, (800) 656-4533 or www.kff.org/hivaids

"HIV/AIDS: The Impact on Hispanics," 1998. National Alliance for Hispanic Health, 1501 16th Street NW, Washington, DC 20036; (202) 387-5000; www.hispanichealth.org

"HIV Infection and Women," 2000. American College of Obstetricians and Gynecologists, P.O. Box 96920, , Washington, DC 20090-6920; (800) 762-2264; www.acog.org

"Lo Que Toda Mujer Embarazada Debería Saber Acerca del VIH y el SIDA: Lo Que Puede Hacer Usted Para Tener Un Bebé Saludable." Spanish language information on HIV and AIDS for pregnant women. AIDS Treatment Information Service, Pediatric AIDS Foundation, Santa Monica, CA.; (800) 342-AIDS (English), (800) 344-7432 (Spanish); hearing impaired, TTY: (800) 243-7889, or ATIS (800) HIV-0440. Other titles include "What Every Pregnant Woman Should Know about HIV and AIDS: What You Can Do to Have a Healthy Baby."

17

Liver Disease

I was not your typical person with liver disease, but then again, perhaps I was. I had always been on the thin side, so I had assumed that the way I was feeling had to do with what I was always doing: I exercised four times a week, went to school part time, and worked at least 8 hours a day. Although I did not have children, I was devoted to my husband and family. As far as anything being wrong with my liver, I do not think I had any real symptoms.

One day I woke up feeling very tired. Not just the kind of tired that we feel when we try to do everything, mind you, but really exhausted. Perhaps because of that, instead of going grocery shopping, I decided to visit my mother.

As soon as she saw me, my mother said, "What is wrong with you? Your eyes are yellow!" I thought that was strange—I knew my apartment was dark, but I would have noticed that. I walked to the bathroom and looked at my face. My mother was right! My eyes were as yellow as a banana.

—Debbie, 26

"*Me duele el hígado*" (my liver hurts) are words some of us heard when we were growing up. It was hard to translate this into English. Saying that your head hurts or your stomach hurts is one thing. To complain that your liver hurts is quite another. And it is not a common complaint in most non-Hispanic households. The fact that we heard it in our Latino homes supports what the recent research says about Hispanics: we tend to have one of the highest rates of liver disease.

Although chronic liver disease and cirrhosis are usually listed among the top ten causes of deaths for non-Hispanic whites, in Hispanic communities liver disease is the third most common disease related to cause of death for Hispanics aged forty-five to sixty-four. The reasons for this remain unclear.

For many of us, when we think of taking care of our bodies, we think about our heart or lungs. The liver is not on our list, but it should be. Not only is the liver one of the most important organs in our bodies, it is also one that is particularly vulnerable in Latinas.

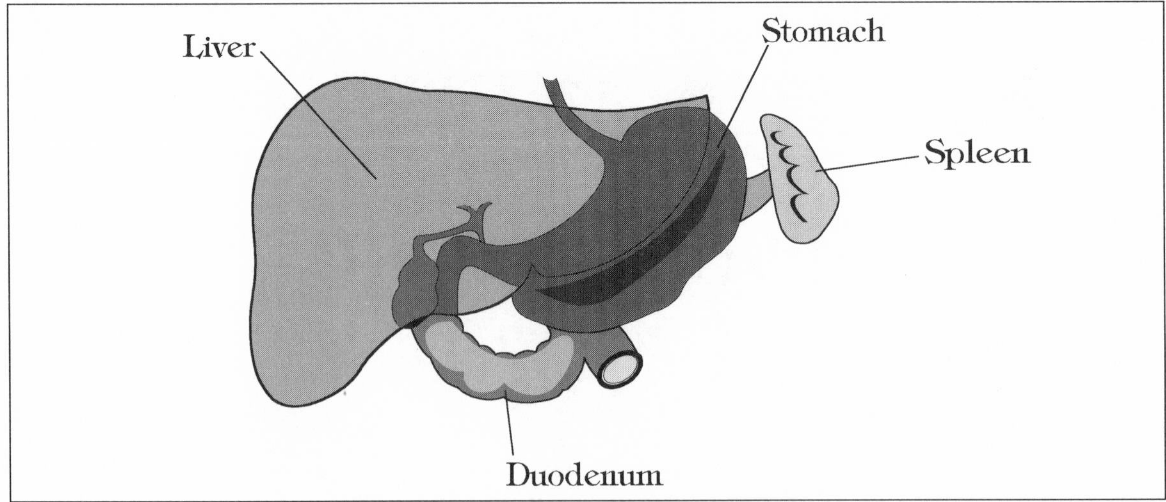

Liver

How the Liver Works

Your liver is located on the lower right side of your chest and extends from the middle of your right breast to the bottom right of your rib cage. It weighs about 3 pounds.

As the largest organ in your body, the liver is sometimes called its processing plant because of the many functions it performs in transforming everything you take in into useful products. These are some of the things the liver does:

- Manufactures new body proteins, bile, and cholesterol
- Stores vitamins, minerals, sugars, and iron
- Regulates blood clotting
- Transports fat stores
- Neutralizes and destroys toxic substances
- Metabolizes alcohol
- Cleanses the blood and removes bacteria
- Maintains hormonal balance
- To some extent, regenerates its own damaged tissue

In adults, there are two major types of liver disease: cirrhosis and viral hepatitis. In addition, autoimmune hepatitis is a special concern for women.

Cirrhosis

Cirrhosis of the liver is a medical condition in which the cells in the liver are damaged and scar tissue forms. When the liver is scarred, it loses its smooth texture and develops a crater-like appearance. This could be due to exces-

Consejos

How to Prevent Liver Disease

1. Have less than two alcoholic drinks a day.
2. Avoid taking alcohol at the same time that you are on any medication (prescription or over-the-counter drugs).
3. Maintain a healthy diet.
4. Get hepatitis B vaccine.
5. Do not share needles from body piercing, tattooing, or injecting drugs with anyone.
6. Practice safe sex.

sive drinking of alcohol as well as the existence of untreated hepatitis B and C viruses. Recent evidence indicates that hepatitis C virus ranks with alcohol as the major cause of chronic liver disease and cirrhosis.

Women seem to be more likely than men to get cirrhosis of the liver. In addition, the disease seems to be particularly aggressive in women. There is neither a cure for cirrhosis nor medication to heal the damaged liver. Treatment is limited to changes in diet, vitamins, diuretics, and total abstinence from alcohol. Transplantation of a new liver may also be considered.

Viral Hepatitis

Hepatitis is inflammation of the liver. This inflammation may be due to viruses, prolonged exposure to environmental toxins, severe reactions to drugs, excessive drinking of alcohol, schistosomiasis (a parasitic disease), immune system malfunctions, accumulation of fat in the liver, or unknown causes.

In viral hepatitis the inflammation is due to a virus. For many years it was thought that viral hepatitis was caused by either the hepatitis A virus or the hepatitis B virus. With time it became obvious that there must be other forms of viral hepatitis. Initially these were referred to as non-A, non-B hepatitis.

Progress in research has led to the identification of five major viruses that are involved in hepatitis: hepatitis A, hepatitis B, hepatitis C, hepatitis D, and hepatitis E. It is also assumed that other viruses (e.g., herpes or mononucleosis) may cause inflammation of the liver.

Routine blood tests can show if there is inflammation of the liver, and more sophisticated blood testing can usually help identify the hepatitis virus that is present. When a diagnosis is still not possible, a small amount of liver tissue will be obtained for more thorough inspection (biopsy).

What Is a Liver Biopsy?

A liver biopsy may be recommended when all other diagnostic tests are inconclusive or negative. It is the only way to diagnose autoimmune hepatitis. A liver biopsy is usually performed in a hospital. Your physician will use ultrasound to select the best place to enter your liver. A local anesthetic will be injected into the skin and surrounding area.

Your physician will insert a long needle for a few seconds and withdraw some tissue from your liver. Most people experience some pain afterward, which may spread to the right shoulder. Fortunately, the pain will last only a few hours to a few days.

The illness may come into full force all of a sudden, with an array of symptoms that is most likely to include fatigue, mild fever, muscle or joint ache, vomiting, loss of appetite, and vague abdominal pain. Some people do not have symptoms until they are in more advanced stages. There is no consistency in how long the symptoms may last: with some people they last a few weeks and with others, several months.

Each of the major kinds of viral hepatitis will be discussed below.

Hepatitis A

When I figured out that I had hepatitis, all I knew then was that it was very contagious. At first I did not tell anyone. I looked at my husband, my mom, my friends, my coworkers to see if they had any signs of illness.

I thought that if it was hepatitis I had to have gotten it from someone who had been near me. I was certain that I would be able to look at them

Consejos

Signs and Symptoms of Liver Disease

1. Abnormally yellow skin tone (jaundice)
2. Urine that is deeper and darker in color
3. Bowel movements that are consistently yellow, gray, or light-colored
4. Nausea, vomiting, and/or loss of appetite
5. Swollen stomach area
6. Itchiness all over the body that stays for a long time
7. An unintentional increase or decrease in weight of 5 percent in less than two months
8. Pain in the stomach area
9. Uneasy sleep
10. Tiredness or fatigue
11. Loss of interest in sex

and know whether they were the ones who had made me sick.

—*Suzanna, 28*

Once known as infectious hepatitis, the hepatitis A virus is found in feces of an infected person. Hepatitis A is most common in children in developing countries and adults in the Western nations. Transmission takes place when food and water contaminated by feces with the virus are swallowed. The virus may be transmitted from person to person and within families.

This is a very hearty virus. It can survive on a surface in a room at normal temperature for long periods. That is why it is often difficult to trace how one was exposed to hepatitis A. Consequently, for more than one-third of persons with hepatitis, the point of transmission is not known.

Prevention

There is a vaccine for hepatitis A that is almost 100 percent effective if taken in two doses six to twelve months apart. Persons traveling to countries where there is hepatitis A are encouraged to be immunized. It is also a good idea to not drink tap water in those countries. Good sanitation practices and personal hygiene are important to prevent the spread of hepatitis A.

Diagnosis

A blood test will determine if you have antibodies for the virus. The antibodies will take four weeks after exposure to appear in your blood.

Treatment

There is no medication to treat hepatitis A. If you are diagnosed with hepatitis A, you will be told to rest for up to one month, eat foods

HOW DO YOU GET VIRAL HEPATITIS?

Mode of transmission	Type of Viral Hepatitis				
	A	B	C	D	E
Food	C	N	N	N	C
Fecal	C	N	N	N	C
Water	C	N	N	N	C
Raw shellfish	C	N	N	N	?
Injecting drugs	U	C	C	C	N
Transfusion	U	C	C	C	U
Sexual	U	C	U	C	U
Anal-oral	C	N	N	N	U
Oral-oral	C	U	N	N	C
Household	C	U	U	U	C
Mother to newborn	U	C	U	C	U

C = Common, U = Uncommon, N = Never, ? = Suspected

Source: Courtesy of American Liver Foundation, 1996.

high in protein, and abstain from sexual activity. It is not known why some people have a relapse after treatment. Usually the virus disappears and you are no longer a carrier, although blood tests will always reveal that you had previous exposure. After exposure there is lifelong immunity.

Hepatitis B

Outside of the United States chronic carriers of Hepatitis B virus (HBV) are very common. It is estimated that close to 200 million people are chronic carriers. Since a percentage of chronic HBV carriers go on to develop cirrhosis, HBV is the most common cause of cirrhosis in the world. In the United States the rate of chronic HBV carriers is much lower. The rate continues to drop as we continue to improve the screening of blood products. Nevertheless, today there are an estimated one million carriers of Hepatitis B in the United States.

This virus is transmitted by contact with blood, semen, saliva, tears, open sores, vaginal fluids, and breast milk from a person who carries HBV. HBV is much easier to contract than HIV. In over one-third of the cases it is not known how the person came in contact with the virus.

Exposure can occur by sharing needles during body piercing, tattooing, or injecting drugs. The virus can also be transmitted during activities in which there is exchange of body fluids (e.g., tongue kissing, genital-genital contact, and oral-genital contact). Infection within a family is likely and also from a mother to child at birth. Some carriers are contagious, and others are not.

Prevention

There is an HBV vaccine. The vaccine is given in three doses: the second dose is given one month after the first dose; the third dose six months after the first. The vaccine effect lasts for at least nine years. The vaccine is recommended for all newborns, infants, children, and sexually active teenagers. It is also recommended for persons considered at high risk of being infected. These include health care workers, emergency workers, military personnel, morticians, embalmers, persons who have multiple sexual partners, persons who live in households with or are the sex partners of HBV carriers, international travelers, patients and staff of institutions for the mentally handicapped, and inmates of long-term correctional institutions.

If you do not want to be immunized, prevention will focus on condom use, wearing rubber gloves to touch any object with body fluid on it, and sterilization of any object used to pierce the skin.

Diagnosis

Most people with HBV have no symptoms. Those who do have symptoms often describe a cluster of complaints that sound like the flu—fever, fatigue, muscle or joint pain, nausea, and vomiting. Only 25 to 35 percent of persons with HBV become jaundiced.

A simple and precise blood test can confirm the diagnosis of HBV.

Treatment

Most adults (90 to 95 percent) recover from HBV within six months. Somehow the body manages to clear itself of the virus. Blood tests will always show that they have been infected with HBV, however, and their blood will not be accepted in blood drives.

The 5 to 10 percent of persons who do not clear the virus from their blood will carry it with them for the rest of their lives. These carriers have no symptoms but are capable of passing HBV to others. A few carriers seem to spontaneously rid the body of HBV, while others deteriorate to cirrhosis of the liver. Chronic HBV is also associated with a high risk for liver cancer.

Medications (interferon alfa–2B, or lamivodine) have been approved for the treatment of persons with chronic HBV. In 35 percent of cases persons treated with interferon alfa-2B are successful in eliminating the virus from the body.

Hepatitis C

Hepatitis C virus (HCV) was first identified in 1989; prior to that it was identified as non-A, non-B hepatitis. There are 3.9 million people in the United States who have chronic HCV infections. Each year there are about 32,500 new cases of HCV, many of which will progress to chronic hepatitis. Up to 80 percent of cases have chronic long-term infection, and it is estimated that half of those are at risk for cirrhosis of the liver. Chronic hepatitis C is also associated with an increased risk of liver cancer.

The disease is spread through contact with infected blood. It is very difficult to track the first exposure to HCV because it can take anywhere from one month to several years after exposure before there are any signs of illness. It is estimated that one-third of cases do not know how they were exposed to HCV.

It is uncommon for the virus to be transmitted through sexual activity, although the Centers for Disease Control (CDC) warns that persons with more than one sexual partner are at risk for HCV.

It is unlikely that a mother can transmit the virus to a child at birth.

Prevention

There is no vaccine for HCV. Because transmission is by exposure to contaminated blood, every effort is made to reduce the likelihood of contact. All blood used for transfusions is tested for HCV. Since 1992, when more sophisticated tests for the hepatitis C antibody (anti-HCV) were developed, only 1 of 6,000 persons who receive a transfusion becomes infected.

Needles used for piercing the skin, tattooing, or injecting drugs can transmit the virus. It is not certain whether the use of condoms prevents transmission of the virus.

Diagnosis

A person can be infected and not know it. There may be no symptoms or mild ones that resemble a stomach flu. Some people have more marked symptoms, including jaundice.

Routine blood tests are the first step in the diagnosis of HCV. Once it is established that there are elevated levels of liver enzymes, a specific blood test for HCV is done.

Treatment

In some cases HCV will clear up. For persons with chronic HCV, interferon alfa–2B and interferon alpha-2A are used. The rate of cure (i.e., long-term remission) is only 10 to 15 percent. New combination therapies are available for HCV, i.e., interferon and the drug ribavirin.

Hepatitis D

Hepatitis D was once known as delta hepatitis. In order to be diagnosed with hepatitis D, a person must first test positive for HBV and then for the hepatitis D antibody. This is most common among injecting drug users and is rare in the United States. Very little is known about this disease. If you are not infected the best prevention is immunization against hepatitis B. Alpha interferon is the only available treatment.

Hepatitis E

Hepatitis E was once known as enteric or epidemic non-A, non-B hepatitis. It is similar to hepatitis A. Transmission is through feces that contaminate the food and water system. Rare in the United States, it is usually found in countries near the Indian Ocean, in Africa, and in underdeveloped countries generally. It is common for the infection to spread within a family.

The best methods of prevention require good sanitation and personal hygiene. You should also avoid tap water when traveling. The course of this disease is still unclear, although it appears to resolve itself within several months.

Autoimmune Hepatitis

Diagnosis was the most difficult part. The blood tests came out negative. I did not have mononucleosis. I was not HIV positive. I did not have viral hepatitis. Still, my liver enzymes were very high. The lupus specialist confirmed that I was fine—or at least that I did not have lupus. For three weeks I stayed in the hospital while they tried to figure out what was wrong with me.

I finally decided that I had had enough and said I wanted to go home. I had to go back to work. So I signed myself out with the condition that I would return to have a liver biopsy. I was not looking forward to that.

The liver biopsy turned out to be the best thing I did. It showed I had autoimmune chronic active hepatitis.

—*Debbie, 33*

This disease was first described in the 1950s as lupoid hepatitis because it seemed to have symptoms similar to those of systemic lupus erythematosus (see Chapter 11). As research continued, it became obvious that it was not like lupus.

Autoimmune hepatitis means that your immune system (i.e., the system that is supposed to protect you from foreign bodies) attacks your liver as if it were a foreign substance. Women make up over two-thirds of the population with autoimmune hepatitis. Some researchers have suggested that there may be a genetic predisposition to this autoimmune disease.

> *Consejos*
>
> **If You Think You Have Been Exposed to Viral Hepatitis**
>
> 1. See your health care provider.
> 2. Take blood tests to determine a diagnosis and identify the type of hepatitis.
> 3. Follow advice on diet and activity.
> 4. Inform those with whom you have been in contact that they may need to be vaccinated or to have injections of gamma (immune) globulin.

Prevention

It is unclear why some young women get this disease. Therefore, it is not known how to prevent it.

Diagnosis

The most frequently reported symptoms are fatigue, aching joints, itching, and jaundice. There may also be signs of more serious complications, similar to those found in more advanced forms of hepatitis, such as fluid in the stomach area. Blood tests are part of the process of establishing a diagnosis. A biopsy is the definitive way to diagnose autoimmune hepatitis.

Treatment

Autoimmune hepatitis is initially treated with medications (prednisone or prednisone with azathioprine). At least two-thirds of patients improve with medication. The medication is continued on a maintenance level for the rest of their lives. Up to 20 percent of patients do not respond to treatment, and for them liver transplantation is the only medical option available.

What does it feel like to have liver disease? One thing is certain—most people get nauseated. The doctors tell us that we are not supposed to feel anything because there are no nerve cells in the liver. But in my support group, many of us know this pain we feel. It is like little sharp needle pains where your liver is. Who knows what that is? Maybe it is from the scarring, or maybe it is some pain you feel through your gallbladder. You almost feel as if your liver had a heartbeat.

At the end of the day you feel very fatigued. You feel great in the morning, but by the afternoon you are exhausted. There is nothing left.

—*Ruth, 31*

What to Do If You Have Hepatitis

• **Be careful about the medications you take.** Because the liver is responsible for processing most medications, you should check with your health care provider before taking even common over-the-counter drugs as well as "natural" substances.

• **Engage in only moderate exercise.** When you exercise vigorously, your system works harder. Such added strain is bad for an organ that is not functioning well. As you feel better and some of the symptoms subside, it is OK to do some light to moderate exercise. Given your level of activity, you are the best judge of what is moderate exercise for you. If you feel you can do some exercise, you should, but do not exercise to the point of exhaustion.

Warning

If you have hepatitis A or E:

Do not prepare meals.

Do not handle food that will be eaten by others.

• **Eat a healthy diet.** Your diet should be well balanced, with added fruit juices and healthy snacks, such as fruit. Because persons with liver disease tend to feel worse as the day progresses, it is a good idea to have a substantial breakfast to carry you through the day.

• **Do not drink alcohol.** When you have hepatitis, your liver has a hard time performing its most basic functions. Drinking alcohol forces your liver to work even harder and will only make it more difficult for your liver to recuperate. When you have recovered from hepatitis, an occasional drink may be acceptable.

Myths and Facts

Myth: If you have hepatitis, you have a contagious disease.

Fact: Hepatitis means inflammation of the liver. This may or may not be contagious, depending on whether it is due to a virus or to an autoimmune problem.

Myth: You can tell when someone has hepatitis because their skin looks yellow.

Fact: Most persons do not develop jaundice. There are five million persons in the United States who have chronic hepatitis B or C, and most do not have any visible symptoms.

Myth: If you are clean, you will not get hepatitis.

Fact: Only hepatitis A and E are prevented by good personal hygiene, but even then, it is not guaranteed that you will not develop either one.

Myth: If I get a transfusion, I will get hepatitis B or C.

Fact: All blood used in transfusions is tested for markers of hepatitis B and hepatitis C.

Myth: Only alcoholics have to worry about damaging their liver.

Fact: Persons who drink socially are also at risk for liver damage.

Myth: Vitamins and other over-the-counter drugs are good for the liver.

Fact: Some of these in excess doses may be dangerous to the liver. Be sure to read the warning labels carefully and check with your health care provider.

Mind

I knew something was wrong, so I went to see my gynecologist. After all, he was the health care provider who knew me best. He had no idea what was wrong with me, but for certain he knew that I was very sick. So he sent me to the emergency room of the hospital.

They thought I had viral hepatitis. The health care workers wanted to know all sorts of things about me. These people I did not know questioned me about my sex life (I told them I was married), whether I used drugs (of course not—I was outraged to even be asked), how often I drank (three drinks a year), was my husband faithful (of course), how did I know he was faithful (how does anyone know what a man does?)—it was so unsettling with all those questions, I began to not trust my family, my friends, or my husband.

As I thought about my hepatitis, I wondered how I could have gotten it and whose fault it was.

—Aida, 28

If we work at healing the body, we also have to work at healing the mind. Part of the treatment for hepatitis is to get lots of rest. But resting the body is sometimes not possible when the mind is not at peace.

When you are first diagnosed with viral hepatitis, you start to retrace your life and try to understand what went wrong and why. It is important to remember that viral hepatitis can be very hardy and that often it is not possible to know how we got it.

Because hepatitis is often transmitted through intimate behavior, some Latinas may feel bad about the choices they have made. For Latinas in a steady relationship, it is only natural for your feelings about yourself and your partner to change. The anger at yourself or the way you became infected must be addressed in a very straightforward way. It can be helpful to seek counseling to address some of these issues.

Consejos

How to Rest Your Mind and Body

1. Watch funny movies or musicals.
2. Listen to your favorite music.
3. Teach yourself deep muscle relaxation.
4. Call a friend.
5. Keep a journal.
6. Take long baths.

For those Latinas who have cirrhosis of the liver, the mental health issues are even more profound. For some, the denial of alcohol abuse continues to be a stumbling block, and despite the importance of immediately ceasing to drink, the alcoholic is not able to. If even their own mortality is not enough to get the alcoholic to seek help, there is little that others can do except to seek professional guidance and support for themselves.

For others who may have hepatitis due to unprotected sexual activity, there is a tremendous amount of guilt, which may inhibit their ability to seek treatment.

Spirit

When I was first on medication I did very well and had few side effects. But after six months, my pancreas was inflamed, I had gained 40 pounds, and I had acne all over my body. The pain in my joints was so severe that I could not even open the door. I think that was the last straw for me. I looked at that door and cried.

I went into the bathroom, and I saw what I had become—someone who needed care, someone who was falling apart. I was completely overwhelmed by the thought of the burden I had become to my family. I was no longer the woman I thought I was to be. Then I remembered what my doctor had told me. I had to be very careful and take my medicines every day, or I would have a brain hemorrhage. That was the answer.

Before I went to sleep, I looked at my pills and set them aside. I took my Bible in my hand and asked God to forgive me, but I was going to stop taking the pills. I went to sleep holding my Bible.

When I woke up the next morning, I was surprised I was still there in my bed, still alive. Maybe God had been somewhere else. So that night I did the same thing. And the following night too. And I kept waking up. I decided that God must have a mission for me after all, and that I should take care of myself.

—*DEBBIE, 30*

As a Latina, how do you deal with an illness that you know is more devastating to Latinas, that may have no symptoms, for which there is no real cure, for which the best treatment is just to rest and eat well, while waiting for your body to cure itself can seem unbearable? What is the best way to handle all the pressures of liver disease?

This is a time when your inner strength is of the utmost importance. Our faith will help some of us during these difficult times. It is not that by praying we are better able to tolerate the fatigue or understand what is going on. It is more that faith can provide a framework in which we can make the best use of the quiet time we have to spend healing and resting.

In most faiths it is accepted that our body is God's temple. Perhaps if we were to accept the value of our body, even the most agnostic among us would at the very least take better care of the health we have.

Resting, eating a healthy diet, not putting toxins into our system—those are the core elements for treating hepatitis. Perhaps what needs to be added to this course of treatment is the pursuit of peace of mind and the nourishment of the soul.

Summary

We do not know why Latinas are especially vulnerable to liver disease. The liver is a major processing plant for the body—it produces what it needs, replenishes what gets used up, and removes what is toxic. When the liver does not work, it may be because we have overloaded it with toxins such as alcohol (cirrhosis), been exposed to a virus (hepatitis A, B, C, D, or E), or simply experienced a malfunction of the body (autoimmune hepatitis). In most cases of viral hepatitis, it is good that the body clears itself of the virus because there is no known cure. Most of the treatment consists of rest, eating well, and eliminating the toxins and in some instances medication.

RESOURCES

Organizations

American Liver Foundation
75 Maiden Lane
New York, NY 10038
(800) 465-4837
www.liverfoundation.org

Hepatitis Foundation International
30 Sunrise Terrace
Cedar Grove, NJ 07009
(800) 891-0707 or (973) 239-1035
www.hepfi.org

Latino Organization for Liver Awareness
PO Box 842
Throggs Neck Station
Bronx, NY 10465
(718) 892-8697 or (888) 367-LOLA
www.lola-national.org

National Digestive Diseases Clearinghouse
2 Information Way
Bethesda, MD 20892-3570
(301) 654-3810
www.niddk.nih.gov/health/digest

Publications and Pamphlets

"Alcohol and the Liver: Myths vs. Facts," August 1997. Information about the effects of alcohol abuse on the liver. American Liver Foundation; (800) 465-4837; www.liverfoundation.org. Other titles include:

"Cirrhosis: Many Causes," September 1996. Information on the conditions that can lead to cirrhosis of the liver (also in Spanish).

"Diet and Your Liver," August 1997. Information on the relationship between nutrition and the liver.

"Facts on Liver Transplantation," March 1997.

"Gallstones: A National Health Problem," July 1996.

"Getting Hip to HEP: What You Should Know about Hepatitis A, B, and C," March 2000. (888) 4-HEP-ABC (888-443-7222).

"Hepatitis A, B, C: Enfermedades Hepáticas Sobre las Que Usted Debe Estar Informado," November 1996. NIH–164/17484109; (888) 4-HEP-ABC (888-443-7222).

"Hepatitis B: Your Child at Risk." Information on immunization for Hepatitis B. (888) 4-HEP-ABC (888-443-7222).

"How Can You Love Me . . . If You Don't Know Me." What to do to maintain a healthy liver. December 1997. (800) GO-LIVER (800-465-4837).

"Viral Hepatitis: Everybody's Problem?" December 1996. Information on the transmission of viral hepatitis. (888) 4-HEP-ABC (888-443-7222).

"What Is Your Risk of Getting AIDS or Hepatitis B on the Job?" Information on the prevalence of hepatitis B. (888) 4-HEP-ABC (888-443-7222).

"Your Liver Lets You Live," August 1997. Information on how the liver functions. (800) GO-LIVER (800-465-4837).

"Datos Sobre el Hígado." Latino Organization for Liver Awareness, P.O. Box 842, Throgs Neck Station, Bronx, NY 10465; (718) 892-8697 or (888) 367-LOLA.

Other titles include (all available in Spanish):

"1 out of every 50 Latinos is Infected with the Hepatitis C Virus"

"Get Tested, Get Treated"

"Autoimmune Hepatitis"

"Liver Donor and Liver Transplant"

"What I Need to Know about Hepatitis A." An introduction to the causes, symptoms, and treatments of hepatitis A (available in Spanish). National Digestive Diseases Clearinghouse. 2 Information Way, Bethesda, MD 20892-3570, (301) 654-3810 www.niddk.nih.gov

"What I Need to Know about Hepatitis B." An introduction to the causes, symptoms, and treatments of hepatitis B (available in Spanish).

"What I Need to Know about Hepatitis C." An introduction to the causes, symptoms, and treatments of hepatitis C (available in Spanish).

18

Sexually Transmitted Diseases

The Silent Epidemic

She had never had a sexually transmitted disease before. She had always associated them with "loose" women, women who were not respectable.

Not only did she have to recover from the physical aspects of her illness, but she had to deal with the dissonance of what it meant to have these diseases. Although cured of the symptoms, she cried, "I am no longer worthy of my husband."

—*Tanya, 48*

Once known as venereal diseases (VD), sexually transmitted diseases (STDs) are a greater problem for Latinas than for non-Latinas. The seriousness of STDs goes beyond immediate discomfort. When undiagnosed or untreated they can cause severe internal damage. Some women may have no symptoms but may discover years later that they are infertile as a result of an untreated STD. This is only one of the reasons that a yearly gynecological exam is so important. We also need to feel comfortable talking to our health care provider about STDs.

It is already difficult for us to talk about our health problems; STDs bring all those taboo topics and behaviors to the surface. To compound the situation, our misconceptions about who gets STDs and why we get them make us embarrassed and unwilling to act when we begin to have symptoms. Most damaging, we refuse to believe that STDs could happen to us.

The fact is that many of us get infected with STDs, often without our knowledge. Complicating the physical problems associated with STDs is the often deep and unrelenting shame we feel because we have an STD. This shame also makes it harder for us to seek the health care we need.

So why do we get STDs? Latinas are taught to be clean. Many of us use bidets or something similar to keep clean "down there." We are generally faithful and monogamous, but despite this we seem to have increasing rates of STDs. The reasons for this increase are clear.

Unfortunately, people do not always tell the truth about what they do or do not do. Not only do we not tell the truth to each other, but sometimes we save the worst and most devastating untruths for ourselves.

As a result, all sorts of people get STDs. Young people get STDs. Older women get STDs. Clean women get STDs. "Nice" women also get STDs. Latinas who choose to be sexually active outside of a long-term, mutually monogamous relationship and do not use condoms are at particularly high risk for an STD. Some Latinas get STDs because they mistakenly believe that they are in a long-term, mutually monogamous relationship when in fact they are not.

The hardest part of accepting that STDs happen to all sorts of Latinas is what it forces us to realize about our relationships. What do we do when we know, suspect, or fear that our partner is not as monogamous as we would like to think? What do we do when we know we have had more partners than we would like for others to know?

Very often what we do is nothing. Our belief is that somehow our partner will act responsibly and do the right thing by us. Yet in our hearts we should know better. We know we are the ones who have to take care of ourselves and make decisions about our sexual relationships.

We may feel uncomfortable having to discuss some of these issues, but we must.

Why Are We at Risk?

When Luz looked at Carlos, all she saw was the love and devotion he had given her these last three years. She felt very lucky. At long last she had found the perfect man. She had gone through her share of lovers, but she knew that she was only the third woman Carlos had known intimately.

She laughed when she thought about this. Here he was, practically as pure as snow, and here she was . . . well, not as pure as she would like to be. Luz felt so complete when they made love. . . .

Then one afternoon he was supposed to come over, but he didn't arrive until very late. When he walked in, his eyes refused to meet hers. As they sat on the couch, he began to speak.

Consejos

Reducing the Risk of STDs in Your Life

1. Limit the number of your sexual partners.
2. Talk to your sexual partner.
3. Always use latex condoms and a spermicide.
4. Look at your body for signs of infection.

It seemed that during the last three years he had been with three other women, and now he was worried that he might have given her something. Luz was astounded. She could not believe what she was hearing. She knew men—Carlos could not have been lying to her all this time. He was pure. She would have known if he had been lying. And what did he mean, that he might have given her something?

There are some steps we can take to reduce the risk of STDs:

1: Limit the number of your sexual partners. STDs have different incubation periods. Thus it is easier to track the source of infection if you limit the number of partners you have. Moreover, the fewer sexual partners you have, the lower the risk that you will be exposed to STDs.

2: Talk to your sexual partner. This can be as difficult for Latinas who believe that one partner is all they need as for Latinas who want to enjoy the banquet of life and feast on all its many pleasures. The first group assumes that it is a matter of respect not to talk about issues such as monogamy, and the second does not want to be intrusive or suspicious. But sexuality and sexual behavior are by their very nature intrusive, and pleasurably so. To have good health, you must be able to talk to your sexual partner.

3: Always use latex condoms and a spermicide. Some Latinas have commented that they do not want to ask a man to use a condom because they think it implies that they do not trust him. Well . . . maybe they should trust their sexual partner and maybe they should not. The facts are that people lie. And they lie about their sexual behavior and sexual partners most of all. If you are not in a long-term, monogamous relationship, using a condom is the first way a partner shows his concern for you. You and your partner have to decide how long to wait before you stop using condoms. Keep in mind that there is great variability in the incubation period before an STD can be identified.

Using a spermicide with nonoxynol 9 offers additional protection against some STDs. This tacitly acknowledges what is a reasonable assumption—that before you were with your partner, at least one of you had a previous sexual relationship. When you are sexually intimate with someone, you become exposed to this person and every other person with whom they have had sexual relations, not to mention every person with whom their previous partners had sexual relations, and so on.

Condoms are used for health reasons—yours and your partner's. The way you use a condom is simple—carefully and consistently (for more about using condoms for birth control, see Chapter 4).

Consejos

If You Choose to Be Sexually Active—

1. Ask your partners if they have had any STDs and if so, which.
2. As part of foreplay, look at your partner's body carefully for signs of STDs. You may be able to see parts of your partner's body that are not as readily visible to them.
3. If you see something that concerns you, do not have sex, and encourage your partners to see their health care provider.
4. Use a latex condom.
5. Use a spermicide with nonoxynol 9.

Warning: Threats of Violence

A few Latinas have expressed concern that their partners might respond violently if they were asked to use a condom. Threats of violence are unacceptable and strongly indicate a dangerous situation. For Latinas who find themselves in this kind of situation, the most immediate concern must be safety and immediate separation from that partner. (See the Resources on page 14.)

4: Look at your body for signs of infection. We need to get better about looking at our bodies. We need to know what we look like when we are healthy and when a pimple is more than just a pimple. With some STDs the first symptoms may be subtle, so we should be careful and check our bodies for any warning signs. Use one mirror or two so that you can see the front and back of your body. Given the information provided below, it is advisable to do this on an ongoing basis. This is especially necessary when you are sexually active and either you or your partner has sexual relationships with other people.

Most Frequent STDs—Causes, Symptoms, Diagnosis, Treatment

There are more than twenty different kinds of STDs. The major ones are HIV/AIDS, chlamydial infections, genital herpes, genital warts, gonorrhea, and syphilis. HIV/AIDS can also be transmitted in other ways and is discussed extensively in Chapter 16. Keep in mind that some STDs have no symptoms and that there is great variability in the treatment for each one. Some can be cured, and others will always be with us.

Chlamydia

Each year four to eight million new people are diagnosed with chlamydia, a curable STD that is now the most common bacterial STD in the United States. Untreated chlamydia results in nearly half of the cases of pelvic inflammatory disease (PID)—an infection of the endometrium, fallopian tubes, and ovaries that is very painful. PID is responsible for infertility (i.e., inability to have children) in 100,000 women each year.

Causal Factors

Chlamydia is caused by the bacterium *Chlamydia trachomatis*. It can also cause an inflamed rectum or "pinkeye" due to inflammation of the lining of the eyes. You may be exposed to the bacterium by engaging in anal intercourse, vaginal intercourse, or oral-genital contact with a partner who is infected with the bacterium.

Symptoms

There is great variability in the symptoms. As many as 85 percent of women with chlamydia have no symptoms or minimal symptoms until the disease is at a fairly advanced stage. When there are symptoms, they usually appear one to three weeks after you have contracted it. These early signs may include a discharge from your vagina or pain during urination, an irritated rectum (proctitis), or inflammation of the lining of the eye (conjunctivitis).

> **Warning**
>
> When taking antibiotics, it is critical that you take the entire course of medicines that has been prescribed to make sure that you have killed all of the harmful bacteria.

Diagnosis

Gonorrhea and chlamydia have similar symptoms and are often found in the same person. Chlamydia is usually diagnosed using special cervical swabs that are analyzed to identify the genes of the discharge, i.e., DNA probe test done on a swab. The test can be done quickly and is as accurate as growing the bacteria in a culture.

Treatment

For seven days, you and your partner will be given an antibiotic such as azithromycin or doxycycline. Penicillin is not effective in the treatment of chlamydia.

If you are pregnant and diagnosed with chlamydia, you must be treated because women can give the bacterium to their babies, causing eye infections or pneumonia. Pregnant women may be treated with erythromycin because doxycycline has adverse effects on pregnant women.

Genital Herpes

There are sixty million persons in the United States with genital herpes. Most people who have genital herpes never have any symptoms, but once you have herpes, the virus is with you for the rest of your life. The virus settles in some of the sensory nerve cells at the end of your spinal cord. Every now and then it may produce symptoms. These are called outbreaks.

While genital herpes is not life-threatening, it can be very severe in persons who have suppressed immune systems. Pregnant women who have an outbreak during vaginal childbirth may pass the virus to the baby. Babies who are exposed to herpes simplex virus (HSV) have serious problems (blindness, brain damage, and in rare cases death).

Causal Factors

There are two kinds of herpes simplex virus (HSV). HSV 1 is the more familiar kind. When you have fever blisters or cold sores on your lips, they are often due to HSV 1. HSV, can also infect the genital area and produce sores there. HSV 2 usually produces sores in your genital area, but they may also occur on your lips and in your mouth. HSV 1 and HSV 2 are different—one cannot change into the other.

In order to become infected with HSV 2, you must have sexual contact with someone who has obvious genital sores. In extremely rare cases, HSV may be spread by contact with a toilet seat or in a hot tub.

Symptoms

Both HSV 1 and HSV 2 may produce sores in your genital area and anal opening and on your thighs and buttocks. If you have open wounds or cuts on other parts of your body, it is possible to have sores there too.

Most people have no symptoms. If you do get symptoms, they are noticeable two to ten days after you contract the virus. The symptoms can last two to three weeks.

In the first few days the symptoms may include an itching or burning sensation, vaginal discharge, a feeling of pressure in the abdominal area, and pain in the legs, buttocks, or genital area. After a few days you may see some small red bumps in the areas where you are infected. These bumps may quickly become open sores (lesions), then crusted on top, and finally heal on their own without leaving a scar.

An HSV infection shows itself in recurrent episodes. During these episodes the virus begins to travel up the nerves to the skin. When the virus is traveling, you may have prodromal symptoms: tingling, itching, or in some cases pain. When it gets to the surface of the skin, the virus creates blisters. These may be very small blisters, but they are enough to infect your sexual partner.

It is not known how often these episodes will recur nor what causes them to occur. Some people have them a couple of times in their life, and others have them several times a year. The mechanism that produces the recurrent episodes is not understood, but we do know that deep emotions and stress may act as a trigger.

Illness, stress, menstruation, and even sunlight have been blamed for these recurrences. The reality is that we do not know. The symptoms and course of the illness show great variability from person to person.

Diagnosis

HSV can only be diagnosed when there are sores. A blood test can tell whether you have been exposed to HSV and developed the antibodies to fight HSV infection. The blood test will not let you know if you are capable of infecting someone else.

Consejos

Staying Comfortable When You Have Sores

- Keep sores clean and dry.
- Avoid touching sores.
- Wash your hands if you have touched sores.
- Avoid sexual contact with other persons until sores have completely healed (i.e., new skin has formed over the sores).

Treatment

There is no cure for herpes. Taking acyclovir within 24 hours of the onset of the first or a recurrent episode can decrease the severity of symptoms. Acyclovir is much more effective when taken orally than when used as an ointment. If an individual is having frequent recurrent attacks of herpes, acyclovir can be used on a regular basis to reduce the number of attacks. Alternative medications to acyclovir include famciclovir and valacyclovir.

Since once infected we always have the virus, genital herpes has an impact on current and future relationships. It is important to decide at what point in a new relationship you will discuss it with your partner.

Human Papillomavirus (HPV) and Genital Warts

There are sixty types of HPV, and about one third of them can be transmitted through sexual contact and live only on genital tissue. Nearly half of the women who have contracted HPV have no symptoms. In the United States, HPV is one of the most common STD, found in as many as 24 million Americans. HPV is responsible for genital warts and has also been the cause of some cases of cervical cancer and other genital cancers (see Chapter 12).

Causal Factors

We don't know what causes HPV. We do know that some HPV is responsible for genital warts while other HPV infections cause warts on the hands and soles of the feet. Genital warts are highly contagious—67 percent of persons who have unprotected sex with someone who has genital warts will become infected.

Symptoms

Within three months of exposure, warts will appear at the point of contact with the infected person—in the vulva, labia (inner and outer), vagina, cervix, anus area, or in rare occasions, the mouth. You may have one tiny wart or several clustered together. If you do not treat them, they will either form fleshy cauliflower-like tissue or in some cases disappear; nevertheless you will still be infected.

Diagnosis

The only way to know if you have genital warts is to have your health care provider look at them. If you do have genital warts, make sure that your health care provider takes a Pap smear to see whether there is evidence of HPV infection of your cervix. HPV infection of the cervix has been found to increase the risk for cervical cancer.

Treatment

There is no cure for genital warts; once you have contracted the virus it remains in your body. Warts may be removed, however, either chemically, by freezing (cryosurgery), by burning them off (electrocautery), by surgery (in the case of larger warts), or by laser. Even though they are removed, they may reappear. They are always contagious.

Gonorrhea

This highly contagious and curable STD often has no symptoms, and it can recur even after treatment if a person is exposed again to the bacterium that causes it. Each year about 400,000 cases are reported in the United States. Untreated gonorrhea can spread through the body, causing pain in the joints and problems in the heart valve and even the brain.

Causal Factors

Gonorrhea is caused by the Neisseria gonorrhoeae bacterium and spreads through genital-genital or oral-genital contact. The moist, warm tissue found in the mouth, cervix, rectum, and urethra encourages the growth of the bacterium. In most women the bacterium settles in the cervix, but if left untreated it will spread to the uterus and fallopian tubes, causing pelvic inflammatory disease (PID).

Symptoms

Most women have mild symptoms. When there are symptoms, they include painful urination, a burning feeling in the vaginal opening, or a vaginal discharge that is yellow or bloody. These symptoms usually appear two to ten days after exposure to the bacterium, although for a few people it may take them several months to appear.

Diagnosis

The presence of the bacterium may be detected through one of three lab techniques; growing the bacteria in a culture, staining biological samples, or detection of bacterial genes. In the first procedure your health care provider obtains a sample of your discharge, places it in a special dish, and allows the bacteria to grow for up to two days. At that time, it is possible to identify the bacterium 90 percent of the time.

Some health care providers find it easier and quicker to use a staining process. In this procedure, a sample of your discharge is placed on a slide and a dye is added. By examining the slide through a microscope, your health care provider can tell you before you leave the office if there is any gonococcus. Unfortunately, this quick method is not completely accurate with women.

Today most providers use cervical swabs as part of a new test that detects the genes of the bacteria. These tests are as accurate as culturing the bacteria if not more so.

A Pap test will not give you any information about gonorrhea.

Treatment

For decades penicillin was the treatment of choice for gonorrhea, but the gonorrhea bacterium has developed antibiotic-resistant strains and so rendered ineffective some of the medicines once used to treat it. Other antibiotics remain effective, however. Some are given by injection (ceftriaxone or spectinomycin), and others are given as pills.

Health care providers usually prescribe a single dose of ceftriaxone, cefixime, ciprofloxacin, or ofloxacin.

Regardless of whether your partner has symptoms, it is critical that he be tested and if necessary treated too.

In February Santina was only thirteen years old, but she knew that she had already become a woman. She was proud of her little breasts and the hair growing between her legs. Even getting her period was an interesting event. It was messy, but she was learning how to keep clean. So when Tomás told her he wanted to show her how much he loved her by having sex with her, she happily said yes.

By August, the pain in her stomach was so intense that she had to be taken to the emergency room. She found out that she had syphilis and gonorrhea. For some time she experienced a great deal of discomfort but was too afraid to tell her parents, so she endured it.

By the time she turned fourteen in December, she had become sterile.

Syphilis

Before the 1900s, syphilis had a long history of ravaging communities. Advances in antibiotics have since brought the disease under control.

Causal Factors

Syphilis is caused by the bacterium *Treponema pallidum*. The bacterium needs a warm, moist environment to survive, such as the mucous membranes of the genitals, mouth, and anus. It is spread from the open sores of someone who is in the primary, secondary, or early latent stage of syphilis to the mucous membranes of their sexual partner. It is possible to become exposed by touching the skin rash of someone in the secondary stage.

It is not spread by touching a toilet seat or towel that has been handled by an infected person.

Symptoms

Untreated syphilis progresses through four stages whose symptoms are explained below.

Primary stage. The first symptom is a painless sore (chancre) in the part of the body that came in contact with the bacterium. There is great individual variability in the length of time between exposure to an infected person and the first symptom. Some may develop symptoms in ten days, while others will have no symptoms for up to three months. For the majority of women, however, the first symptom occurs two to six weeks after exposure. This first symptom is hard to detect because it may be painless or occur inside our body. An untreated person may infect others throughout this stage. Regional lymph node enlargement usually accompanies this lesion.

Secondary stage. About three to six weeks after a chancre appears you will have a skin rash, either all over your body or in the palms of your hands, on the bottom of your feet, or in some other area. It may take from several weeks to several months for the rash to heal. Throughout this time, any contact with the broken skin of the infected person will spread the disease. Other symptoms of this stage include mild fever, fatigue, headache, sore throat, swelling of the lymph nodes, and hair loss. If left undiagnosed and untreated, these symptoms may recur over a two-year period.

Latent stage. If syphilis is left undiagnosed and untreated, it eventually enters a latent stage. In this stage there are no overt symptoms, and the disease is not contagious. One-third of the persons who reach this stage deteriorate to the tertiary stage of syphilis.

Tertiary (late) phase. When it reaches this stage, the disease causes serious problems: mental disorders, blindness, heart abnormalities, and neurological disorders. In this stage, an infected person can no longer transmit the bacterium to others, but the degenerative changes often lead to death.

Diagnosis

It is very hard to diagnose syphilis in the early stages because the symptoms are common to many other diseases. A diagnosis of syphilis is based on three things: the clinical judgment of your health care provider, examination of samples from a sore under a microscope, and either the Venereal Disease Research Laboratory (VDRL) test or the rapid plasma reagin (RPR) test. These two tests are blood tests that may mistakenly indicate the presence of syphilis when the person actually has another viral or autoimmune disorder. Consequently, a positive result on the VDRL or RPR test is followed by a fluorescent treponemal antibody-absorption (FTA-ABS) test or a *Treponema pallidum* hemaglutination assay (TPHA).

While these tests are helpful, they have some drawbacks. In the first place, with the VDRL and RPR it may take up to three months after exposure for a positive result to be detected. Secondly, FTA-ABS and TPHA may not pick up whether you have been reinfected with a new syphilis infection.

The only way to know for certain whether the bacterium is in the nervous system is by a spinal tap. This is usually done only with persons who are in the latent or late stages of the disease to confirm a diagnosis so as to ensure the proper treatment.

Treatment

Penicillin by injection offers quick results. Within 24 hours of the injection, most people will no longer transmit the virus. Although treatment is effective in all but the late stages, and offers a cure, it is often not possible to repair damage to organs. Moreover, the antibodies that are produced may not protect from future infections.

Facts and Myths

Myth: You can tell when someone has an STD.
Fact: You cannot tell when someone has an STD. The person may not have symptoms and may not even know they have an STD.
Myth: STDs cause fewer problems for women than for men.
Fact: Because women sometimes do not have symptoms until the infection is very serious, they have more severe problems than men.
Myth: There are cures for all STDs.
Fact: There are cures for some STDs. There is treatment but no cure for genital herpes, HPV, and HIV/AIDS.
Myth: Gonorrhea is easily treated.
Fact: There are new types of gonorrhea that are not responding to treatment.
Myth: If you keep yourself very clean, you will not get an STD.
Fact: STDs are not related to personal hygiene.
Myth: If you have no symptoms, you do not have an STD.
Fact: You can have an STD and have no symptoms.
Myth: You can get an STD from masturbating.
Fact: You must have contact with an infected person to get an STD.

What Do You Do If You Have an STD?

1: Tell your partner. The reason you need to tell your partner is that often both of you will have to be treated. It is advisable not to use this discussion of your physical health to address other issues in the relationship. It is a good idea to stick to the facts about the STD. Questions of trust, fidelity, and other related issues should be addressed at a separate time.

If you have had more than one partner and feel uncomfortable sharing this information with them, you may want to send an anonymous letter recommending that they see their health care provider.

2: Take all of your medicines. Regardless of whether you are feeling better, you need to take the full course of the medicines you are given. Especially with antibiotics, it is the cumulative effect of the full dose that is the treatment.

3: Do not have sex while you are being treated. Your body needs to heal and rest. You also do not want to run the risk of being reinfected or of infecting someone else.

4: Plan follow-up visits to your health care provider. With some STDs, it is important for your health care provider to monitor your progress.

Consejos

If You Have an STD—

1. Tell your partner.
2. Take all of your medicines.
3. Do not have sex while you are being treated.
4. Plan follow-up visits to your health care provider.
5. Consider what you should do to avoid a recurrence.

5: Consider what you should do to avoid a recurrence. After we are diagnosed and treated for an STD, we often begin to rethink our relationships and the kinds of physical intimacy we share. Since some STDs can only be treated and not cured, we have to consider different ways our sexuality can be safely expressed.

Some of us may feel that total sexual abstinence is the only way to stay free of STDs, but we have to be careful to balance our negative experience with our human need to express our sexuality. Hugging, kissing, giving and receiving massages, and stroking are all ways to show affection. It may be that we decide to wait a little longer before we allow someone to be sexually intimate with us.

Mind and Spirit

STDs are very difficult for us to talk about. The physical aspects of recognizing symptoms are straightforward, and the treatments are fairly simple. Perhaps the difficult part is understanding what it means to have an STD.

Are we being punished for something we did? Does this mean that we are with the wrong partner? To look into illness trying to find some hidden intent or meaning is detrimental. If we have an STD that was diagnosed and treated, it should only mean that we were exposed to an illness and were fortunate enough to go for treatment and care at an early stage.

It is natural, though, to try to understand what happened. It is also natural to ask ourselves how this could have happened to us. The issue of infidelity may need to be considered. In cases where we thought we were in a long-term, monogamous relationship, we may ask ourselves how we managed to so seriously misjudge the situation. Very often, in the process of pondering these things, we end up blaming ourselves for what was not fully under our control. We need to remember that we all make mistakes—we misjudge, we do not have all the information we need, we are vulnerable after the breakup of a marriage or relationship, we may have been deliberately deceived.

In the end, STDs make us come face to face with the most intimate expressions of our sexuality in our relationships. If we are not able to talk to our partner about these things, are we really ready for sexual intimacy? We must think about this.

STDs happen to at least 1 out of 4 people, yet we act as if nobody we know will have an STD. Perhaps if we talked about sex a little more with our friends and sexual partners and were more relaxed about sex, we could be more honest and could truly prevent STDs.

Summary

If we are not 100-percent successful in preventing STDs, we must be able to recognize the symptoms so that we can obtain proper treatment. There are over twenty types of STDs, each with its respective symptoms, diagnosis, and treatment. Chlamydia, HPV, genital herpes, gonorrhea, and syphilis are the most common. Some cannot be cured, but all can be treated.

The earlier you begin treatment, the better the outcome. Because there may be no symptoms, you must be smart about your sexual behavior and honest about your partner. Because of the type of activity in which you or your partner engaged, even though you have no symptoms, it is often a good idea to seek evaluation for the possible presence of an STD.

STDs force us to acknowledge and confront many of our cultural taboos. To get past them, we must engage in frank and candid discussions with those we love. And that is good, because true love in a relationship is about caring for each other's health and well-being.

RESOURCES

Organizations

Alan Guttmacher Institute
1120 Connecticut Avenue NW, Suite 460
Washington, DC 20036
(202) 296-4012
www.agi_usa.org

American Social Health Association
P.O. Box 13827
Research Triangle Park, NC 27709
(919) 361-8400 or (800) 230-6039
www.ashastd.org

Amigas Latinas en Acción Pro-Salud
240A Elm Street
Somerville, MA 02144
(617) 776-4161

National Institute of Allergy and Infectious Diseases
Building 31, Room 7A50
31 Center Dr. MSC 2520
Bethesda, MD 20892-2520
(301) 496-5717
www.niaid.nih.gov

National Public Health Information Coalition
604 Lullingstone Dr.
Marietta, GA 30067
(770) 509-5555
www.nphic.org

National Women's Health Network
514 10th Street NW, Suite 400
Washington, DC 20004
(202) 347-1140
www.womenshealthnetwork.org

Planned Parenthood Federation of America
810 Seventh Avenue
New York, NY 10019
(212) 541-7800
www.plannedparenthood.org

Hotlines

American Liver Foundation Hotline
(800) 465-4837

Herpes Resource Center Order Line
(800) 230-6039

CDC National AIDS Hotline
(800) 342-2437 (English) or (800) 344-7432 (Spanish)

National Herpes Hotline
(919) 361-8488
9 a.m. to 7 p.m. Eastern Time, Monday through Friday

National HPV Hotline
(877) 478-5868

National STD Hotline (Centers for Disease Control)
(800) 227-8922

Sexually Transmitted Diseases Information Line
(202) 832-7000

Publications and Pamphlets

"Gonorrhea and Chlamydia," September 2000. Pamphlet No. 12345/98765. Patient Education series. American College of Obstetricians and Gynecologists; (800) 762-2264. Other titles include "How to Prevent Sexually Transmitted Diseases," Sept. 2000. Pamphlet No. 4567/7654.

"Herpes: What It Is and How to Deal with It," 1999. Pamphlet No. 1520. Family AAFP Health Facts series. American

Academy of Family Physicians, 11400 Tomahawk Creek Pkwy, Leawood, KS 66211-2672; (800) 944-0000. Other titles include "STDs: Common STDs and Tips on Prevention," 1994. Pamphlet No. 1565.

"STD's; What You Need to Know." American Social Health Association; (800) 783-9877. Many other titles are available.

PART IV

Para Vivir Bien . . . Living Well

19

Eating for Health and Pleasure

Salud con Gusto . . . Health with Pleasure

María was talking to her best friend, Hortensia, about how she wanted to eat a healthier diet. She knew that she should eat more fruit, but she really did not like apples and oranges. They just did not appeal to her. Hortensia seemed surprised when María said she did not like fruit.

"But you always have tomatoes and avocados in your house," Hortensia said.

"Of course!" María answered.

"Well," said Hortensia, "those are fruits too, and as Latinas we cook with those a lot. You also eat mangos, bananas, and melons," added Hortensia, having gone out to eat with María many times. "Fruit is more than just apples!"

Good News, Bad News

First there is the good news for Latinas. We have healthier eating habits than non-Latinas—we just did not know it. We eat less fat, more fruit, more vegetables, and more fiber. Research shows that this healthy diet is found even among Latinas who have recently arrived in the United States and are on limited incomes.

This is surprising to many of us. Too often the messages we get make us believe that our "different" diet is "bad" or "not as good." But what we know about our diet is relatively new.

The problem has often been that research on nutrition focused on food items that were on the typical nonethnic menu. Many of the foods that we eat at home, especially the ones we make with fresh ingredients, were not included in food charts or tables. As Hispanic foods have become more popular, nutrition experts have responded by beginning to study some of the more common foods we eat.

Unfortunately, some glaring distortions have been made by well-intentioned researchers who were not culturally proficient. For example, the Center for Science in the Public Interest published a report, which the press picked up, declaring that Mexican food is not healthy. What they should have said was that the food they chose to study at commercial fast food Mexican restaurants was not healthy. We know that the food we prepare at home is quite different.

MYTHS AND FACTS ABOUT WHAT LATINAS EAT

Myth: Latinas eat a lot of fat.

Fact: Latinas eat lower levels of fat than other women do.

Myth: Latinas use a lot of lard.

Fact: Focus groups with Latinas have shown that in the United States even recently arrived Hispanic immigrants are unlikely to use lard.

Myth: Latinas do not eat fruits or vegetables.

Fact: Latinas are more likely to eat fruits and vegetables than other women are.

Then there is the bad news. The lives we lead today have been changing the way we eat for the worse. We are eating more like mainstream non-Latinas—and that is not good. Latinas who accept the typical American diet end up eating less fruit, more fat, and less fiber. These Latinas are also drinking more alcohol and smoking more too.

I always thought that when I had a home of my own, my kitchen would be like my mom's and that I would prepare all the foods I grew up eating. The house would be full of great smells—onions sizzling, beans simmering, chicken roasting. But my mother's job was to stay home and take care of the family. I work full-time, and cooking the way she did just doesn't fit into my life. Now I pick up pizza or some other easy-to-prepare food at the supermarket. This isn't the way I thought things would be. It isn't healthy either, but I don't know what else to do.

Food in Our Daily Lives

Tengo mucho que hacer (I have a lot to do). The pace of our daily lives, compounded by our many responsibilities, forces us to make choices about eating that are based on ease and speed rather than nutrition or pleasure. Our meals are based on how easily and quickly we can prepare what we are going to eat and how quickly we can eat it.

Our lives are often much more demanding than our mothers' as we juggle all the pressures of working and caring for our families. Things are not the way we imagined they would be. We do not have the time to shop every day for fresh foods or to cook using those ingredients on a daily basis. Too often we find ourselves alone in the kitchen without any other helping hands, throwing a meal together based on what is in the cabinets and refrigerator—whatever is least objectionable and easiest to prepare. And eating itself no longer takes place at a time set aside for talking with family and friends but is rather an activity piggybacked onto other activities, like watching television.

We eat in between activities or as part of other activities. The epitome of this is the microwaved TV dinner. It is quick to prepare, easy to eat, and even if you have minimum abilities of balance and coordination, it allows you to do other things as you prepare and eat it. Eating is no longer a primary activity. It is not surprising that we are not thoughtful about what we eat, because we just want to finish eating so we can move on.

For too many of us, breakfast has become an impediment to getting on with the things that really matter. So we rush through our first meal by popping some prepackaged breakfast food into the toaster and grabbing it as we run out of the house. Lunch has become the time when we catch up with errands, and once again eating must be quick and easy. We send our children to school with lunches that are prepackaged and highly processed, and our children feel the need to keep up with the other children by bringing the current "in" packaged lunch food.

We adults sometimes just "do lunch." That means that we have lunch with someone as part of conducting business. This requires that in between bites of food we do work and look good. For those meals where we want to make a good impression, we choose what we will eat strategically, usually focused on neatness rather than nutrition. Eating a balanced meal takes a back seat to being able to project the right impression. It is no surprise that by dinner time we are so tired that we find it easier to order pizza, buy an already roasted chicken, or pick up some fast food.

Although when we were growing up our families focused on fresh foods, we are too often left with a time crunch between work and sleep that only allows for packaged and quickly prepared foods. Thus time has become our most precious gift, which is sliced away from our lives at every turn, often without regard to our needs. The opportunity to linger over meals and discuss events is more and more frequently reserved for fantasies and for new lovers.

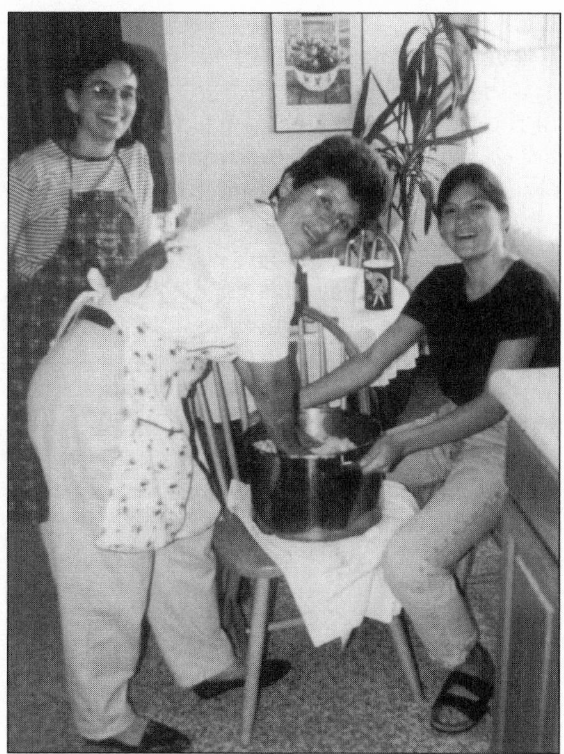

We enjoy cooking together.

Making Time

1. Make soup stock once a month and freeze it into small cubes for use in recipes.
2. Marinate several meats at a time. (Maximum storage time: pork and lamb, three days; chicken, two days; and beef, two days.) Remember not to add garlic to chicken and beef until the day of cooking.
3. Invest in a rice cooker.
4. Cook beans and keep them in the refrigerator to reheat during the week or freeze for later use.
5. Freeze fresh berries and bananas for future use in "smoothies."
6. Buy fruits at different stages of ripening to last you all week.
7. Keep bread in the refrigerator and freeze tortillas.
8. Make meals for the week and freeze in meal-size containers.
9. Shop for greens twice a week and keep them well wrapped in a crisper.
10. Peel a week's worth of garlic and refrigerate it in a closed glass jar.

Our challenge is to combine the reality of life today with what we know about food and nutrition.

Knowing the Effect of Food

Food is the fuel our body needs to function properly. And the best way to provide fuel to our body is by eating a healthy diet. The vitamins, minerals, fiber, and other nutrients that we get from food all benefit the body in specific ways. Only two vitamins are produced by the body—vitamin D, when the skin is in sunlight, and vitamin K, made in the intestine. Some vitamins enable the body to make better use of the other substances it needs. For example, we know that vitamin C helps the body absorb iron.

The body also stores vitamins in water (e.g., vitamins C, B1, B2, B3, B6, folic acid, B12, biotin, and pantothenic acid) or in fat (e.g., vitamins A, D, E, and K). While the water-soluble vitamins are lost through urine, perspiration, and other bodily fluids, fat-soluble vitamins may be stored and can build up to toxic levels if too many are taken.

We know that sugar and fat affect the biochemistry of the body and brain. In moderate quantities they make us feel good. For most of us, even caffeine in moderation is acceptable. The key is to learn what substances your body needs and how your body reacts to them. Think about how what you eat will be used by your body—how it will help or hurt your body, mind, and spirit.

We may think that we have to drink milk because milk is good for us. Yet drinking milk may be a problem for those of us with lactose intolerance, a condition in which our digestive system says no to milk and some milk products. Specifically, we may get gas or stomach aches or may feel nauseated. When lactose intolerance is a problem, we have to be creative and find other ways to obtain the calcium we need, perhaps by eating *quesadillas*, tamales, and desserts with milk in them. There are also a variety of lactose-free milk products available, although at a somewhat higher price.

Consejos

When Too Much of a Good Thing Is Not Good

Toxicity results from more than:

Vitamin A	25,000 IUs a day for several months
Vitamin B6	500 mg (250 times the recommended daily allowance) or even 50 mg a day
Iron	200 mg doses have been fatal to young children

Consejos

Drink Lots of Water

Nearly two-thirds of your body is water. Water is essential for your body to function well, and that includes every process from absorption to elimination. It is a good idea to drink eight 8-ounce glasses of clean water each day (see Chapter 24).

Feeling that we need to lift our spirits, we may have a drink, forgetting that—regardless of the way it may make us feel initially—alcohol is a depressant. Moreover, alcohol in the form of wine, beer, or mixed drinks is a source of "empty calories." Some Latinas fool themselves into thinking they can make alcohol healthy by adding orange juice or tomato juice to a mixed drink, but this gesture is of marginal benefit.

We need to be very thoughtful about how food affects us. Sometimes we want to eat foods that contain fat, cholesterol, sugar, and salt because we like the way they taste, but we have to remain aware that in excess these are unhealthy choices.

Making Choices

Every Saturday my mom would take us food shopping. We would fill our shopping cart with the different ingredients she would need. She never bought canned foods or prepared foods. Every-

thing had to be made fresh for her family. She knew it was important to use the right ingredients. Throughout the store she would focus on what made each food special. The melons had to smell sweet. The colors had to be just right too. A chicken had to have a nice golden tone to its skin.

Let's begin by focusing on traditional foods—rice, beans, chicken, salad, and tortillas are all good. To eat well means that you eat the right food, not that you deny yourself food or lose weight. Many of the staples in the Hispanic diet are both tasty and good for you, providing the minerals, vitamins, fiber, and other substances that our bodies need. These foods include:

- Fruits (mango, papaya, bananas, and tomatoes) and vegetables (yucca, *malanga*, carrots, and *nopalitos*).
- Beans—black, pinto, red, navy, and pigeon. These are among the healthiest foods we can eat, and their popularity has made them easier to find.
- The combination of rice and beans, which provides all the amino acids our bodies need to produce the proteins that are essential for our health.
- Corn and flour tortillas, which provide whole grains.
- Chicken, fish, and meat, which are used in moderation as in *carnitas*, *carne asada*, *arroz con pollo*, soup, *picadillo*, and *guisados*.
- Adequate servings of milk and dairy products, as in *batidos de fruta*, *flan*, and *queso*.

All of these foods provide the body with the nutrients needed for good health. Healthy eating means that we are attentive to what our bodies need. (You will notice that in this chapter we deal only with good nutrition. Issues related to weight are extensively discussed in the following chapter.)

To help us understand what it means to eat well, experts from two government agencies—the U.S. Department of Agriculture and the U.S. Department of Health and Human Services—have worked together to develop nutritional guidelines. Rather than focusing on specific foods or weight goals, these broad guidelines recommend the following:

- Eat a variety of foods.
- Balance the food you eat with physical activity to maintain or improve your weight.
- Choose a diet with plenty of grain products, vegetables, and fruits.
- Choose a diet low in saturated fat and cholesterol, and moderate in monounsaturated fat.
- Choose a diet moderate in sugars.
- Choose a diet moderate in salt and sodium.
- If you drink alcoholic beverages, do so in moderation.

What does all this mean? It means that we have to think about what we eat so that we can eat for health and pleasure. The key word is *moderation*. The concept of moderation implies that you do something but not to excess. As Latinas, we are raised in very rule-bound communities where everything we do is compared to a community norm. Rules tend to be binary (i.e., yes—no, stop—go) in order to make decisions and actions clear. It is therefore difficult for many of us to understand that moderation as a goal means that it is, to a certain extent, up to us to determine how much of a particular food or beverage is healthy for our bodies.

When it comes to good nutrition, we have to drop our binary thinking and consider eating as a continuum, with the effect of good or bad eating as cumulative. We neither have to give up salt nor add salt to everything. We have to be very much aware of what our bodies need to function well—and customize our eating patterns to match.

Every country wants their people to be healthy and so it should not be surprising to find out that most countries develop their own set of nutritional guidelines. A few examples from our hemisphere are listed below:

- Argentina's consumers are encouraged to cook and eat at home with family members and drink plenty of nonalcoholic beverages. The guidelines also use the opportunity to communicate, "If you smoke, stop as soon as possible."
- Chile uses the pyramid to communicate their nutritional messages and has separate guidelines for seniors, children, and women of child-bearing age.
- Costa Rica uses a plate to show the four main food groups. Consumers are told that food is best in the most natural form possible.
- Guatemala uses the familiar bean pot to deliver the dietary messages which includes the recommendation to add one egg or piece of cheese at least once a week to balance the meals and also at least once a week to add liver or meat to your diet to strengthen your body.
- Mexico uses a pyramid to depict their guidelines and also recommends that consumers keep the salt shaker off the table, reduce the amount of sugar in drinks, and limit eating foods with additives or dyes.

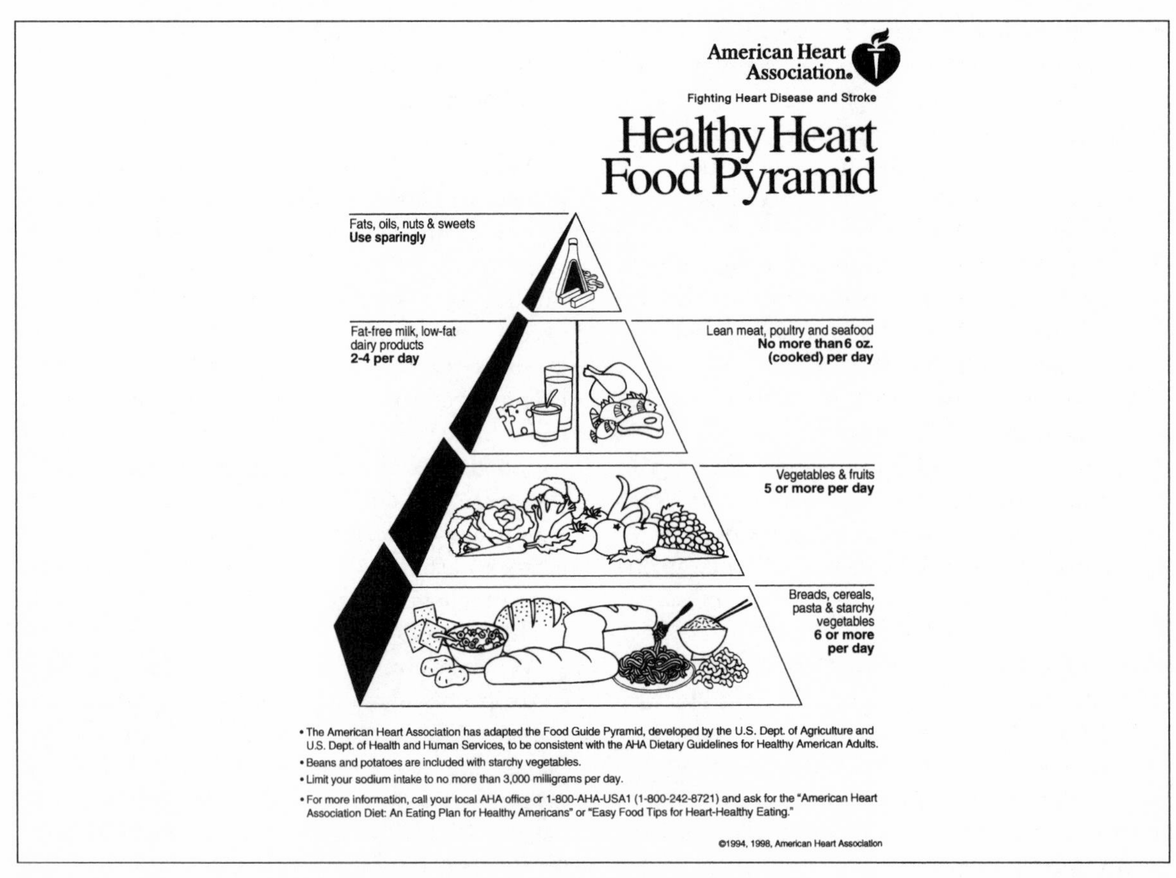

American Heart Association Food Pyramid

In 1992 the U.S. Department of Agriculture released it's first "Food Pyramid" and since then there have been a variety of adaptations to better communicate what is meant by healthy eating. For Latinas, the American Heart Association's food pyramid seems to be the most helpful and consistent with our eating habits. The AHA version differs from the USDA guidelines in a variety of ways, e.g., beans and potatoes are included with starchy vegetables instead of with meat, poultry, and fish; nuts are included with fats and oils rather than meat.

Keep in mind that no one food gives you all the nutrients you need to stay healthy, so it is best to eat a variety of different foods every day. But what is a variety of food? The best way to think of what you should eat is to look at the food pyramid.

It is hard to be exact about what we eat because planning meals for the day is often beyond our control. Instead of thinking of what you will eat for each meal, think about what your typical day is like and try to keep the food pyramid in mind. For instance, if you eat two cups of rice at lunch, you may want to skip those extra slices of bread at dinner.

Most of your meals should be made up of the items at the bottom of the pyramid—breads, cereals, rice, beans, potatoes, and pasta. You then need to eat slightly fewer portions of vegetables and fruit. Remember what a serving of food is and that you should limit your lean meat, poultry, and seafood to no more than 6 oz. (cooked) per day. The beef burrito or cheeseburger you have for lunch may use up your allotment in the meat category for the day.

Finally, you need to eat very small amounts of fats, oils, nuts, and sweets, the foods at the top of the pyramid. Keep in mind that many of the foods we eat already have fats, oils, and sweets added to them (e.g., chips, chocolate, and packaged pancake mixes).

Of just as great importance is understanding what counts as a serving of food. The chart on the next page gives you an idea of what a portion is.

Food Labels at a Glance

When most of us look at a food label, what we see is a lot of numbers and inaccessible information. The challenge is to make it work for you. Remember that the Percent Daily Values are based on a 2,000-calorie diet. To help guide you in reading the label, here are five basic things for you to look at carefully:

1: Contents. It may say apple juice in big print on the label, but when you look at the contents you may find that it also has grape juice and corn syrup.

2: Portion. The first thing to do is to look at what the label says is a typical portion. Then estimate what a typical portion would be for you, which may be either more or less than the amount given. For example, if your typical portion is two times the portion given, you will have to multiply by 2 to get the amount of calories, fat, and vitamins that you will realistically be eating.

3: Fat Content. Next look at the fat content and the calories from fat to get a sense of how much of your daily fat allowance is in a portion. Dietary guidelines recommend that we get less than 30 percent of our daily calories from fat, with no more than 10 percent saturated fat.

4: Calories. Most of us have been counting calories since we were small, so we all know what they are. The essential question to ask yourself is whether the food is worth the calories you consume. Look carefully at the portion size relative to calories. For example, the

How Much Is in a Portion?

BREADS, CEREALS, RICE, BEANS, AND PASTA

One slice of bread
One 7-inch tortilla
1 ounce of ready-to-eat cereal
½ cup of cooked cereal, rice, or pasta
l cup of cooked dry beans

VEGETABLES

1 cup of raw leafy vegetables
½ cup of other vegetables—cooked, chopped, or raw
¾ cup of vegetable juice

FRUIT

One medium banana, mango, orange, or apple
½ cup of chopped, cooked, or canned fruit (without syrup)
¾ cup of fruit juice

MILK, YOGURT, AND CHEESE

l cup of whole milk or yogurt
l½ ounces of natural cheese
2 ounces of processed cheese

label on a bag of pretzels (minimal fat) may say that it contains four servings of 50 calories each. But when we look at the bag it is best to be honest. Acknowledge that the bag may contain someone else's idea of four portions, but the reality is that it is more like one portion, which in all likelihood you will eat in one sitting. Therefore that 50 calories per portion is closer to 200 real calories.

5: Other nutrients. Finally, take a look at all the other nutrients listed and make sure you are meeting your nutritional needs.

Eating well means making healthy food choices most of the time, not all the time. For example, you will probably feel better about your improved eating habits if you allow yourself a few high-fat and high-sugar foods occasionally rather than denying yourself these foods altogether. When you completely deny yourself a favorite food, you are likely to crave it and eventually break down and eat it in large quantities.

Additionally, be aware that since 2001 the USDA set a standard for what is "organic". All products that meet the standard will be allowed to put the USDA seal on their label.

The Facts about Fat

Many of us love chocolate but are worried about eating it because chocolate is supposed to be bad for us. Many of us believe it is because of all the sugar, so we buy chocolate made with a sugar substitute. Or we buy bittersweet chocolate because we know if it is bittersweet it has less sugar.

Taking the sweet out of chocolate makes us feel that we are being good. But although bittersweet chocolate may be more bitter, it still has the same nutritional culprit—fat.

When you switch to a chocolate or candy made with a sugar substitute, you have reduced your caloric intake by only a small amount. It is not the sugar but the fat and other emulsifiers that give chocolate the richness we sometimes crave. So the next time you feel you need chocolate to lift your spirits, remember that most of the calories are coming from fat. The same thing is true of most cakes and piecrusts—it is the fat that is the major culprit in making them unhealthy.

Fat does make food taste better. If it did not, it would be easy to reduce the amount of fat we eat. Fat is also a nutrient that provides energy to the body. Our bodies need fat to help us efficiently metabolize cholesterol into estrogen and carry vitamins A, D, E, and K throughout the body. But while the body needs fat to function properly, much of what we need is manufactured by our own bodies and can be found naturally in the foods we eat. It is rarely necessary to add fat to our food.

Eating too much fat can lead to excessive weight gain, which can damage our health by increasing the risks of high blood pressure, gallbladder disease, and joint problems. In addition, high fat intake is associated with a greater likelihood of fat building up in the coronary arteries, leading to heart disease.

Consejos

How to Make Meals Healthier

1. Think of meat as a flavoring and you will eat less of it.
2. Pork tenderloin has less fat than other cuts of pork.
3. Select cuts of meat cost less than Choice or Prime and have less fat. Prime meat tends to have fat that is marbleized throughout and is more difficult to cut off.
4. Remove the skin and visible fat from chicken. This is especially helpful for increasing the health value of chicken thighs.
5. Salmon and tuna soufflés (made from egg whites) are easy to make, glorious to serve, and healthy to eat.
6. Use olive oil instead of lard to make your cooking base or *sofrito*.
7. Build your dinner around rice and beans.
8. Eat more red sauces instead of white sauces (which have more fat) with your pasta.
9. Eat dark green vegetables (e.g., broccoli, spinach), which are more nutritious than lighter green vegetables.

Fat is found in two different forms: hard (saturated) and liquid (polyunsaturated and monounsaturated). **Saturated fat** (hard) is found in meat, poultry, dairy products, lard, and certain vegetable oils such as palm, palm kernel, and coconut oil. When hydrogen is added to vegetable oil to make it solid we have created transfat. Hydrogenated vegetable oil and partially hydrogenated oils should be avoided. **Monounsaturated fat** (liquid) is found in olive and canola oil. **Polyunsaturated fat** (liquid) is found in safflower, corn, and soybean oil. It is also found to a lesser degree in some fish.

Hard fat is more likely to increase the risk of heart disease and raise cholesterol levels, but because fat is so high in calories, all fats cause weight gain when eaten in excess. If you are concerned about your health or want to change your weight, eating less fat is one important change that you can make.

Which foods are high in fat? Butter, oil, cheese, cream, margarine, lard, ground meat, chicken skin, many cuts of beef and pork, fried foods, mayonnaise, *churritos*, bacon, salad dressing, *chorizo*, and pork rinds are all high in fat. Which foods contain fat that is not so obvious? Chocolate, nuts, baked goods, cookies, milk, refried beans, crackers, peanut butter, and gravy.

How is more fat added to foods? By frying, adding bacon or *chorizo*, adding butter or margarine, using drippings for cooking, adding mayonnaise or salad dressing.

The healthy thing to do is to eat less of all fats. When fat is used, it is better to use small amounts of monounsaturated or polyunsaturated vegetable oils, especially olive oil, rather than lard or butter.

What Is Cholesterol?

Cholesterol and fat are not the same thing. Cholesterol is a waxlike material found only in animal products such as beef, pork, poultry, fish, lard, milk and milk products, and egg yolks. Fruits (including bananas, avocados, and mangos), vegetables, and grains have *no* cholesterol. Cholesterol is needed by the body for good health, but many people eat more than the body needs.

Too much cholesterol in the body can lead to heart disease. Foods rich in cholesterol include dairy products, eggs, organ meats, beef, pork, chicken, and shell fish. Some animal products contain more cholesterol than others. Foods lower in cholesterol include lean cuts of beef and pork, chicken and turkey white meat with no skin, fish, and low-fat dairy products.

About Sugar

Contrary to what is frequently believed, sugar does not cause diabetes. However, people who have diabetes need to control the amount of sugar they eat because their bodies cannot properly metabolize it. Neither does sugar actually cause tooth decay. Tooth decay is caused by bacteria that feed on sugar. Teeth that have not been cleaned properly are subject to decay.

Some examples of foods high in sugar are cakes, regular soda, cookies, Kool-Aid, Tang, alcoholic drinks with added sugar, and candy. Some examples of sweet foods low in sugar are fruits, animal crackers, vanilla wafers, and plain graham crackers.

Consejos

Using Herbs and Spices

1. Use lemon juice and lime juice as a base for all marinades (excluding pork).
2. Use apple cider vinegar as a base for pork marinade.
3. Use oregano, cumin, onions, and garlic to enhance flavors of meats.
4. Use unfinished bottles of red wine and white wine for marinades.
5. Squeeze lemon on your corn-on-the-cob instead of butter.
6. Adapt most recipes by reducing salt to half of what is recommended and doubling the amounts of onions and garlic used for seasoning.

Consejos

The Story on Fat Substitutes

The research jury is still out on many fat substitutes, including margarine. Wait and see whether they have any positive effects. In the meantime use monounsaturated or polyunsaturated oils. Even small amounts of butter may be better than margarine.

About Salt and Sodium

The connection between salt and sodium is often misunderstood. Sodium is an element that, along with chloride, makes up salt.

Sodium (40 percent) + Chloride (60 percent) = Salt

Our bodies need only about ⅛ teaspoon of salt (300 mg of sodium) every day to be healthy. Since sodium is so common in the foods we eat, however, it is difficult to eat only 300 mg per day. The recommended amount of sodium per day is 2,400 mg (1 teaspoon of salt). Many people eat 7,000 mg or more of sodium per day. This is more than twenty-three times the amount our bodies need.

The good news about eating less salt is that you can easily get used to the taste of low-salt foods. It takes only two weeks for your taste buds to make the adjustment, and then you won't even notice that you are eating less salt.

Consejos

Recipe Modifications

1. When making *flan*, substitute fat free evaporated milk for regular evaporated milk.
2. When frying eggs, use a nonstick pan and (because all nonstick pans are not totally nonstick) add a few drops of olive oil.
3. Serve dressings, syrup, and sauces on the side to encourage dipping food instead of soaking food in them. This applies to maple syrup too.
4. Reduce the amount of *chorizo* you use in recipes by half so that the *chorizo* becomes a flavor enhancer rather than the main dish.
5. Plantains are delicious when roasted rather than fried in fat. Wrap them in foil and put them in the oven at 350 degrees for 1 hour for an easy and tasty treat. You can also wrap them in microwaveable plastic wrap and microwave them for a few minutes on high.
6. Use chicken broth for mashed potatoes instead of butter.

And there is ample incentive for reducing the salt in our diets. A diet that is high in salt can cause high blood pressure, heart problems, kidney disease, and stroke.

Sodium is found in:

• Fresh foods—Small amounts of sodium are found naturally in almost all foods. For instance:

1 medium tomato	=	10 mg sodium
1 cup black beans	=	6 mg sodium
1 medium boiled potato	=	16 mg sodium
1 medium mango	=	4 mg sodium

• Processed and packaged foods—Salt and sodium are used as a preservative and flavoring in many processed and packaged foods. These additives include sodium benzoate, sodium nitrate, and monosodium glutamate (MSG). Processed and packaged foods include canned products, cheese, frozen meals, processed meats (such as Spam), and instant foods such as breakfast cereals and precooked rice.

1 cup canned tomato juice	=	486 mg sodium
1 cup canned black beans	=	922 mg sodium
½ cup instant potatoes	=	340 mg sodium
1 cube chicken bouillon	=	1,152 mg sodium

When food is processed, the sodium content increases. People who eat many processed and packaged foods as well as fast foods often find that they eat more sodium than they need.

Examples of foods high in salt and sodium are chicken bouillon, canned foods, cheese, frozen meals, lunch meats, instant breakfast cereals, precooked rice, *saladitos*, potato chips, tortilla chips, crackers, and salted nuts. Foods low in salt include fresh fruits, fresh vegetables, dry (not canned) beans, grains, most breads, fresh meat, poultry, and fish.

Fiber

Fiber promotes digestion and assuming that we need to eat more fiber, we should:

- Eat beans and peas several times a week.
- Add rice, vegetables, beans, and peas to soup.
- Eat corn and whole-wheat flour tortillas instead of white flour tortillas.
- Eat whole-grain bread rather than white bread.
- Leave the skin on potatoes instead of peeling them.

- Eat oatmeal and whole-grain ready-to-eat cereals several times a week.
- Eat fruits like guava, apples, pears, and plums with their skins.

Nowadays there are many good cookbooks that can help us prepare tasty and healthy meals. The resources that follow will help you eat healthy meals.

Summary

Rethinking the foods we eat is one of the easiest and most dramatic changes we can make in our lives. The results can change how we feel and look and benefit our overall health. The key is to become aware of how our bodies use food and of what foods our bodies need. While we may get most of our nutrients from a balanced diet, the demands of our lives may also make it necessary for us to take vitamins.

We have to learn what nutrients we need and build on the benefits that accumulate from the traditional Hispanic diet. Eating well-belanced meals does not mean that we never have chocolate or that we do not eat the things we enjoy the most. Rather, we must learn that moderation is the key to eating in a way that is nutritionally sound.

RESOURCES

Organizations

American Anorexia/Bulimia Association, Inc.
165 W. 46th St., Ste. 1108
New York, NY 10036
(212) 575-6200
www.aabainc.org

American Dietetic Association
216 West Jackson Boulevard
Chicago, IL 60606
(800) 366-1655 or (312) 899-0040
www.eatright.org

American Heart Association
7272 Greenville Avenue
Dallas, TX 75231-4596
(800) 242-8721 or (214) 706-1220
www.americanheart.org

American Stroke Association
7272 Greenville Avenue
Dallas, TX 75231-4596
(214) 706-1525
www.strokeassociation.org

Center for Nutrition Policy and Promotion
U.S. Dept. of Agriculture
1120 20th Street NW, Suite 200, North Lobby
Washington, DC 20036
(202) 418-2312
www.usda.gov/cnpp

Food and Drug Administration Office of Consumer Affairs
Parklawn Building, Room 1685
5600 Fishers Lane
Rockville, MD 20857
(301) 827-5006 or (888) 463-6332
www.fda.gov/oca/oca.htm

Food and Nutrition Information Center
U.S. Dept. of Agriculture/National Agricultural Library, Rm 364
10301 Baltimore Ave.
Beltsville, MD 20705-2351
(301) 504-5719
www.nal.usda.gov/fnic

National Cancer Institute Cancer Information Service
Building 31, Room 10A03
31 Center Dr. MSC 2580
Bethesda, MD 20892-2580
(800) 4CANCER (800-422-6237)
www.cancernet.nci.nih.gov/ncipubs/

Hotlines

American Dietetic Association Consumer Nutrition Hotline
(800) 366-1655 (English)

Books

The PDR Family Guide to Nutrition and Health. Montvale, NJ: Medical Economics Data, 1995.

Somer, Elizabeth. *The Essential Guide to Vitamins and Minerals.* New York: HarperCollins, 1996.

Somer, Elizabeth. *Nutrition for Women: The Complete Guide.* New York: Henry Holt, 1995.

Publications and Pamphlets

"Action Guide for Healthy Eating," 1995. NIH Publication No. 95-3877. Tips on low-fat, high-fiber eating. National Cancer Institute Cancer Information Service, www.cissecure.nci.nih.gov.nicpw; (800) 422-6237. Other titles include:

"Celebre la Cocina Hispana," 1995. NIH Publication No. 95-3906(s). Healthy Hispanic recipes.

"Eat Less Fat," 1996. NIH Publication No. 95-3910. Tips on reducing fat intake (also available in Spanish).

"The Food Pyramid," 1996. Publication No. HG-252. How to choose what and how much to eat from each food group (also available in Spanish). Center for Nutrition Policy and Promotion, U.S. Department of Agriculture, 1120 20th Street NW, Suite 200, Washington, DC 20036; (202) 208-2417.

20

The Body We Have . . . The Body We Want

Sonia shook her head as she looked at herself in the mirror. She was so disappointed with the image she saw. Her breasts were the wrong size, her waist was too big, and her legs were too short. It was hard to look at that image and feel good. To make matters worse, she was beginning to see that the smiles she had cherished were beginning to leave little lines on her face. So she put more makeup on to cover the lines and covered her body with a baggy sweater so that no one would notice all the things she did not want anyone to notice.

Too often when we look in the mirror we are not pleased with the woman who looks back at us. Some of us stare at the image and want to lose weight; others want to gain weight; an ever-increasing number of us want to make surgical changes in our appearance; and some of us just look away in disgust, knowing we will never be able to make the changes we feel are needed. But the changes we want to make may have little to do with what we really need to do and even less with what is healthy.

Through the variety of sources of information that help form our self-image, we have learned that if we look a certain way we will get the affection and nurturance we desire. Some of us use an unattractive appearance to insulate ourselves from the affection that others of us seek. The consequences of the way we feel about how we look are far reaching. Too often they invade the depths of our souls and temper every smile that slips through.

Regardless of the changes we think we should make, our goal must be to make healthy changes that balance our body, mind, and spirit. Too many of us focus on looking good and forget that what we really need is to be healthy. If we are healthy, we will naturally look good and feel good. Our new *dicho* (saying) should be "Feel good, look good."

Most women are taught to be critical of themselves. In addition, as Latinas, in our commitment to take care of others we often abandon ourselves to suffer from what can best be called benign neglect. But neglecting ourselves is never benign.

The challenge that faces us, as Latinas, is to find a way to be happy with who we are and to integrate the different messages we get from society.

*When I was a kid, my mother would kiss me good-bye every morning when I left for school. Her words were always the same: "*Te adoro, mi gordita*" (I cherish you, my little chubby one). In my family,* mi gordita *was an endearment. I knew I was loved and that being* gordita *meant I was especially cute. In another culture, I might have been teased about my weight, but I was a happy kid. I was in college before I began to feel that* gordita *wasn't necessarily what I wanted to be.*

—*Julia, 56*

When we see ourselves, we see *una gordita* (a chubby one) or *la flaca* (the thin one). *Gordita* can be an endearing term for many Latinas, but *la flaca* is never said in an endearing way. Whether you are *gordita* or *flaca*, though, the first step is to recognize what standard you are using to determine what you want to be.

From movies to television to magazines to CD-ROMs, the images of Latinas are few and far between. As a result, too often we end up inundated with images of women who are very different from most of us. These women have lighter complexions and are taller and weigh less than most Latinas. Most important, these images are not of women who are managing real lives but of women who are trying to sell a product or an idea. So, how will each one of us decide what we want to look like?

We need to develop a realistic image of our body. But the problem is that we often develop images that do not address our body.

To help us achieve American culture's ideal figure, entire industries have sprung to life. They advise millions of women to spend billions of dollars on diet foods, weight-loss and weight-gain programs, and food supplements. We buy books because their titles tell us we will be able to lose in thirty days the pounds it took ten years to accumulate.

The effect of the "never too thin" and "ideal weight" messages has been girls who begin to diet in elementary school, grown women who obsess about every extra ounce, women who shroud their bodies in layers of oversized clothing to hide how thin they are, and women whose self-esteem is undermined because they do not meet the ideal. Ironically, the "never too thin" messages have not resulted in weight loss. In fact, data on non-Hispanic women in America show a trend toward increasing weight. This increase may be due at least in part to the second message women get—that it is good to eat and that food is best when it is easy to prepare, convenient, and abundant.

The United States is the birthplace of fast food, 24-hour diners, and three square meals a day. We are taught that we should eat whenever we want and at a pace that practically insures indigestion. At the same time that we get the "thin, thin, thin" message, we also get the message to "eat, eat, eat" and to do so quickly. And if you are too thin, you are accused of having an eating disorder, when in fact you may be struggling to gain weight. How can we reconcile these conflicting messages?

Consejos

How to Make Your Body the Best for You

1. Understand how you think about your body.
2. Change how you think about eating and food.
3. Understand weight, fat, muscle, and metabolism.
4. Change your activity level.
5. Eat healthy food.

The first step is to understand ourselves better. Some of us may have to come to terms with obstacles we cannot surmount. We may always have short legs, or we may always be too tall to be considered "petite." Others of us need to address aspects of ourselves that we can change. For example, because we know that it isn't healthy to be too heavy, some of us must lose weight.

1: Understand how you think about your body. Hispanic culture does not subscribe to the American view that a woman can never be too thin, nor does it focus on an ideal weight. In fact, among Latinas it is often acceptable, if not desirable, for a women to be a bit . . . *gordita*. As Latinas, although we may share these values, we live in American society, which gives women strong negative messages about being *gordita* and drives each one of us toward an ideal often quite different from the way we actually look. Others of us may struggle to gain weight in order to be more appealing.

2: Change how you think about eating and food. Eating. It is what we do to celebrate. It is what we do when we gather together to talk with our *comadres*. And it is one of the major activities that brings families together. We grow up thinking of eating as one of the most important activities we share with those we love. And it is not just the eating that is important to us but every part of the sitting down to a meal.

When we Latinas were growing up, meals were more than a time set aside to nourish our bodies. They were times for *la familia* (the family). We worked together to prepare the meal and set the table. Each of us would then sit in our place, and the table would bubble with the details of our day. The food scenes in the movie *Like Water for Chocolate* detail the familiar passions involved in the selection of ingredients, the preparation of food, the serving of food, and the way food affects our every mood.

We learned how to mix the right blend of olive oil, garlic, cumin, oregano, and onions to prepare a basic *sofrito*. We learned that the preparation of food, with all of its technical aspects, was how love could be shown.

I would always ask my mother how she knew what to put in all her different soups. She would smile and say that you know by the smell. She encouraged me to smell the vapors and enjoy the different scents of the vegetables and spices.

I remember shaking my head and saying that I could not smell the difference. To me it was just vapors. Living by myself, years later, I found that when I would make my soup, I would smell the vapors as they rose above the pot. And somehow I knew that I had put just the right mix of things in the pot. I guess I really could tell the difference . . .

—Cassandra, 35

How do we know how much spice to put in? Do we measure with tablespoons and measuring cups? Most of the time we do not. We put a little of this, a fistful of that, blend it together, inhale the scent, and know if it is right. Food preparation becomes a component of eating that goes beyond a recipe and involves all the senses.

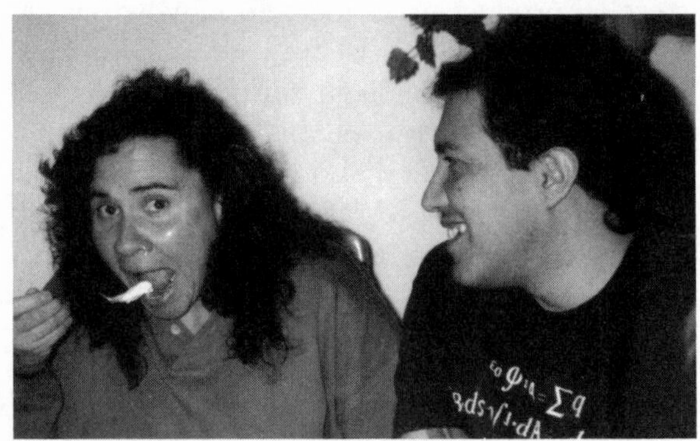

We like to eat!

In many ways our relationship with food goes back to some of our spiritual roots—being grateful for the food before us and being thankful for the love shared between us as we sit around the table. We appreciate the food before us because we know the effort and love that went into making it.

I remember the first time I had dinner with one of my non-Latina friends. We entered her dining room and everyone sat down to eat. The only time people spoke was when they asked for food to be passed to them. It was so strange for me. In that family, dinner was a quiet time, and you only spoke if you were spoken to. How different it was from mealtime in my home! Some of us would work in the kitchen preparing the food, while others would set the table—we each had our chores. We would chatter away about our day and our plans. I understood much better why my non-Hispanic friends liked to eat at my house. It was more than the delicious food my mom always managed to prepare. Dinner at my house was alive with the stories that each person shared of the day's events.

Our lives have changed, and too often meals have become subordinate to other activities, so that while we may have fond memories of meals past, our present realities place us in a different setting. Still, food memories are an important part of our lives, and the exercise of will power alone will not change any unhealthy behavior we have developed. To change how we eat, we have to change how we think about food. Eating in our community is an emotional activity, and we can make our values work for us.

3: Understand weight, fat, muscle, and metabolism. New medical evidence indicates that some Hispanic body types were designed to carry more weight than the "ideal weight" tables would indicate. Other findings suggest that some of us Latinas have weight problems because we metabolize fats differently than non-Hispanics do. We each have to decide what's right for ourselves as Latinas and as healthy women.

I am sure you know how much you weigh. In all likelihood you weighed yourself in the past month at least once. The reason we focus on weight as the major indicator of how we look is that it is the simplest thing to measure.

Increasingly, however, we are focusing not just on weight as a measure of health but on where we carry that weight. For instance, persons who carry their weight in the stomach area are much more prone to heart attacks than persons who carry their weight on their hips, thighs, and buttocks. Consequently, the apple-shaped person seems more at risk of a heart attack than the pear-shaped one.

Consejos

To Reduce Saturated Fat

1. Make rice and beans the central part of your meal.
2. Use meat for flavor rather than as the major part of the meal.
3. Use olive oil instead of butter.
4. Instead of adding butter to pasta, add chicken broth.
5. For sandwiches use mustard instead of mayonnaise.
6. Do not add cheese to sandwiches.
7. Eat pancakes with syrup on the side and no butter.
8. Remove skin and all visible fat from chicken.
9. Avoid cream or butter sauces.
10. Check the nutritional content on the labels of everything you eat or cook with.

As for fat and muscle, a pound of fat takes up more space than a pound of muscle. Moreover, a pound of muscle burns more energy than a pound of fat. That means that a muscular person can consume more calories than a person whose weight comes mostly from fat.

Two Latinas can be the same height and weight but if their weight is based on different percentages of body fat, their appearance can vary greatly. At 5 feet 3 inches, a 200-pound woman who has only 24 percent body fat will look very different from a woman of the same height and weight who has 44 percent body fat. Not only will the women look different, but the woman with less body fat will also be able to eat more. And more fat instead of muscle translates into larger clothing sizes too.

Finally, I am sure that many times you have been surprised at how different people can be—some are unable to gain weight no matter how much they try, while others only have to look at a tamale and it goes right to their hips. How fast your metabolism works determines how efficiently you burn or store food. Regular exercise increases your metablism.

4: Change your activity level. In order to be healthy we must be active. Chapter 21 provides extensive information on how to be physically fit through exercise. Whether your goal is to increase or decrease your body size, exercise is a key ingredient to your health.

5: Eat healthy foods. The first thing to keep in mind is that we need to maintain many aspects of our traditional diet. In Chapter 19 we discussed the beneficial aspects of the diverse Hispanic foods. Our traditional foods are rich in flavor and texture and a delight to the senses as well. The challenge is to combine our Hispanic view about food and the foods that are part of our traditions with some of the healthier components of the dominant American diet.

Setting Healthy Goals

How do you decide what is the right goal for you? First, instead of being driven by a specific number, try to think of a weight range where you would like to be. Today the trend is to use Body Mass Index (BMI) as one of the measures to determine a person's health. Keep in mind that BMI is not a measure of the percentage of body fat. Moreover, since BMI is based on overall norms it may not be as directly applicable to Latinas. To calculate your BMI you can use the table on the next page or one of the formulas below:

Your weight in pounds ÷ your height in inches ÷ your height in inches × 703

OR

Your weight in kilos ÷ your height in cm ÷ your height in cm × 10,000

Once you know your BMI you may use the guidelines below to help you decide what to do to be more healthy.

Category	Guideline (regardless of age or sex)
Underweight	less than 18.5
Healthy weight	18.5 to 24.9
Overweight	25 to 29.9
Obese	over 30

Here are some key questions to ask yourself to help set healthy and realistic goals.

1: How much did you weigh the last time you felt comfortable with your weight? And I mean *comfortable*. The important goal is that you feel good and be able to do the things that make you happy. Perhaps you have never felt very comfortable with yourself. If that is the case, focusing on your weight may not be the best place to start.

BODY MASS INDEX (BMI) TABLE

BMI	19	20	21	22	23	24	25	26	27	28	29	30	31	32	33	34	35
Height	**Weight (in pounds)**																
4′10″ or 58″	91	96	100	105	110	115	119	124	129	134	138	143	148	153	158	162	167
4′11″ or 59″	94	99	104	109	114	119	124	128	133	138	143	148	153	158	163	168	173
5′ or 60″	97	102	107	112	118	123	128	133	138	143	148	153	158	163	168	174	179
5′1″ or 61″	100	106	111	116	122	127	132	137	143	148	153	158	164	169	174	180	185
5′2″ or 62″	104	109	115	120	126	131	136	142	147	153	158	164	169	175	180	186	191
5′3″ or 63″	107	113	118	124	130	135	141	146	152	158	163	169	175	180	186	191	197
5′4″ or 64″	110	116	122	128	134	140	145	151	157	163	169	174	180	186	192	197	204
5′5″ or 65″	114	120	126	132	138	144	150	156	162	168	174	180	186	192	198	204	210
5′6″ or 66″	118	124	130	136	142	148	155	161	167	173	179	186	192	198	204	210	216
5′7″ or 67″	121	127	134	140	146	153	159	166	172	178	185	191	198	204	211	217	223
5′8″ or 68″	125	131	138	144	151	158	164	171	177	184	190	197	203	210	216	223	230
5′9″ or 69″	128	135	142	149	155	162	169	176	182	189	196	203	209	216	223	230	236
5′10″ or 70″	132	139	146	153	160	167	174	181	188	195	202	209	216	222	229	236	243
5′11″ or 71″	136	143	150	157	165	172	179	186	193	200	208	215	222	229	236	243	250
6′ or 72″	140	147	154	162	169	177	184	191	199	206	213	221	228	235	242	250	258
6′1″ or 73″	144	151	159	166	174	182	189	197	204	212	219	227	235	242	250	257	265
6′2″ or 74″	148	155	163	171	179	186	194	202	210	218	225	233	241	249	256	264	272
6′3″ or 75″	152	160	168	176	184	192	200	208	216	224	232	240	248	256	264	272	279

Source: Evidence Report of Clinical Guidelines on the Identification, Evaluation, and Treatment of Overweight and Obesity in Adults, 1998, NIH/National Heart, Lung, and Blood Institute (NHLBI)

Issues of self-esteem are too often wrapped up in our body image. And as Latinas, the messages we have received from the dominant culture in the United States too often emphasize those things we are not and cannot be.

2: How many years ago was that? Remember that as you get older your body shifts and your metabolism slows down, and that makes it harder to lose weight. Those of us trying to gain weight may find that after menopause it becomes easier. It is natural, normal, and good for a woman's body to be different from a girl's body.

3: Has there been any change in your health status? Sometimes the shape of our bodies may be a natural result of changes in our health. If we begin to take hormones as part of our attempt to control our fertility or in order to help our bodies adjust to menopause, our bodies may change. Also after pregnancy our bodies may be different.

4: Do most of your clothes fit? Fitting means more than just getting your clothes on. Fitting means that you can breathe, walk, sit, stand, and engage in normal day-to-day activity without having to worry about the positioning of your attire. Sometimes we squeeze

Six Questions to Help Set Your Weight Target

1. How much did you weigh the last time you felt comfortable with your weight?
2. How many years ago was that?
3. Has there been any change in your health status?
4. Do most of your clothes fit?
5. Are you able to walk up two flights of steps without being out of breath?
6. Can you walk 1 mile in 20 minutes or less?

ourselves into clothes and get the *salchicha* (sausage) look, believing that if we can get into an outfit that is really too small for us we are OK. Others get lost in layers of clothing as they try to conceal the shape of their body. The reality is that clothes that fit comfortably are the most attractive. Evaluate the clothes in your closet by fit, not size.

When I think of my closet I think that someone should fine manufacturers for failure to provide truth in labeling. I mean all that business of "one size fits all." Who on earth ever came up with that concept?

While men's clothes are tailored down to the sleeve length, I am supposed to believe that my 5 foot 11 inch friend, Debbie, who weighs all of 140 pounds, and I, with my 5 foot 2 inch (minus) and 185 pound (plus) figure, will both be able to wear the same blouse. At the very least the label should say, "one size fits most."

—*DORA, 38*

While Seventh Avenue uses as its ideal a size 6 or size 8 mannequin, the fact is that half of all women in the United States wear size 14 or larger. One of the most revealing articles I have read in a woman's magazine showed a size 10 model trying on various size 10 dresses, skirts, and tops. The photographs showed that only one brand fit her well. Although in all the pictures she wore clothing labeled size 10, some items were too big, some too small, and only a few were just right. So do not judge your size by the size of clothing. Try on several items and check how they fit. Then decide when was the last time they fit well.

5: Are you able to walk up two flights of steps without being out of breath? If you cannot do this, exercising is an important thing to consider. You should discuss any changes in diet or exercise you plan to make with your health care provider so that you get a good sense of what you should be capable of doing. Additionally, when you exercise you should be able to speak without huffing and puffing. If you cannot speak, you are overdoing it.

6: Can you walk one mile in 20 minutes or less? It is not necessary to be able to run a mile or to have great speed. The goal is to be able to move at a moderate pace for an extended period of time. One mile in 20 minutes is a good pace. If you are able to do this then you are on your way to health. If you cannot do this, then it is time to start a walking program.

Before you know it you will be able to walk one mile in 20 minutes.

Latinas come in all sizes and shapes. The important thing is to recognize what is right for you and to know how much change is realistic for you. Too often weight becomes just one more external pressure pushing us away from the woman we really are. There is no use trying to be somebody that you were never meant to be.

Losing Weight

Several years ago I discovered the secret to weight loss. To lose weight you have to do

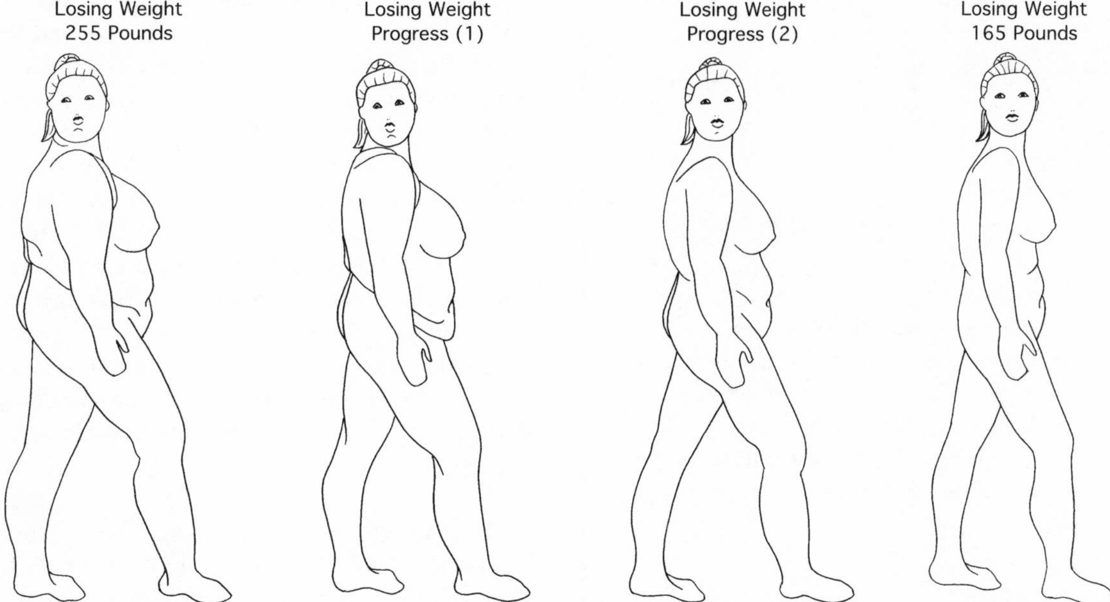

three things: (1) eat healthy foods—which sometimes means eating less fatty foods and more fruits and vegetables, (2) increase your activity, and (3) be patient. In short, the amount of food you put into your body has to be less than the energy you put out, and you have to give yourself time to lose weight or you will give up. While packaged diets and diet foods are tools that theoretically help some of us to lose weight, the reality is that for most of us they are often just a waste of money. We just have to change the way we do things.

I wish there were some other way, but those three steps are what will work best. What you need to do is find the combination of foods that makes you feel most satisfied and provides the best nutrition. In order to inspire you in this process in a realistic manner, the drawings above are of a real woman in her mid-thirties who went from 255 pounds to 165 pounds.

There are so many diets that it is hard to tell which one will work for you. While one Latina will do well by joining a group and meeting on a regular basis, another Latina would rather simply cut back on her desserts.

Myths and Facts

Myth: If I eat a low-fat diet, I can lose weight and eat everything I want.

Fact: A low-fat diet may be good for your heart, but if you eat more in calories than you expend, you will not lose weight.

Myth: There is a great diet where you lose 5 to 10 pounds in five days.

Fact: To keep off the weight you lose, you should lose weight slowly (about 1 pound a week or less).

Myth: I cannot change my weight.

Fact: You can change your weight if you follow the steps in this chapter.

Myth: I can eat margarine instead of butter and lose weight.

Fact: Margarine and butter have the same amount of fat and calories.

Consejos

For Your Body, Mind, and Spirit

1. Be healthy. You are getting healthier because you are working toward your goal.
2. Be realistic. You will probably not look like a fashion model.
3. Be patient. Take it slowly. You did not get to your size in one day, so give yourself time. Weight is more likely to stay off if you change your eating habits slowly and permanently.
4. Be forgiving. One day off your plan does not mean that you are off the plan permanently.
5. Be active.
6. Be happy.
7. Be at peace with yourself.

Healthy eating means more than counting calories or fat grams. It means that we eat to nourish our bodies. There are three important things to do:

1. Eat when you are hungry.
2. Eat what you want.
3. Stop when you are satisfied.

1: Eat when you are hungry. In other words, eat when you feel hungry. To eat in a healthy way means that you do not eat by the clock or let other people's needs determine when you eat. If someone else is hungry but you are not, do not feel that you have to eat. By the same token, if you are trying to eat less, do not wait until you are painfully hungry to eat, because this will only encourage overeating.

As a first step you have to understand that it takes skill and practice to listen to your body.

2: Eat what you want to eat. To say that you will never have *flan* again is not realistic. It is more important to eat less of it and keep it for special occasions than to deny yourself completely. If you totally deny yourself something you consider a true pleasure, you increase the chances that you will engage in binge eating. Remember, however, that if you do go on a binge, you can always go back to your healthy eating program. Don't use one slip as an excuse to quit.

If you are trying to eat more, make sure you eat foods you enjoy. High-calorie foods that you do not like will not make eating pleasurable for you.

3: Stop when you are satisfied. This is the hardest part. Most of us do not know what it means to be satisfied. We pile our plate with food the way we did when we were younger, even though as we get older we metabolize our food more slowly and need to eat less. Many of us eat until we are bloated. Sometimes we feel that to show our appreciation for a meal we have to eat everything in large quantities. But this is not good for anyone. You have to teach yourself to eat what you need and recognize when you are satisfied.

What does it mean to be satisfied? Using a 7-point scale, with 1 being totally starving and

Consejos

Eating Scale—Goal Is 4

7 = Extremely full
6 = Moderately full
5 = Somewhat full
4 = Satisfied
3 = Somewhat hungry
2 = Moderately hungry
1 = Extremely hungry

7 being that bloated, uncomfortable feeling when you have overeaten, try to focus on being at level 4—right in the middle. It should feel comfortable.

Maintaining Your Goal

The first thing you have to remember is that as you get older your metabolism slows down. This is good for those of us who need to gain weight. For most of us, however, it explains why we have trouble maintaining our weight even though we eat much less than we did when we were younger. What follows is a healthy eating program that, when combined with daily vitamins and exercise, will help most Latinas increase their fitness.

A HEALTHY EATING PROGRAM

First Meal	Calories
Coffee, 1 Tbs. milk, 2 tsp. sugar	72
Orange juice (4 oz.)	50
One egg (any style)	110
2 pieces of toast or 1 bagel or 2 tortillas	200
Total	432
OR	
Various fruits (banana, apple, or orange)	100
Dry cereal (check package)	130
2% milk (one cup)	110
Total	340
OR	
Hot oatmeal made with 2% milk	200
2 tsp. sugar	32
Total	232
OR	
Three 6″ pancakes	180
2 Tbs. syrup (no butter)	120
Fruit	100
Coffee (black)	0
Total	400

Main Meal	Calories
1 cup rice or pasta	200
½ cup beans or red sauce	100
4 oz. lean meat or 6 oz. fish	300
2 cups leafy vegetables or salad	100
Total	700
OR	
¼ lb. lean ground meat	400
Bread or tortilla	200
1 Tbs. salsa/ketchup	50
Lettuce, tomatoes, and pickles	75
Total	725
OR	
Grilled chicken breast	250
Bun	200
1 Tbs. mayonnaise	100
Lettuce, tomatoes, and pickles	75
Total	625

Second Daily Meal	
1 cup rice or pasta	200
½ cup beans or red sauce	100
2 cups leafy vegetables or salad	100
Total	400

Two Snacks (During the Day or with Meal)	
1 mango	100
⅛ piece of fruit pie (do not eat crust)	100
Total	200

Plastic Surgery

I had not seen Patricia since she had the bags under her eyes removed. I remember when I spoke to her soon after the surgery. She talked about the pain and how when she first looked at herself in the mirror, she was horrified at how she looked and began to cry. But she soon learned not to cry because her tears made her eyelashes stick together and it was even more painful to open her eyes.

When we sat down for lunch I tried not to stare at her. She looked the same to me—just a tiny bit fresher. For all that money, risk, and pain I thought

I would see some major difference. But what I thought did not matter. Patricia felt that after all she had gone through with her divorce, her plastic surgery gave her a new lease on life. And what was I to say? When I looked at her I smiled and, as only a friend would, said, "You look great!"

—Biba, 48

Some Latinas decide to change their appearance surgically. While some of these procedures may seem minor and commonplace, very often they involve complicated matters related to self-esteem and other psychological issues that deserve extensive discussion. To insure the best outcomes, it is strongly recommended that a Latina considering major cosmetic surgery discuss her rationale with a mental health professional. If she still chooses to pursue surgery, the best advice is to:

- Have reasonable expectations about the outcomes, both cosmetically and in your life.
- Remember that surgery always involves some risk.
- Make sure you have a reputable surgeon who is skilled and board-certified. (Contact the Information Service of the American Society of Plastic and Reconstructive Surgeons at 444 E. Algonquin Road, Dept. P, Arlington Heights, IL 60005.)
- Ask to see some pictures of your surgeon's successes with your skin tone. Remember that women with darker skins may not heal as well as women with fair complexions.
- Make sure that the operating area is board-certified if the procedure will be done in the surgeon's office by an organization such as the Accreditation Association for Ambulatory Health Care (847-676-9610).
- Be prepared for a recuperation period that is longer than you are told it will be.
- Know that you will probably have to repeat the procedure in a few years.
- Realize that liposuction should be avoided because of its long-term effects.

To provide you with more information on related topics, there is an extensive list of publications below.

Summary

The ideal self that we imagine is often not only inconsistent with our body but a product of marketing techniques designed to sell us products to make our bodies different than they are. For most people, maintaining a healthy self-image requires understanding how we think about our body and setting realistic goals for things we may want to change.

Fundamentally, we need to understand the role of weight, fat, muscle, and metabolism in the body we have. There are many myths about these critical factors, which need to be dispelled so that we can plan to shape our bodies in the way we desire within our biological limits.

RESOURCES

Organizations

American Anorexia/Bulimia Association, Inc.
165 W. 46th St., Ste 1103
New York, NY 10036
(212) 575-6200
www.aabainc.org

American Dietetic Association
National Center for Nutrition and Dietetics
216 West Jackson Boulevard
Chicago, IL 60606-6995
(800) 366-1655 or (312) 899-0040 ext. 4653
www.eatright.org

American Heart Association
7272 Greenville Avenue
Dallas, TX 75231-4596
(800) 242-8721 or (214) 706-1220
www.americanheart.org

National Health Information Center
P.O. Box 1133
Washington, DC 20013-1133
(800) 336-4797

Books

Cash, Thomas F. *What Do You See When You Look in the Mirror? Helping Yourself to a Positive Body Image.* New York: Bantam, 1995.

Hirschmann, Jane R. *When Women Stop Hating Their Bodies: Freeing Yourself from Food and Weight Obsession.* New York: Fawcett, 1995.

Patterson, Catherine M., and others. *Nutrition and Eating Disorders: Guidelines for the Patient with Anorexia Nervosa and Bulimia Nervosa*. Van Nuys, CA: PM, 1992.

Wolfe, Naomi. *The Beauty Myth: How Images of Beauty Are Used against Women.* New York: Doubleday, 1992.

Publications and Pamphlets

"Eating Disorders." National Women's Health Network, 514 10th Street NW, Suite 400, Washington, DC 20004; (202) 628-7814.

"Eat Less Fat," 1995. NIH Publication No. 93-3910. Tips on reducing fat intake (also available in Spanish). National Institutes of Health, National Cancer Institute, Washington, DC; (800) 422-6237.

"Exercise and Weight Control." Diet and nutrition information while on a fitness program. President's Council on Physical Fitness and Sports, Washington, DC 20201; (202) 272-3421.

"Get Fit, Trim Down: Managing Weight and Following the Dietary Guidelines to Lower Cancer Risk," April 1995. Pamphlet No. E54-TD/E38AICR. Information Series Part III. American Institute for Cancer Research, Washington, DC; (800) 843-8114.

"Lean Toward Health," 1995. Includes ways to reduce the fat in your diet. American Dietetic Association National Center for Nutrition and Dietetics, 216 West Jackson Boulevard, Chicago, IL 60606-6995; (312) 899-0040 ext. 4653.

"Weight Control: Losing Weight and Keeping It Off," 1999. Pamphlet No. 1522. American Academy of Family Physicians, 11400 Tomahawk Creek Pkwy, Leawood, KS 66211-2672; (800) 944-0000.

PLASTIC SURGERY

Organizations

American Academy of Facial Plastic and Reconstructive Surgery
310 S. Henry Street
Alexandria, VA 22314
(800) 332-FACE (800-332-3223) or (703) 299-9291
Not all members are certified by the American Board of Plastic Surgery.
www.aafprs.org

American Society of Plastic and Reconstructive Surgeons
444 E. Algonquin Road
Arlington Heights, IL 60005
(800) 635-0635 (information service) or 847-228-9900 or (888) 4-PLASTIC
www.plasticsurgery.org
All members are certified by the American Board of Plastic Surgery

Hotlines

Plastic Surgery Information Service
American Society of Plastic and Reconstructive Surgeons
(800) 635-0635
Call to receive a list of five active ASPRS members in your area, free brochures, and verification of a physician's certification in plastic surgery.

Publications and Pamphlets

"Facial Peels and Laser Surgery," 2000. Basic facts about chemical peeling. American

Academy of Facial and Reconstructive Surgery, Washington, DC; (800) 332-FACE (800-332-3223). www.aafprs.org Other titles include:

"Facelift," 1994. Basic facts about facelift surgery.

"Facial Scar Revision," 1993. Basic facts about facial scars and the methods available to treat them.

"Plastic Surgery of the Chin," 1993. Basic facts about chin augmentation and chin reduction surgery.

"Plastic Surgery of the Ear," 1994. Basic facts about cosmetic surgery of the ear.

"Plastic Surgery of the Eyebrows and Forehead," 1994. Basic facts about plastic surgery of the upper face.

"Plastic Surgery of the Eyelids," 1994. Basic facts about plastic surgery of the upper face.

"Plastic Surgery of the Nose," 1994. Basic facts about cosmetic and functional surgery of the nose.

"Hair Replacement," 1984. Basic facts about surgical treatment of hair loss.

"What is a Facial Plastic Surgeon?" 1994. Tips on selecting the right surgeon for you.

21

Exercises Are a Must-Do

"Tengo Que Hacerlo" . . . "I Have to Do It"

The track had been something she always walked by. After all, the high school was nearby. And somehow, after all those years of being her local landmark, it had become a part of her regular activities.

Every morning Henrietta would wake up, put on her sweats and walking shoes, and go to the track. She could not help but smile at the thought of herself walking around the track in her baggy pants and sweatshirt. This was not how she ever thought she would spend her mornings.

But Henrietta was getting used to going there and doing it at her own pace. She neither ran nor walked fast. She just walked. And although the first time she tried, she could barely make it one time around the track, she was now able to go around the track three times.

Without even noticing when it had happened, she knew her legs and heart had grown stronger.

The research indicates that Latinas do not exercise as much as other women. That is no surprise to us—we do not need data to tell us what is abundantly clear by just being with each other. For too many of us, exercise has become the thing we do *si sobra tiempo* (if there is leftover time).

There are many reasons why we do not exercise: some of us do not like competition; others believe that exercise is inspired by vanity and self-indulgence; and then there are those with a litany of excuses—no time, too tired, no place, no one to do it with, wrong clothes, too expensive, or whatever. Still others find exercising just plain boring.

Exercising, however, is something that we need to incorporate into our lives because it makes us stronger and therefore happier. It's not simply a matter of looking better, but of enabling ourselves to manage our lives better, with greater energy and vitality. And we all want that.

Rocío thought to herself, "This time I am going to exercise for me."

She had exercised to attract a new partner. She had exercised to fit into a dress she wanted to wear. She had exercised so that wearing her bathing suit did not make her feel so bad. Rocío had worked hard to get into shape most of her life.

Every summer it was a struggle to be fit.

But now she was in her fifties. Her forties had freed her of many of the excesses of her younger years. Now when she looked at her body she did so in a different way. Her body really was God's temple, and it was time she took care of it because it was the right thing to do.

Doing It—From Getting Started to Keeping It Going

How often do we exercise? It varies. Some Latinas may just be getting started, while others already have an ongoing exercise plan that is fulfilling and fun. To sustain our exercise program we need to understand the underlying factors: motivation, scheduling, choice of activities, level of effort, and support. If you have health problems, and even if you do not it is a good idea to talk to your health care provider before starting an exercise program.

Motivation—From Decision to Commitment

For many of us the idea of having to wake up and exercise every morning is enough to make us roll over, pull the covers over our head, and go back to catching those extra minutes of sleep before another long day. It seems impossible to add another activity to our life. This is the hardest part of exercising—deciding to begin. It is much easier to push our need to exercise to the bottom of our "To Dos," which are already compressing our time.

The best way to start is by deciding that you will do as much as you *can*. That means that although some days you may not exercise, your goal is to gradually make exercise a part of your life. Start where you can, even if it is only once a week. Then increase your exercise time to three nonconsecutive days a week, and if you want to, every other day.

Exercise is not something we do for a little while, or for the summer, or for a trip, or to attract or keep that special someone, or to fit into an outfit for a particular occasion. For exercise to be effective over the long run, we need to see it as an essential part of our lives, as natural a part of our day as brushing our teeth.

Exercising should not be an add-on to our lives. It must be something we do as surely as we put clothes on before we go outside or as regularly as we eat our meals. Just as we do not usually go more than a day without eating, we should not go without exercise on a regular basis.

Consejos

Understand Yourself and Your Exercise Plan

Factor	Getting Started	Ongoing
Motivation	Decision	Commitment
Scheduling	Plan	Integrate
Choice of activities	Favorite	Diverse
Level of effort	Minimal time	Making time
Support	External	Internal

Scheduling—From Planning to Integrating

When you begin your exercise program, it will seem as if you have to make extra time in your day, but there are several things you can do to make new time, such as shortening your shopping trips or watching a little less television. The good news is that you will soon have some new time added to your day. Once you start exercising regularly, your body will function better and you will be more energetic and effective when you are awake.

As you get accustomed to exercising, you will integrate the activity into your schedule. So, instead of driving you may decide to walk, or instead of shopping you may go on a bicycle ride or to a dance class. Although exercise might begin as an activity that you reluctantly schedule in, it will become an activity that you schedule around.

Choice of Activities—From Favorite to Diverse

Raisa hated to exercise. That was the truth. She never liked it and she never wanted to do it. It all seemed so unappealing. She knew she would never be like the women on television or in magazines—and she did not care. So what if her stomach would never be perfectly flat? Even when she was a teenager she always had a little pancita *(belly).*

One day Raisa noticed a sign in the grocery store that announced a jazz class to be held at the local community center. She had always wanted to learn those smooth moves. As she signed up for the class she knew that this was going to be fun. Jazz had always been something that made her insides sizzle.

Ask a Latina what comes to mind when she thinks of exercise, and the image will include a class of relatively lean women bouncing around wearing tight clothes. And with that thought, she may decide that if that's what it takes to improve her breathing and her heart, well . . . maybe she will just pass on it.

Keep in mind, though, that every time we move we are exercising some part of our body. One of the benefits of exercise is burning calories and revving up our metabolism. Calories are a good measure of how much energy we use in our daily activities. The following list shows some of our most common activities and how many calories we use. Some of these activities may not sound like anything we would do, but the fact is that we already engage in exercise—we just have to be more conscious of opportunities to do so and find more of them.

USE IT AND LOSE IT

Activities	Calories Burned Per Hour*
Sitting quietly	80
Standing quietly	95
Light activity	240
Office work	
Cleaning house	
Playing golf	
Moderate activity	370
Walking briskly (3.5 mph)	
Gardening	
Bicycling (5.5 mph)	
Dancing	
Strenuous activity	580
Jogging (9 min. per mile)	
Swimming	
Very strenuous activity	740
Running (7 min. per mile)	
Racquetball	
Skiing	

*For a healthy 140-pound woman. If you weigh more than 140 pounds, you will probably burn more calories per hour. If you weigh less, you will probably burn fewer calories per hour.

Source: Dietary Guidelines for Americans, U.S. Department of Agriculture/U.S. Department of Health and Human Services, 1990.

When we do anything there are ways to move *more* and ways to move *less*. Exercise requires that we move more of whatever we are moving and/or keep moving for a longer period of time. This may mean that we repeat the same motion several times. To exercise may require that we walk a little farther, walk up or down steps, or just take longer and/or faster strides as we walk.

To begin an exercise program, it is a good idea to do an activity that you enjoy. Some Latinas think that exercising means they should run or jog, when they really do not like to do either.

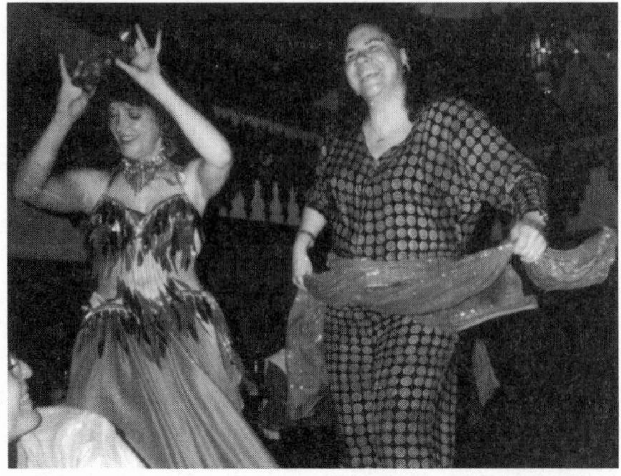

There are many ways to keep active and exercise.

But exercise can be whatever appeals to you that raises your heart rate. If you like to walk, for instance, you should begin your exercise program by walking.

When exercise has become something you do on a regular basis, you should start thinking about what other benefits exercise might bring. It is important to know how the exercise you are doing helps your body. For example, some movements are good for your heart, others make you more flexible, and others make you stronger. If you would like more strength, perhaps you should add weights to your program. If you want more flexibility, perhaps you should stretch more or sign up for a dance class, which can also help reduce your stress levels (a positive side effect of any exercise).

One reason for having a diverse program is to keep you interested, so that boredom alone doesn't encourage you to quit. There are plenty of enjoyable ways to get more exercise, so if you're not having fun with your regimen, perhaps you just need to try another one.

The best exercise programs are comprehensive: they build your cardiorespiratory endurance, muscular strength and endurance, and flexibility. They also sufficiently diverse to maintain your interest.

You are the best judge not only of which exercise program gives you the most benefit but also which one you are most likely to maintain.

PERCENT OF TIME BY GOAL AND TYPE OF ACTIVITY

Goal	Aerobic	Strengthening	Flexibility
Lose weight	50%	50%	
Look toning	20%	80%	
Be healthy	35%	35%	30%
More energy	80%	20%	

Level of Effort—From Minimal Time to Making Time

Magda was making breakfast as she watched the exercise show on television. She shrugged her shoulders as she thought, none of the women look like they have to work out at all. Why don't you ever see overweight women exercising? Magda could not imagine getting undressed and then getting into a shiny leotard and tights.

Besides, a lot of the exercises were just too strenuous and difficult for larger women. And forget the time. After a long day at work she barely had the energy to make dinner.

Exercise was good to do, but she just could not fit it into her life.

At the start of your program you should plan to increase the time and strenuousness of your activities slowly so that your body and your schedule can adjust. One day of sore muscles can discourage anyone who is trying to make an honest beginning to exercising, as can an exercise schedule that is overly ambitious. You may want to start at three 10- to 15-minute sessions and build your time up slowly to 45 or 60 minutes.

If you want to feel healthy, three 30-minute

SAMPLE EXERCISE PROGRAM

Exercise	Day						
	1	2	3	4	5	6	7
5 to 10 minutes of stretching or warm-up	X		X		X		X
10 minutes of strengthening			X				X
20 minutes of aerobic	X		X				X
20 minutes of endurance	X		X		X		X
10 to 12 minutes of stretching or cool-down	X		X		X		X
Estimated Total Minutes	60		70		40		70

sessions a week will make you feel healthier in three weeks. To lose weight and see results, it will take six to eight weeks if you exercise 45 minutes three days a week; if you exercise five days a week you should see results in four to six weeks. The frequency of exercise will help determine how soon you begin to see changes. While you can do aerobic exercises on practically a daily basis, it is important to give your muscles at least 24 hours of rest in between strengthening exercises.

Over time your body will enjoy exercising. You will become used to it and find that you just do not feel the same without it.

Support—From External to Internal

We all need support to start our exercise program. In the beginning it may be useful to exercise with a friend or in a class. The support of family and friends also makes it easier for us to engage in these activities because they may volunteer to do some chores that may have occupied our time.

But while it may be nice to have someone encouraging us to exercise, the important fact is that exercise is something we do for ourselves because it helps us stay healthy and fit. We also have a sense of mastery once we are able to do something that we were unable to do before. By keeping a record of your accomplishment you will be able to see how you are moving along.

Perhaps even more important than the physical benefits, though, we may find after a while that exercise provides us the opportunity to focus on our innermost thoughts. Latinas who walk or run or ride a bicycle often say that the truly precious benefit of exercise is its effectiveness as a stress reducer and an opportunity to clear the mind.

Given all these factors, what are the best exercises for us to do? What follows is the best of the best, keeping in mind that these exercises do not require lots of special equipment.

The Best to Do

Walking Is Aerobic

While running may be fun for some people, the most appealing exercise for most people is walking. Walking does not require special clothes or equipment—all we need is a comfortable pair of shoes.

Most of us walk every day. The best way to make walking into exercise is by (1) increasing the distance we walk, (2) increasing the steepness of the area where we walk, and (3) increasing our speed.

1: Increase the distance. This means that perhaps instead of having your lunch at your desk you walk to a place that is farther away and have your lunch there. You do not have to increase the distance all at once. You may even choose to walk around one block and increase how many times you go around it every month.

SAMPLE WALKING PROGRAM

	Warm-Up	Target Zone	Cool-Down	Total
	Walk Normally	Walk Briskly	Walk Normally	
Week 1	5 min.	5 min.	5 min.	15 min.
Week 2	5 min.	7 min.	5 min.	17 min.
Week 3	5 min.	9 min.	5 min.	19 min.
Week 4	5 min.	11 min.	5 min.	21 min.
Week 5	5 min.	13 min.	5 min.	23 min.
Week 6	5 min.	15 min.	5 min.	25 min.
Week 7	5 min.	18 min.	5 min.	28 min.
Week 8	5 min.	20 min.	5 min.	30 min.
Week 9	5 min.	23 min.	5 min.	33 min.
Week 10	5 min.	26 min.	5 min.	36 min.
Week 11	5 min.	28 min.	5 min.	38 min.
Week 12	5 min.	30 min.	5 min.	40 min.

2: Increase the steepness (incline). When we have to go up stairs or climb a hill, we use up more calories. When doing any kind of exercises on a staircase, however, make sure that you do not have problems with your knees or if you do that your health care provider has approved the activity.

3: Increase the speed. The faster you walk the more aerobic exercise you get. You do not have to run or power-walk, you just have to walk at a brisker pace. This may mean that a walk you would normally take in 20 minutes you reduce to 19 or 18 minutes. Increases in speed do not have to be dramatic to have an impact.

Where you walk may be important for your safety. Here are some good ideas.

- During the day, walk on the local school track when it is not in use.
- Do laps in a large indoor mall.
- Try walking in place in your own apartment or house.

To help you monitor your progress, you should keep a chart of when you walk, how long you walk, and how far you walk. You will be surprised at how soon you will be able to walk a greater distance and for a longer period of time.

The chart below tells you what your target heart rate should be when walking. As soon as you are done exercising, put your finger on

YOUR TARGET HEART RATE

Age	Target Heart Rate Zone (beats per minute)	Average Maximum Heart Rate (beats per minute)
	50%–75%	*100%*
20 years	100-150	200
25 years	98-146	195
30 years	95-142	190
35 years	93-138	185
40 years	90-135	180
45 years	88-131	175
50 years	85-127	170
55 years	83-123	165
60 years	80-120	160
65 years	78-116	155
70 years	75-113	150

Your maximum heart rate is approximately 220 minus your age. The above figures are averages and should be used as general guidelines only.

your pulse (wrist or neck) and count your pulse beats for 10 seconds. Take that number and multiply it by 6 to calculate your heart rate. It is very important to stay within your target heart zone. If you go higher, you begin to strain your heart and may in fact hurt it more than you help it.

Keep in mind that you calculate your maximum heart rate by subtracting your age from 220. If you are thirty, your maximum heart rate would be 190; it would be 180 for a forty-year-old.

Floor Exercises for Flexibility and Endurance

For many years Latinas have shared with me and with each other their experiences with good exercise that did not cause too much wear and tear on the body and at the same time seemed to work on the right parts. What follows is a series of exercises drawn from those experiences, which you may find helpful. They were developed keeping in mind that some of us may be larger than others and that some of us have delicate backs. The exercises begin and end with stretches. The flexibility and toning that good stretches produce is essential so that we do not hurt ourselves.

It is very helpful in terms of your motivation to keep a journal of how many exercises you do each day. You should eventually work up to more sets of exercises. Track your progress and you will be pleasantly surprised.

In general, breathe out (exhale) when you exert yourself, and breathe in when you do the less strenuous part of an exercise. Diagrams are provided to show you how to do the exercises correctly. As always, make sure to check with your health care provider before you begin this or any exercise program.

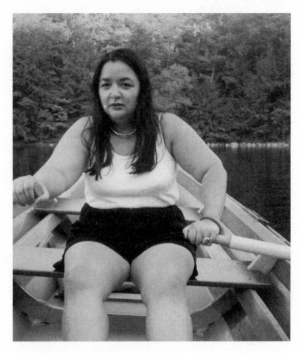

Latinas enjoy all types of sports.

STRETCHING

1. Reach to Ceiling—rope climbing in place

Stand with your arms at your sides.
Stretch your arms above your head.
Reach for the ceiling as if you were climbing a rope for at least 10 seconds.

2. Neck Rolls

Stand with your arms at your sides.
Let your neck relax.
Take 8 counts to roll your neck around in one smooth, slow motion.

> *Consejos*
>
> **"No Pain No Gain" Is Wrong**
>
> Exercising should not hurt you. If you overdo it, you have to give your muscles time to recuperate. To prevent pain and injury, you should ease into any exercise program.

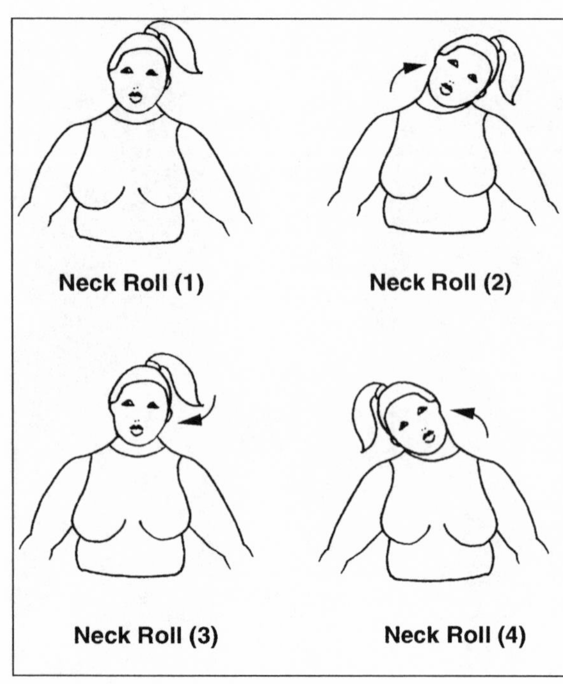

Neck Rolls

Stop for a count of 3 when you get to the beginning position.
Repeat three times.
Take 8 counts to roll your neck around in one smooth, slow motion in the other direction.
Stop for a count of 3 when you get to the beginning position.
Repeat three times.

3. Side Stretch (good for waist)
Stand with your arms above your head.
Slowly stretch to the right and hold for 4 counts (do not bounce).
Slowly stand upright and hold for 4 counts.
Slowly stretch to the left and hold for 4 counts (do not bounce).
Repeat at least four times to each side.

4. Stretch
Lie on your back on the floor.

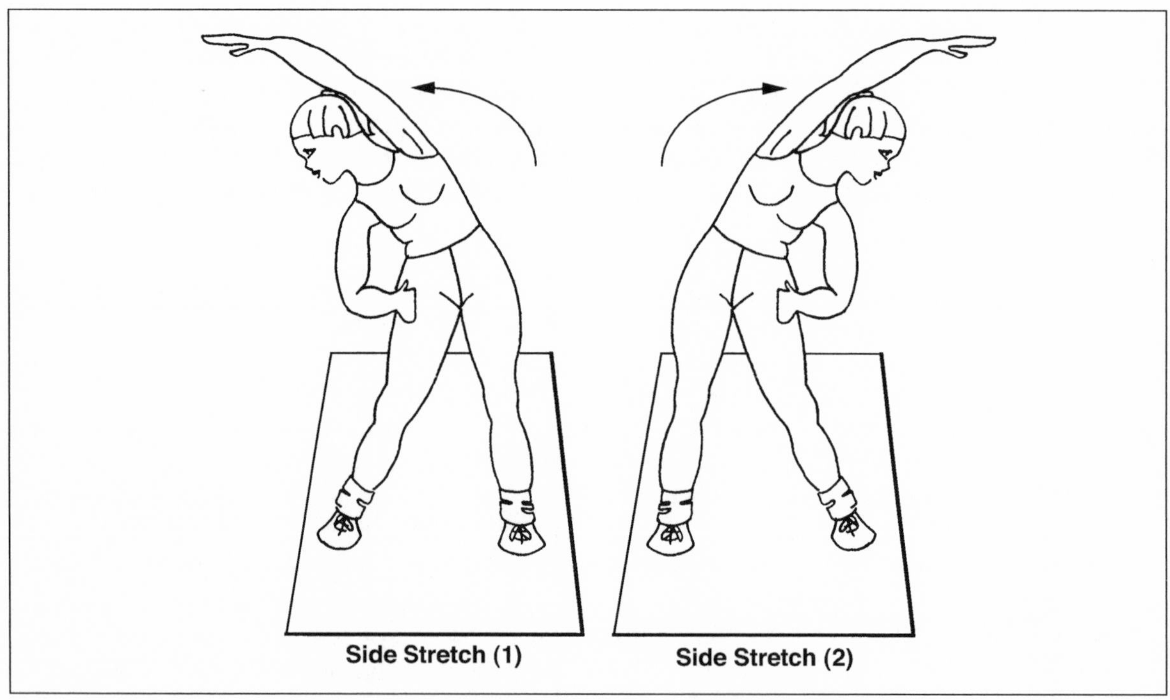

Side Stretch

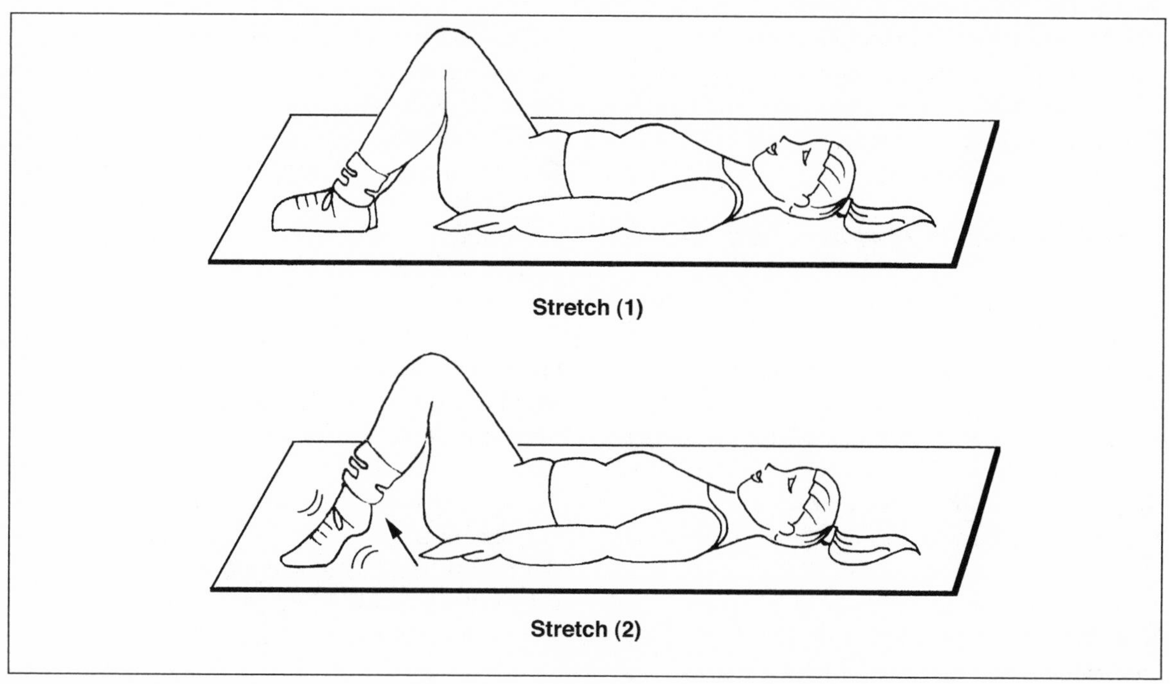

Stretch

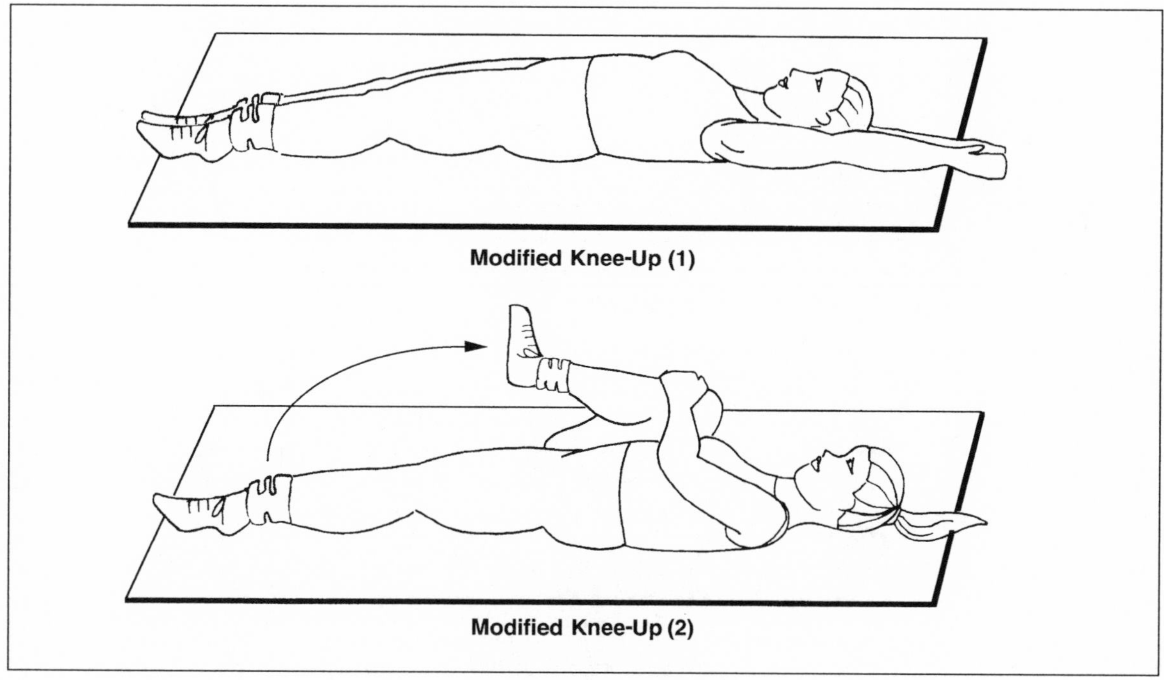

Modified Knee-Ups

Bend your knees while keeping your feet flat.
Lift your feet, point your toes down, and hold for 4 counts.
Repeat at least four times.

MUSCLE TONE

1. Modified Knee-Up (good for stomach and buttocks)
Lie on your back on the floor with arms at your sides.
Slowly bring your bent left knee up to your chest.
Hold for 4 counts. (In the beginning you may want to use your hands to hold the knee up.)
Slowly bring your left leg down.
Slowly bring your bent right knee up to your chest.
Hold for 4 counts.
Slowly bring your right leg down.
Repeat at least four times for each leg.

2. Modified Sit-Up (good for stomach)
Lie with your back on the floor and knees bent.
Place your hands on sides of head by ears. (This should be a light touch.)
Roll shoulders and upper back forward and off the ground. (Feel the pull in your stomach. It doesn't matter if your shoulders are only a few inches off the floor. Make sure that you feel the exercise in your stomach.)
Hold for 4 counts.
Roll back down slowly.
Repeat at least four times.

3. Modified Hip-Up (good for stomach and butt)
Lie flat on the floor.
Bend both knees and keep feet flat on floor.
Lift butt up and hold up for count of 4.
Repeat at least four times.

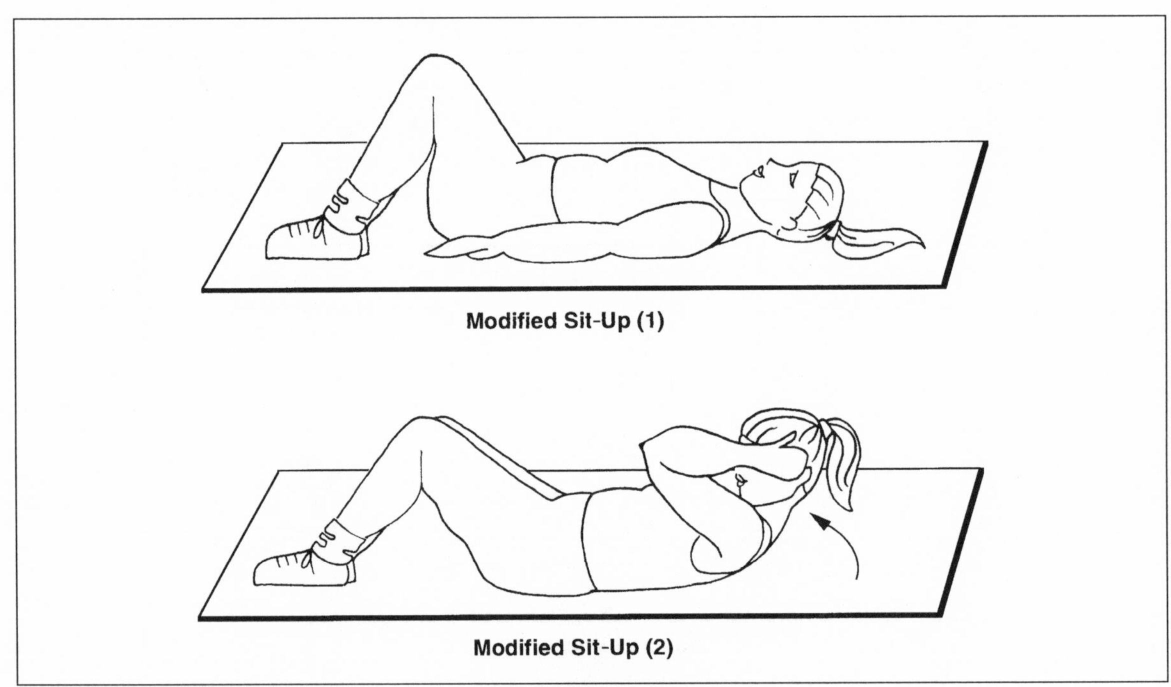

Modified Sit-Up (1)

Modified Sit-Up (2)

Modified Hip-Up

Consejos

You Are Doing Sit-Ups the Wrong Way If—

- The back of your neck hurts.
- You are pulling yourself up by your head.
- You feel the exertion in your shoulders.

You are doing them the right way if the only muscles you feel being worked are your stomach muscles.

4. Making a U (good for stomach)

Lie on floor with hands above your head flat on the floor and your feet together.

At the same time, slowly raise your arms, lift your shoulders up, and raise your feet. (It will probably take you a long time to make a U or V because you may only be able to lift yourself up a few inches. That is a good start. You should feel this in your stomach and not in your neck.)

Hold for a count of 4.

Slowly come down.

Repeat at least four times.

STRETCHING

Repeat stretches 1 through 4 above.

Feet Up on the Wall

Lie on the floor near a wall.

Lift feet up on wall.

Lie quietly with feet on the wall for at least 2 minutes.

Think quietly to yourself about how your body feels.

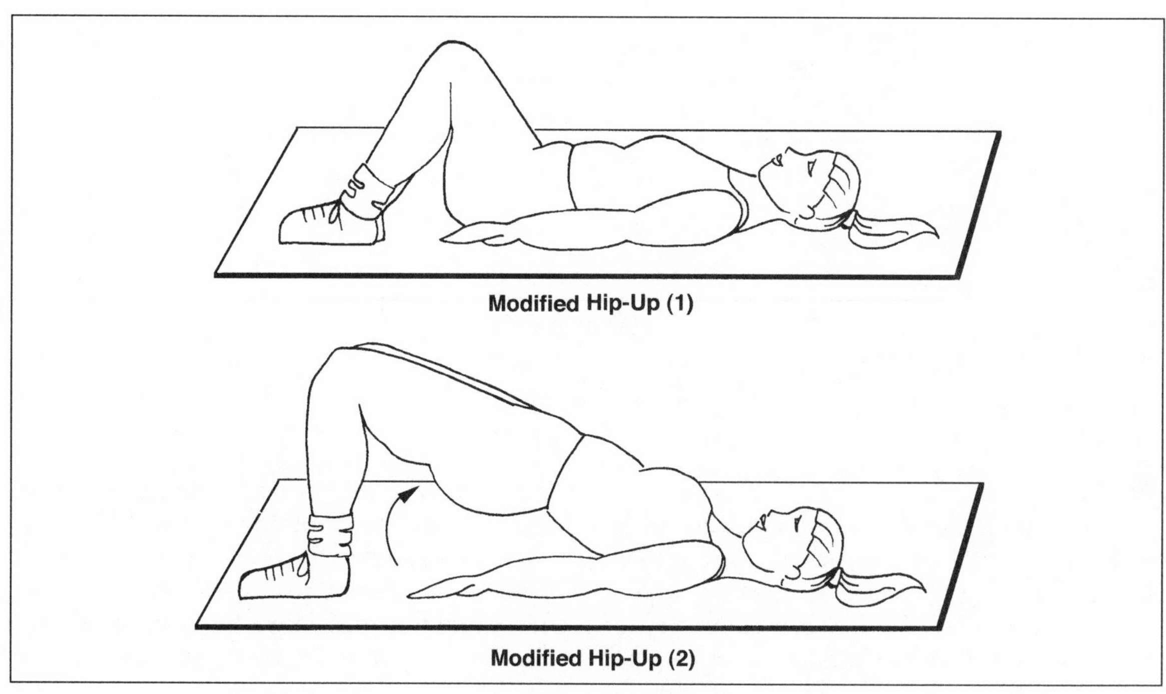

Modified Hip-Up

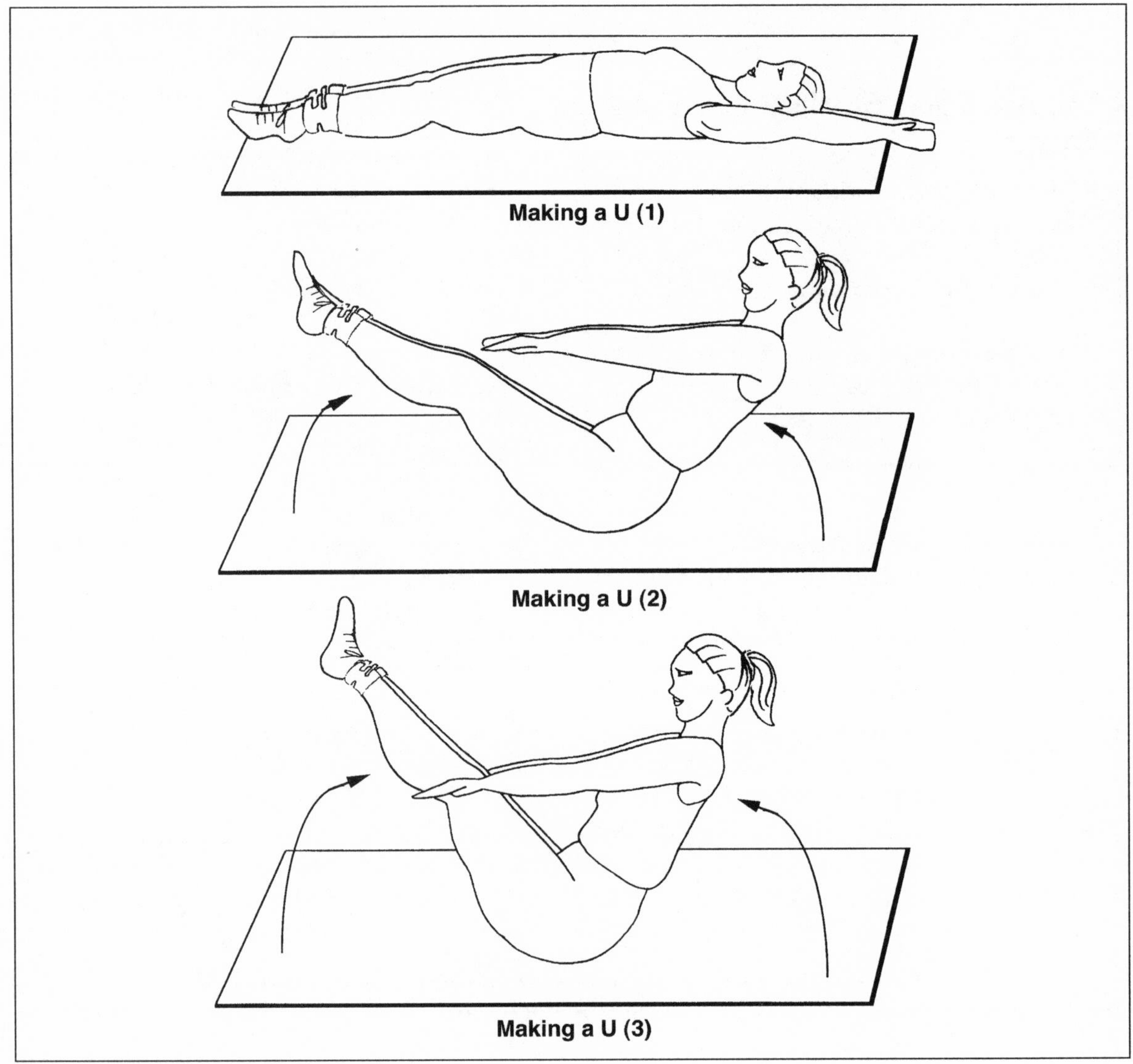

Making a U

Strength

Even though most of us do not want to be and will not be body builders, it is still important for us to strengthen our muscles. Using free weights is easy to do in the privacy of your own home. While joining a gym may get us access to more sophisticated equipment, the fact is that most of us do not keep going to the gym for long periods of time. Nevertheless, free weights (not ankle or wrist weights) are very important for several reasons. First, it is good for us to be strong. Second, with each new pound of muscle we burn 30 to 40 extra calories a day. Finally, we tighten our muscles and look better toned.

Many women have the mistaken impression that lifting weights will make them big. Unless you're very thin, though, lifting weights will make you smaller, not bigger.

You may want to begin with 3-pound weights and gradually work up to 5-pound weights. Some women may want to lift more weight, but all this should be very carefully supervised because you can injure yourself by the inappropriate choice and handling of weights.

Make sure you speak to an instructor who will guide you in the proper choice and handling of weights. Give yourself a 1-minute rest between exercises. Strengthening exercises should be done no more than every other day.

MYTHS AND FACTS

Myth: If I exercise, I will lose weight.

Fact: If you exercise, you will become more fit. You may or may not lose weight.

Myth: If I develop more muscle, I will lose weight.

Fact: When you develop muscle, you lose fat. Fat is bulkier than muscle, so you may be leaner looking but actually weigh more.

Myth: I have to exercise every day for at least an hour.

Fact: Moderate exercise (30 minutes) at least three times a week is very beneficial.

Mind and Spirit

Lourdes wondered whether she would be able to swim a mile again.

As she looked at the pool, she knew what the pattern would be. The first few laps would be a struggle. Then she would finally get to the quarter-mile point. Her body would be exhausted and her throat would hurt from the chlorine, but she would press on because she knew she had been able to do so before.

Soon she found herself reaching the half-mile mark, and just about then she knew she was OK because now she was getting closer to the end. As she let her body cut through the water, she felt her mind wandering less to the other people in the pool as she became more a part of the water around her.

At the three-quarter mile mark, Lourdes knew she was going to make it. The last quarter-mile was always the best and somehow the easiest. Her body no longer seemed to fight the water but rather floated in it as she moved forward.

This must have been what it was like in the womb, she thought to herself. With each stroke her mind became calmer, and her spirit felt a oneness with her surroundings that she could not duplicate in anything else she did.

Lourdes finished the mile. And as she pulled herself up from the ladder she felt great!

Although to most people exercise seems to be of primary benefit to the body, it has a perhaps even more important impact on our mind and spirit. Whether experiencing a runner's high or that moment of surpassing what we thought we could do, those of us who exercise regularly feel calmer and happier because of our activities, and this is what keeps us doing them regularly. As stressful as life can be, exercise is a tool at our very fingertips that can ease our minds, increase our energy, and help us feel and look our best. Don't pass up the opportunity.

Summary

Exercise is good for us. Our hearts pump more efficiently and our lungs function better as they work together to carry the nutrients in our blood throughout our bodies and then take away the wastes and toxins. We become stronger, not just because we can lift heavy weights but because as we move our muscles and use our bodies we expand the limits of our abilities.

Exercise literally makes us feel happier because it makes our bodies produce more endorphins, a hormone that produces natural feelings of well-being while it reduces pain. When we make time for exercising, soon we find that our lives fall into place around this activity, which becomes as essential to us as brushing our teeth.

RESOURCES

Organizations

American Heart Association
7272 Greenville Avenue
Dallas, TX 75231-4596
(800) 242-8721 or (214) 706-1220
www.americanheart.org

Melpomene Institute
1010 University Avenue
St. Paul, MN 55104
(651) 642-1951
www.melpomene.org

National Health Information Center
P.O. Box 1133
Washington, DC 20013-1133
(800) 336-4797

National Women's Health Resource Center
5255 Loughsboro Rd.
Washington, DC 20016
(877) 986-9472
www.healthywomen.org

President's Council on Physical Fitness and Sports
200 Independence Avenue SW
Washington, DC 20201
(202) 690-9000
www.fitness.gov

Hotlines

Aerobics and Fitness Association of America Hotline
(800) 445-5950

Publications and Pamphlets

"Aqua Dynamics: Water Exercises Are the New Way to Stay in Shape." President's Council on Physical Fitness and Sports, 200 Independence Avenue SW, Washington, DC 20201; (202) 690-9000. Other titles include:

"Fitness Fundamentals: Guidelines for Personal Exercise Programs." US GPO No. 1990-279-047-814/21139.

"The Nolan Ryan Fitness Guide." Exercise tips from one of baseball's major league players. Advil Forum on Health Education.

"Exercise: A Healthy Habit to Start and Keep," 1999. Pamphlet No. 1564. Health Notes from AAFP Family Health Facts series. Information on how to exercise to improve your health. American Academy of Family Physicians, 11400 Tomahawk Creek Pkwy, Leawood, KS 66211-2672; (800) 944-0000.

"Exercise and Your Heart: A Guide to Physical Activity." Information on how exercise can be good for your heart rate and overall health. American Heart Association, 7320 Greenville Avenue, Dallas, TX 75231-4599; (800) 242-8721; www.americanheart.org

"General Fitness Resource Packet," June 1999. General information on how women can be more physically fit. Women's Sports Foundation, Eisenhower Park, East Meadow, NY; (800) 227-3988. Other titles include:

"Fact Sheet," March 11, 1996. Information on physical fitness benefits for women.

"The Balancing Act: A Womans Guide to Sports and Fitness." Information on fitness for women.

"Diet and Health Recommendations for Cancer Prevention," 1998. AICR Information Series Part III. American Institute for Cancer Research, Washington, D.C.; (800) 843-8114.

"Facts about Heart Disease and Women: Be Physically Active," August 1995. NIH Publication No. 95-3656. U.S. Department of Health and Human Services, National Institutes of Health, National Heart, Lung, and Blood Institute, Bethesda, MD; (301) 251-1222.

"How to Be a Fat-Burning Machine," October 1995. *Glamour Magazine*, p. 232.

"Pep Up Your Life: A Fitness Book for Mid-Life and Older Persons." Pamphlet No. PF 3248(1193)-D549. American Association for Retired Persons and the President's Council on Physical Fitness and Sports, Washington, DC; (202) 640-9000; www.fitness.gov

"Weightlifting for Weight Loss," October 29, 1996, *Washington Post* Health, p. 20.

"Fitness & Exercise" (#305). "Eating Right" (#304). Stay Well series. Information on how to be physically fit. MetLife Insurance Company Medical Department, Health and Safety Education Division, One Madison Avenue, New York, NY 10010-3690; (800) MetLife

"Your Ideal Workout: How Much, How Hard, How Fast, How Often?" September 1996. *Glamour Magazine*, p. 298.

22

The Best Medicines

It was such a waste of time to go to the doctor just to get the same pills.

Since childhood Iris had suffered from very bad sore throats. As an adult she was always ready for her next one. To take care of any problems, she always kept a bottle of antibiotics around. Iris knew that all she had to do was take the antibiotics for a few days and the sore throat would go away.

So whenever she got a prescription, she took just half and saved the rest for the next time she got sick. She did not have the luxury of taking time off from work if she was sick. She had to work.

Luz said that she did not take any medication. She did not like it. She did not trust it. All those chemicals in the body did not sound good for her. Luz wanted only natural medicine. Luz would take cough syrup—but that was different. She had always found that it worked.

What does Rx mean to you? Originally it represented the astrological sign of Jupiter. In ancient times the symbol was added to every prescription so that Jupiter would use his power to bless the medicine, so that the medicine would then cure the patient. It was well known that there would be no cure of the body unless the Gods willed it.

This view of body and spirit as inextricably linked permeated every aspect of ancient medicine. In most early cultures the health care provider and religious leader were often the same person. These were the healers on whom communities depended to cure whatever ailed the body, mind, and spirit.

Since medicine and science have progressed, what Latinas face is an age of specialization, where each part of our being is cared for by a different profession. The body is attended to by health care providers; the mind is healed by mental health professionals; and the spirit is left to the care of whatever religious or secular healer we choose.

Latinas know that healing is more than a science. When we take medicines, for instance, we realize that at least part of their effectiveness stems from our belief that they will help us. Latinas need an even better understanding of medicines, however. Knowing how medicines work and what effect they have on us is critical. Although some of us tend to be deferential to our health care providers and take whatever they prescribe, others seem to need more information about the medicines to fully accept using them.

What is a medicine? Very few of us have been told what has to happen before something is labeled a medicine, to be sold either by prescription only, through specially designated health care providers, or over the counter without a prescription. Even fewer of us are aware of what the difference is between generic and brand-name drugs—aside from the price to the consumer.

Modern Medicine

In the early 1900s, most of the medicines we took were limited to natural products and their derivatives, and even young, healthy people died from illnesses and infections that are now easily treatable with currently available medications. With the discovery of penicillin in 1929, the treatment of disease with medicines began to change by leaps and bounds. The therapeutic revolution that followed has progressed from medicines discovered by chance, to medicines that were discovered by a deeper scientific understanding of the pharmacologic principles of the way chemicals conduct messages around the body, to current medications evolving from a better understanding of our genetic and cellular makeup.

In 2000 there were over 1,700 new drugs being developed. Pharmaceutical companies are quick to point out that they spend an average of $359 million on each new drug before they bring it to market. This takes into account that for every product that makes it to the shelf to be sold, 5,000 other products did not make it.

Yet little of this research has been performed on Latinas or with women's particular health concerns in mind. Through the early 1990s, the bulk of pharmaceutical research did not include women of childbearing age because of concerns about possible fetal injury. Although in 1993 the Food and Drug Administration adopted rules strongly recommending that manufacturers provide drug trial data by race and ethnicity, these data are not required. So what we know about Latinas and drugs is very limited, but what we do know is cause for alarm.

> *Alert*
>
> Federal legislation passed in 1994 freed supplements from most Federal regulation. Sold as foods, supplements which include vitamins, minerals, herbal and amino acids do not have to prove to the FDA that they are either safe or effective.

In 1993 Dr. Richard Levy did a study that addressed the concern that Hispanics and other subpopulations responded to medications differently from the general population. While his data were not specific to Latinas, he did document that for Hispanics there were factors, which could probably be attributed to inherited metabolic differences, that impacted the way the body used medication.

Add to this finding the increasing evidence that women differ from men in the way they metabolize drugs, and it is evident that the Latina response to common medications will be different if not unique. At the moment the details of the Latina response are largely uncharted, although we do know that with respect to antidepressants, Hispanics require lower doses and tend to have more side effects. Given the high rate of depression among Latinas, this finding is very important.

Our struggle, as Latinas, is to be better

informed about the medicines we take. The first step is to know how they got on the shelf.

Getting to Market

The process of discovering that a certain chemical—either made in the laboratory or found in nature—can be made into a specific medicine to treat a certain illness is long and grueling. It used to take up to twelve years to bring a medicine to market, but recent changes have made it possible to bring new medicines to the consumer faster. Sometimes the time from discovery to your home is only eight years.

That may sound like a long time, especially if you have an illness for which there is currently no approved treatment or cure. But the process, which has been fine-tuned over the past fifty years, has been developed to make sure that only safe and effective medicines are available for us to use.

How does a manufacturer spend so much money on research and development? The answer is simple—clinical trials.

Clinical Trials

We often hear that a drug is in clinical treatment trials. All that means is that they are starting to give that drug to people as part of a research project to see what effects the drug has and to make sure that the drug is safe. A clinical trial does three major things: (1) tests a new approach, (2) answers questions about the safety and effectiveness of the drug, and (3) determines whether there should be further testing.

For each clinical trial there must be a plan or blueprint that describes the purpose of the trial and specifies the number of volunteers that will be needed, their characteristics, and how care will be provided for them. This entire plan is called a protocol.

Volunteers are assigned to a control group or an intervention group. The control group usually gets the best available treatment, and the intervention group gets the new treatment. Strong ethical guidelines prohibit trials from withholding treatment from a patient for the sake of research except when it is anticipated that withholding treatment will neither cause permanent injury nor diminish survival times.

To make sure that a volunteer has an equal chance of being in either group, volunteers are assigned at random, by computer, to one group or another. When the volunteers do not know what group they are in, it is called a single-blind study. In a double-blind study, neither the volunteers nor the attending health care providers know the group to which the volunteer has been assigned.

Regardless of whether you are in the control or intervention group, people who volunteer to serve in clinical trials are often offered free ongoing monitoring of their health. Of course, the volunteers have no control over which group they are placed in. Some people prefer to be in the intervention group because it involves the newer treatment, but there are instances in which the control group has better results.

Most clinical trials require the following steps to insure that volunteers have the maximum protection.

- Nonhuman testing. Testing in people does not occur until there has been extensive testing in the laboratory and in animals.
- Peer review. Every publicly funded institution has an Institutional Review Board (IRB), which is supposed to make sure that patient safety and ethical issues are addressed. If there are questions about either safety or ethics, an IRB can stop a trial from taking place.
- Ongoing audits. Throughout the trial there is a series of checks and balances to make sure that the protocol is being followed.

Warning: Informed Consent Is Sometimes Not Informed

Before you agree to be part of a clinical trial, you will be asked to sign a form which states that you have been informed of and understand the risks of being part of the clinical trial.

One of the major problems with informed consent is that too often the volunteer signs the form without truly being aware of all the risks. A contributing factor is that in an effort to provide all the details of the research program, the descriptions are sometimes so technical that it is hard to understand to what you are actually agreeing.

If you do not understand the clinical trial or feel in any way coerced into participating, you should neither sign the form nor participate in the trial.

- Informed consent process. Before agreeing to serve as a volunteer, individuals are given as much information as possible about the risks, benefits, and procedures of the clinical trial. After being informed, they are asked to sign a form that states that they have been informed and gives their consent to be in the trial.
- Ongoing monitoring. The health status of volunteers is monitored on an ongoing basis.
- At-will withdrawal. A volunteer may withdraw from participation in a clinical trial whenever he or she chooses.

For Latinas, participating in a clinical trial will not only provide state-of-the-art treatment and monitoring at minimal or no cost, but it will also help advance scientific knowledge about the effect of a medicine or treatment with Latinas. This is very important because, while many of the medicines might be used by Latinas, the bulk of clinical trials have not included Latinas and have often specifically excluded all women of childbearing age.

Clinical trials are divided into three phases. The goals of Phase I are to determine that a treatment is not harmful and to learn the effects of the treatment and the best way to give the treatment (pill, injection, patch). The goal of Phase II is to establish that the treatment has the effect intended. Phase III involves comparisons of one approach to another to determine the most effective way to proceed.

Consejos

If a Drug Is Not Approved in the United States

Sometimes drugs are available in other countries before they are available in the United States. This is because other countries may allow a company to sell a drug after the clinical trials pertaining to Phase II. Countries that do this then track patients to see if they have adverse reactions to the drugs. If there are reports of negative effects, the drug is removed from the market.

The FDA process may take longer, but it is considered the gold standard for drug approval worldwide. The FDA advises consumers to purchase drugs that are FDA approved because the agency's thorough review process has determined the drugs to be safe, effective, and produced in facilities that are clean and capable of producing a consistent, standardized product.

Think about it before you take a drug that does not have FDA approval.

National Institutes of Health (NIH) Clinical Trials

(800) 411-1222

As of 1997, NIH had some 1,000 active clinical research protocols. Patients are admitted to the NIH Clinical Center only on referral by a physician or dentist. A physician who feels that a patient may be suitable for a study at NIH may submit the patient's diagnosis and medical history to:

Patient Referral Service
Clinical Center
Building 10, Room 1C255
10 Center Drive, MSC 1170
Bethesda, MD 20892-1170
(800) 411-1222 or (301) 496-4891
(bilingual reference specialists available)

If a patient is accepted, the Clinical Center will correspond with the patient's physician and often with the patient, to arrange when the patient will come to the hospital. Accepted patients are not charged for care at the Clinical Center but may be responsible for transportation costs.

Areas of clinical study include aging, alcohol abuse and alcoholism, allergy, arthritis, musculoskeletal and skin diseases, cancer, child health, chronic pain, deafness and other communication disorders, dental and orofacial disorders, diabetes, digestive and kidney diseases, eye disorders, heart, lung, and blood diseases, infectious diseases, medical genetics, mental health, neurological disorders, and stroke.

Throughout each phase of the clinical trials, the Food and Drug Administration (FDA) works with the manufacturer to ensure that the best and most meaningful information is collected. When all three phases have been completed, all the information is submitted for formal review by the FDA. If either the FDA or the manufacturer is not certain of some of the results, it may be necessary to do more tests. When all of the questions are answered, the FDA decides whether to approve the drug.

Brand Name (Pioneer) or Generic

It was difficult for Mara to buy her medicines. She was taking five different pills a day, and Medicare did not cover them. On her last visit to the pharmacist, she had been amazed at how arrogant he was. He had tried to give her a generic medicine!

She had looked at the pills and said, "These are not the ones I get." The pharmacist had answered, "Yes, these are slightly less expensive because they are generic."

"I do not want the generic drug. I want the brand kind," Mara had said. The pharmacist had looked at her in exasperation and said, "A generic and a brand drug are basically the same thing. The only difference is that the generic kind is cheaper."

At this point Mara had had enough. She had looked at him and, with the controlled anger that gave her a special dignity, said, "Sir, I take the brand drug because it works for me. The other one does not. Don't you think I would like to have the cheaper one? But it does not work for me. It does not matter to me if it is a generic or a brand, but to my insides it does!"

To encourage manufacturers to engage in the decade of research it takes to bring a new drug (also called a pioneer drug) to market, they are given a patent for up to twenty years so that they are the only ones who can make the product. As the sole manufacturer of the drug, a company usually sets a price that will help it recoup its investment in research, continue to fund new research, and make a profit.

Once that time has expired, other manufac-

Consejos

What Does It Mean That a Generic Drug Is Bioequivalent to a Pioneer (Brand) Drug?

Bioequivalency means that two drugs are within the same range. The bioequivalent range is 80 to 125 percent of the pharmakinetic parameters based on the concentration of the drug in blood samples.

turers are allowed to make the drug using the same compounds. These drugs are called generics. Major health plans encourage their members to use generic drugs because they are usually cheaper. Since 50 percent of generics are produced by major drug manufacturers, the assumption is that the ingredients are the same but without the fancy label or packaging.

We are all aware of the effect a brand name has on the consumer. For example, there are seemingly countless numbers of blue jeans manufacturers, and there is every reason to believe that the only difference between the expensive brands and the cheaper brands is the label. But we also know that not all blue jeans are the same. Sometimes the cheaper ones may look the same and be 100 percent cotton, but they do not last as long or hold their shape as well. By the same token, certain inexpensive brands are sturdier than more expensive ones. Each one of us has to find the blue jeans that fit our form, shape, and pocketbook. Similarly, when it comes to the medicines we take, we must find the medicine that works for us and not just decide based on the label, i.e, brand or generic.

According to the FDA, a generic drug is "a version of a drug product that is equivalent to the pioneer or brand-name drug and is not marketed until the pioneer drug's patent exclusivity has expired." A generic drug must contain the same active ingredients as the pioneer drug; be identical in strength and dosage; be taken the same way; have the same indications and other labeling instructions; be bioequivalent; meet the same batch-to-batch requirements for identity, strength, purity, and quality; and be manufactured under the same strict standards as pioneer drug products.

Nevertheless, it should be up to you and your health care provider to decide whether you are better off taking the brand or generic version of a medicine. Unfortunately, health plans often limit the ability of health care providers to prescribe the drug that they believe to be more effective.

Given the potential differences, always be sure to ask your health care providers whether they are prescribing a generic or brand (pioneer) drug, and don't hesitate to ask why they decided to prescribe that particular drug.

Over-the-Counter Drugs

When the pharmacist gives me that long printout about the medicines, I don't know why they even bother. Those things are too long and too technical. It only makes me feel that I should not take the medicine. And then the information that is in the box is so tiny and tells you too many things that you will never use. I just throw it out.

Anyway, the outside of the prescription bottle tells you everything you need to know—when to take it and how much.

In the United States there are laws limiting the types of medicines that can be bought without having a prescription from a health care provider. These over-the-counter (OTC) drugs are generally low in toxicity, have a low potential for harm, and are not habit-forming, and their conditions for use are easily understood.

Since 1980 more than eighty-five drugs

Consejos

Questions to Ask Your Health Care Provider

1. What is the name and dose of the drug I am taking?
2. What should this drug do?
3. When should I take the drug?
4. How should I take this drug? May I take it with food, alcohol, or OTC medications?
5. Are there any side effects I need to look out for?
6. Are there any special storage requirements?

have made the switch from prescription to OTC. Given our increased emphasis on self-care, there will probably be many more.

Taking OTC drugs requires that we know our diagnosis. In many cases, although the drug is available without a prescription, it is advisable to check with your health care provider before using it to treat your condition. One concern is that OTC drugs may mask symptoms and make us feel more comfortable when we may have some underlying condition that should be attended to. The best way to proceed is to follow the directions on the label and contact your health care provider if your symptoms persist or worsen, particularly if you have never experienced the symptoms before.

Being an Educated Patient

You should ask your health care provider the following questions:

1: What is the name and dose of the drug I am taking? It can be difficult to listen closely to our health care provider when a medicine is being prescribed. Often our minds are focusing on our condition and on how we will have to rearrange our lives in order to get better. Nevertheless, we always need to know the name and the dose of the drug we are taking.

You should feel comfortable asking your health care provider for the spelling, especially if you cannot read the name on the handwritten prescription. Particularly when we are being treated for several conditions, it is best to write down all of the medicines and *remedios* we are taking (prescription, OTC, teas, etc.) and share them with our health care provider. This is important because some drugs interact with others and may either cancel out the positive effects of the new medications or create additional problems.

2: What should this drug do? Make sure you know what the medicines are supposed to do, how long it will take for the desired effect to begin, and how long it will be before you begin to feel better. Although your health care provider cannot guarantee that you will feel better in a specific number of days, it is good to have an idea of how the treatment should progress. In most cases the effect is not as immediate as we would like it to be.

3: When should I take the drug? How often have we heard a health care provider say that all we have to do is take a drug four times a day? The reality is that some drugs have to be taken four times during your waking hours, and others need to be taken four times during a 24-hour cycle.

Many Latinas who have been hospitalized have commented that they did not like it when the nurses woke them in what seemed like the middle of the night to give them a pill. However, with certain drugs this is necessary. Ask your health care provider how evenly spaced your doses should be and whether you might need to set an alarm to take a nighttime dosage.

4: How should I take this drug? May I take it with food, alcohol, or OTC medications? Many of us have become so accustomed to the little stickers with recommendations that are placed on prescription bottles or boxes that we rely on them alone to guide us. That is not enough. It is best to talk to your health care provider and, whenever possible, to the pharmacist about the medications we are taking. Be sure to mention other drugs or *remedios* that you are taking, because they may change the impact of the medication.

5: Are there any side effects I need to look out for? There was a time when health care providers were reluctant to discuss side effects because they believed such information would predispose patients to exhibit the symptoms. In this view the patient was not seen as a partner in her health care but rather as someone who had to be protected. These days most responsible health care providers will warn you of potential side effects so that you can be prepared to handle them. Some pharmacists also provide this information.

> *Consejos*
>
> Encourage your health care professional to call (800) FDA-1088 to let the FDA know about any adverse effects you have.

6: Are there any special storage requirements? Some medicines need special storage in order to keep their integrity. You may have to refrigerate the medicine or keep it away from direct light.

How to Read Your Prescription

How many times have you received a prescription and wondered what all the letters

PRESCRIPTIONS: CLEARING UP CONFUSION

Script	Latin	Abbreviation	English
ac	ante cibum	ac	Before meals
bid	bis in die	bid	Twice a day
c		c	With
caps		caps	Capsule
disp #60		disp #60	Dispense 60 pills
disp #30		disp #30	Dispense 30 pills
gt	gutta	gt	Drop
hs	hora somni	hs	At bedtime
pc	post cibum	pc	After meals
po	per os	po	By mouth
prn	pro re nata	prn	As needed
q4h	quaque 4 hora	q4h	Every 4 hours
q6h	quaque 6 hora	q6h	Every 6 hours
qd	quaque die	qd	Every day
qid	quater in die	qid	Four times a day
Rx		Rx	Take
Sig:		Sig:	Directions to patient:
tab		tab	tablet
tid	ter in die	tid	Three times a day
top		top	Topically

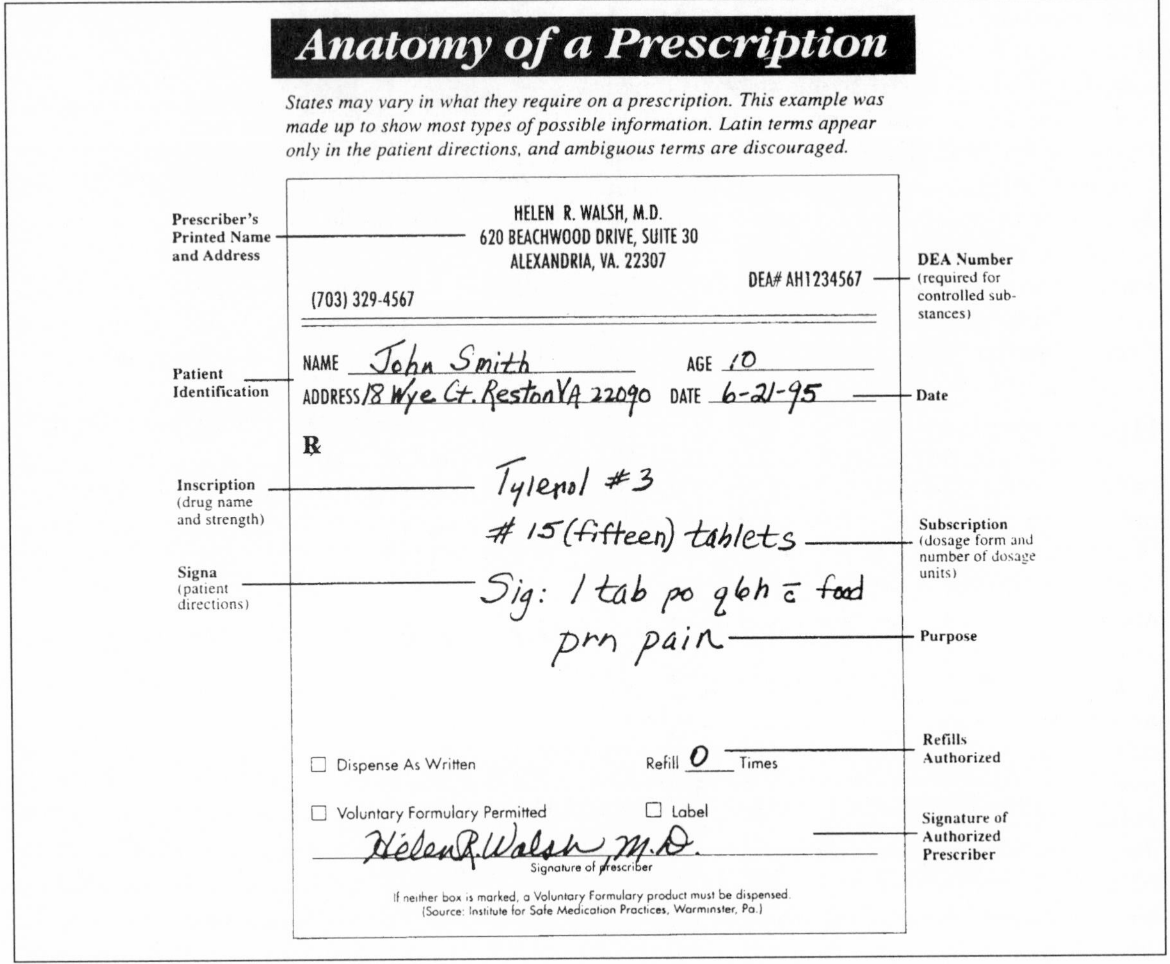

and scribbles meant? Even when you could make them out, they still seemed unintelligible. Somehow we assume that the pharmacist will be able to read the prescription and dispense it from the many drugs in the cabinets. However, to be a partner in your health care requires that you know what a prescription says. So if you see "*Sig: Tab qid pc & hs*," you will know, from asking your health care provider, that it means "Directions to patient: Take tablet four times a day after meals and at bedtime."

Anatomy of a Prescription
States may vary in what they require on a prescription. This example was made up to show most types of possible information. Latin terms appear only in the patient directions, and ambiguous terms are discouraged.
Prescriber's Printed Name and Address
HELEN R. WALSH, M.D.
620 BEACHWOOD DRIVE, SUITE 30
ALEXANDRIA, VA. 22307
DEA# AH1234567
DEA Number (required for controlled substances)
(703) 329-4567
Patient Identification
NAME John Smith
AGE 10
ADDRESS 18 Wye Ct. Reston VA 22090
DATE 6-21-95
Date
℞
Inscription (drug name and strength)
Tylenol #3
15 (fifteen) tablets
Subscription (dosage form and number of dosage units)
Signa (patient directions)
Sig: 1 tab po q6h c̄ food
prn pain
Purpose
Dispense As Written
Refill 0 Times
Refills Authorized
Voluntary Formulary Permitted
Label
Helen R. Walsh, M.D.
Signature of prescriber
Signature of Authorized Prescriber
If neither box is marked, a Voluntary Formulary product must be dispensed.
(Source: Institute for Safe Medication Practices, Warminster, Pa.)

Myths and Facts

Myth: Natural products are healthier for you.
Fact: Some natural products are healthy for you; others are untested and not FDA approved and should be approached with caution.
Myth: If I take more vitamins I will feel better.
Fact: You can take too much of a vitamin (see Chapter 19), with serious negative effects.
Myth: All you need to know is that a medicine or treatment has been approved by the FDA.

Fact: Although all medicines are regulated by the FDA, they differ in the amount of scrutiny they receive. Vitamins, supplements, and many natural treatments are not subjected to vigilant research procedures, which include clinical trials.

Myth: Vitamins and supplements are regulated just like any medicine.

Fact: Vitamins and supplements do not have to go through clinical trials or prove their effectiveness.

Consejos

What Is Health Fraud?

Most cases of health fraud are attempts to coerce consumers to spend money for products that have no clinical or scientific evidence to support their claims. If it sounds too good to be true, it usually is not true. To report products that you are concerned about, call the Health Fraud Coordinator in your area (see the resource section).

Home Remedies

I didn't have a good relationship with my mother, but when I was sick she would take very good care of me and would always call the doctor right away. That might be the reason I got sick quite often, because I liked to have the doctor come to see me at our house.

Even when I was a child, I enjoyed listening to the doctor talking and explaining what he was going to do to make me feel better. I can still smell the teas my mother gave me to take with my pills, the sobaditas *(rubbings) of the lady who gave me my shot, while the syringes and needles were being sterilized in boiling water. She would make me believe I was getting a shot without the needle. It was magic! I can still smell the* cataplasmas con alcanfor *(camphor poultice) and I don't know what else, but it smelled so good, it gave me much relief when I had the mumps. I wish I knew what it was. All that special care and attention made me feel so much better.*

—Ana, 59

Each Latina has her very special memories of medicines, treatments, and mixtures that we ate or drank to make us feel better. For many of us, these *remedios* were something we used but did not talk to anyone else about. We felt that others would not understand.

Today, with increasing interest in what are called alternative treatments, some of our *remedios* are being recast in words and wisdom that are more acceptable to mainstream medicine and culture. So the *sobaditas* of pressure points to alleviate illness are now discussed in terms of acupressure and reflexology. Some of the herbs that we used for tea are now being investigated for their medicinal properties. The natural medicines we have always valued, which have often been the major care available to us, are now more widely used.

The fact to keep in mind is that many of our home medicines and treatments work for reasons that are not easily documented and have been dismissed for too long by the scientific literature. As more medicines are being derived from natural remedies (foxglove, Mexican yam), there will be increased research to understand the biochemistry of these substances at the molecular level.

In the meantime it is wise not to waste your money on medicines whose effectiveness is only demonstrated through testimonials. First, these testimonials are not necessarily true. And second, a medicine that has a good effect on one person may not have the same effect on another. Most manufacturers with legitimate claims that their products are good for everyone are more than willing to go through clinical trials to show that they are safe and effective. If someone is selling a special cure or remedy without research on its effectiveness, you may want to reconsider what you are buying.

Summary

To be an effective consumer of medicines requires that we understand what medicines we are taking, engage in meaningful dialogue with our health care provider and pharmacist, and use home remedies appropriately.

Medicines (over-the-counter and prescription) travel a long and costly route to get from the laboratory to the medicine cabinet. Unfortunately, the process has usually not included Latinas, so that much of what we know about the effects of drugs on Latinas is relatively new. We do know that Latinas metabolize some drugs differently from other people.

There are many ways to heal our bodies. Medicines that are consistent with our mind and spirit will always work the best.

RESOURCES

Organizations

American Medical Association
515 North State Street
Chicago, IL 60610
(312) 464-5374
www.ama-assn.org

Food and Drug Administration
Office of Consumer Affairs
Parklawn Building-Room 16–85
5600 Fishers Lane
Rockville, MD 20857
(301) 827-5006 or (888) 463-6332
www.fda.gov/oca

FDA/NIH Council
426 C Street NE
Washington, DC 20002
(202) 544-1880

Institute for Safe Medication Practices
1800 Byberry Rd.
Huntingdon Valley, PA 19006
(215) 942-7797
www.ismp-org

National Consumers League
1701 K Street NW, Suite 1201
Washington, DC 20006
(202) 835-3323
www.natlconsumersleague.org

National Council on Patient Information and Education
4915 St. Elmo Ave., Ste 500
Bethesda, MD
(301) 656-8565
www.talkaboutRx.org

Books

Mastroianni, Anna C., Ruth Faden, and Daniel Federman, eds. *Women and Health Research: Ethical and Legal Issues of Including Women in Clinical Studies.* Vol. 1. Washington, DC: Institute of Medicine, National Academy Press, 1994.

The PDR Family Guide to Women's Health and Prescription Drugs. Montvale, N.J.: Medical Economics Data, 1994.

The PDR Family Guide to Prescription Drugs. Montvale, N.J.: Medical Economics Data, 1999.

Publications and Pamphlets

"FDA Tips for Taking Medicines," Pamphlet No. 98-3221. Food and Drug Administration, HFD-8, 5600 Fishers Lane, Rockville, MD 20857; call your local FDA office or (888) 463-6332. Other titles include:

"Fraudulent Health Claims: Don't be Fooled." (Internet Only).

"Use Medicine Safely," 1992. Pamphlet No. FDA 93-3201.

"The Miracle and Promise of Vaccines." FDA Council, 426 C Street NE, Washington, DC 20002; (202) 544-1880. Other titles include "The Immune System: The Body's Symphony Conductor" and "Infectious Diseases: What Will Tomorrow Be Like without Penicillin?"

"Taking Part in Clinical Trials." A booklet for patients with cancer (also available in Spanish). National Cancer Institute, Bethesda, MD 20892; (800) 422-6237 or 301-496-6667. www.cissure.nci.nih.gov/ncipubs

"Food and Drug Interactions." National Consumers League, 1701 K Street NW Suite 1200, Washington, DC 20006; (202) 835-3323 ($2.00 for nonmembers of NCL). Download free at www.nclnet.org

District Health Fraud Coordinators

NORTHEAST REGION

New England District
Joseph Raulinaitis
Food and Drug Administration
44 Front Street, Suite 380
Worcester, MA 01608
(508) 793-0422
FAX: (508) 793-0456
E-Mail: *jraulina@ora.fda.gov*

New York District (Downstate)
Lisa Utz
Food and Drug Administration
850 Third Avenue
Brooklyn, NY 11232
(716) 551-4461 ext. 3165
FAX: (716) 551-4499
E-Mail: *lutz@ora.fda.gov*

New York District (Upstate)
Joan B. Trankle
Food and Drug Administration
300 Pear St., Suite 100
Buffalo, NY 14202
(716) 551-4461 ext. 3171
FAX: (716) 551-4499
E-Mail: *jtrankle@ora.fda.gov*

CENTRAL REGION

Cincinnati District
Lawrence E. Boyd
Food and Drug Administration
6751 Steger Drive
Cincinnati, OH 45237-3097
(513) 679-2700 ext. 167
FAX: (513) 679-2773
E-Mail: *lboyd@ora.fda.gov*

Baltimore District
Karen S. Anthony
Food and Drug Administration
10710 Midlothian Turnpike, Suite 424
Richmond, VA 23235
(804) 379-1627
FAX: (804) 379-2968
E-Mail: *kanthony@ora.fda.gov*

Chicago District
Kathleen Haas
Food and Drug Administration
300 S. Riverside Plaza, Suite 550
South Chicago, IL 60606
(312) 353-7840
FAX: (312) 353-0947
E-Mail: *khaas@ora.fda.gov*

Detroit District
Evelyn DeNike
Food and Drug Administration
1560 East Jefferson Avenue
Detroit, MI 48207
(313) 226-6158
FAX: (313) 226-3076
E-Mail: *edenike@ora.fda.gov*

Philadelphia District
Anitra Brown-Reed
Food and Drug Administration
U.S. Customhouse, Room 900
Second and Chestnut Streets
Philadelphia, PA 19106
(215) 597-4390 ext. 4548
FAX: (215) 597-0875
E-Mail: *abrown-r@ora.fda.gov*

New Jersey District
Mercedes Mota
Food and Drug Administration
10 Waterview Blvd., 3rd Floor
Parsippany, NJ 07054
(973) 526-6009
FAX: (973) 526-6069
E-Mail: *mmota@ora.fda.gov*

Minneapolis District
Frank Sedzielarz
Food and Drug Administration
240 Hennepin Avenue
Minneapolis, MN 55401
(612) 334-4100 ext. 193
FAX: (612) 334-4134
E-Mail: *fsedziel@ora.fda.gov*

SOUTHEAST REGION

Atlanta District
Myla Chapman
Food and Drug Administration
60 Eighth Street, NE
Atlanta, GA 30309
(404) 347-4001 ext. 5346
FAX: (404) 347-1913
E-Mail: *mchapman@ora.fda.gov*

Florida District
Martin Katz
Food and Drug Administration
555 Winderley Place, Suite 200
Maitland, FL 32751
(407) 475-4729
FAX: (407) 475-4769
E-Mail: *mkatz@ora.fda.gov*

San Juan District
Nilda Villegas
Food and Drug Administration
#466 Fernandez Juncos Avenue
San Juan, PR 00901-3223
(787) 729-6852
FAX: (787) 729-6847
E-Mail: *nvillega@ora.fda.gov*

Nashville District
Sandra Baxter
Food and Drug Administration
297 Plus Park Blvd.
Nashville, TN 37217
(615) 781-5385 ext. 122
FAX: (615) 781-5383
E-Mail: *sbaxter@ora.fda.gov*

Lynne C. Isaacs
Food and Drug Administration
555 Winderley Place, Suite 200
Maitland, FL 32751
(407) 475-4704
FAX: (407) 475-4768
E-Mail: *lisaacs@ora.fda.gov*

New Orleans District
Marie Fink
Food and Drug Administration
4298 Elysian Fields Avenue
New Orleans, LA 70122
(504) 253-4542
FAX: (504) 253-4560
E-Mail: *mfink@ora.fda.gov*

SOUTHWEST REGION

Denver District
Shelly Maifarth
Food and Drug Administration
Denver Federal Center
Building 20, Entrance W-10
Denver, CO 80225
(303) 236-3046
FAX: (303) 236-3551
E-Mail: *smaifart@ora.fda.gov*

Dallas District
Reynold Rodriguez
Food and Drug Administration
3310 Live Oak Street, Room 514
Dallas, TX 75204
(214) 655-5317 ext. 514
FAX: (214) 655-5220 or (214) 655-5331
E-Mail: *rrodrig1@ora.fda.gov*

Kansas City District
Mary H. Woleske
Food and Drug Administration
P.O. Box 15905
Lenexa, KS 66285-5905
(913) 752-2423

FAX: (913) 752-2413
E-Mail: *mwoleske@ora.fda.gov*
PACIFIC REGION
Seattle District
Connie Rezendes
Food and Drug Administration
22201 23rd Drive S.E.
P.O. Box 3012
Bothell, WA 98041-3012
(425) 402-3178
FAX: (425) 483-4996
E-Mail: *crezende@ora.fda.gov*
Mihaly Ligmond
Food and Drug Administration
22201 23rd Drive S.E.
P.O. Box 3012
Bothell, WA 98041-3012
(425) 483-4895
FAX: (425) 483-4996
E-Mail: *mligmond@ora.fda.gov*

San Francisco District
Jeff Watson
Food and Drug Administration
1431 Harbor Bay Parkway
Alameda, CA 94502-7070
(510) 337-6879
FAX: (510) 337-6702
E-Mail: *jwatson@ora.fda.gov*
Los Angeles District
John Nicholson
Food and Drug Administration
4615 East Elwood Street, Suite 200
Phoenix, AZ 85040
(602) 829-7396 ext. 223
FAX: (602) 379-4646
E-Mail: *jnichols@ora.fda.gov*

23

Taking Care of Our Families

Nuestras Familias . . . Our Families

Once again Mari found herself having to take care of her mother. They had gone through so much together in the last few years. Her mother's illness had not been an easy adjustment for either one of them.

They had had to overcome much of their past so that they could confide in one another—their hopes but also their disappointments. It was hard to find the words in English to capture the essence of the relationship or the changes it had undergone.

When Mari thought about mother or family, *the words did not seem to capture the depth of the commitment. As a Latina, her relationship with her mother and family defined so much of who she was and what she did. . . .*

Mari thought about how complex it was to be a Latina. Her non-Latina friends also had a mother and a family, but it was different. The American nuclear family was a vision—that had apparently failed.

Mari knew that her family had endured because it was much more than a nuclear family. Family was all those people who were related by blood or by life. The ties that bound her to her mother and to each family member made her responsibility to them more than she could sometimes handle. And yet, at times like this, it was because of that sense of responsibility that somehow she managed to do the things she had to do.

With that thought Mari closed her eyes, taking a deep breath to reach deep inside herself and draw inner strength from her Latina spirit once again.

Latinas are more likely to have a parent living with them than are other women. However, as families increasingly move geographically apart due to jobs, education, and other demands, caring for a parent in the parent's home or one's own home is becoming less of an option for many Hispanic families. Even when the parent maintains an independent living arrangement, it is usually up to us to make the *arreglos* (arrangements) when they become ill. And although we do what we have to do, often without hesitation or complaint, caring for a parent brings up many complicated issues.

The need to care for a parent often comes at a time in our lives when we think we have finally finished taking care of the family we raised. Instead of finding the relief we have anticipated, we find ourselves caring for the family that raised us. Others of us find that the health of a parent deteriorates just when we are starting to create our own lives separate from them. This is part of life, and regardless of how well we map out other aspects of our lives, we do not get to choose when the responsibility to take care of a parent will begin.

Most of what has preceded this chapter is about how to take care of ourselves. As Latinas, though, we accept that an important part of our lives involves taking care of others. In order to meet the often conflicting demands of our lives and those of our parents, we must be proactive. We must know what living arrangements are options for our parents, how to structure the health care services they need, and what our role in each of these situations will be.

Living Arrangements

When Dolores called me the other day, she sounded very tired. Her mother had to have surgery—again. I knew what that meant—that her mother would be staying at her house until she had fully recuperated.

That was not easy on Dolores. The few times I had visited the house when her mother was there, I was surprised to find her so demanding. Their relationship had not been the very best, but what else was Dolores to do? As Dolores's friend I knew she didn't have any choice.

For the next few months Dolores would put her life on hold, restructure her home, and organize all of her activities for the purpose of helping her mother get better. Miguel, Dolores's older brother, was no help during these times. He always managed not to do his part by saying that he did not have space.

Dolores never complained. She knew this was her responsibility as surely as she knew she was her mother's daughter.

Consejos

Steps for Planning a Parent's Living Arrangements

1. Discuss with your parent who will be responsible for him or her.
2. Discuss the matter with your family.
3. Discuss the matter with your extended family.
4. Make adjustments for physical limitations.
5. Review all essential financial and legal records.

The best time to talk about living arrangements is before they are necessary. As much as we may not like to admit it, there will come a time when our parents or older relatives are unable to care for themselves. How that is handled should be addressed by following some key steps.

1: Discuss with your parent who will be responsible for him or her. This is probably the most difficult conversation you will ever have with your parent because it acknowledges that life for all of you is changing. For parents who have been independent their entire life, it may seem that the discussion is premature. Yet by discussing these things in advance and remaining flexible, it will be easier to address other issues as they arise.

In most families there is one obvious person, usually a daughter, who will take primary care of the parent. Some of the other children may also want to have a role, even when the parent may not want them to be involved. It is best if everyone is given a role that is agreeable to all.

There are several arrangements that may be considered:

• Living by themselves with assistance from others. In this situation the parent lives in their own house or apartment. You may be able to obtain regular assistance through Meals on Wheels, the Visiting Nurse Association, chore services provided for older adults, or other arrangements.

• Living with you. The parent lives with you and your family. Usually at least one room is made available for them. In other instances it may be possible to provide the parent with more private space. These options include converting a detached garage or space within a home into an "in-law" apartment or placing an "ECHO" home (a prefabricated small, portable cottage) in the back or side yard of a single family home.

• Living with another family member. The parent lives in the home of another family member. Sometimes several older members of a family choose to live together and share care and other household responsibilities.

• Living with a non-family member. Elderly are increasingly looking to homesharing as a way of increasing social interaction, home chore assistance, and safety. In some instances, elderly may share a home with an acquaintance or some elderly and religious groups now sponsor roommate finder services and shared homes. Of course, it is important to know who you are sharing a home with before entering into such a situation.

• Living in an assisted-living facility. In this situation the housing ranges from one room to an apartment in a facility. The facility usually provides meals or dining facilities as well as other services to assist each resident. Many facilities also provide recreational activities. The services can range from independent living with only some chore support to twenty-four-hour skilled nursing care. Some facilities offer the ability to change up to increasing levels of support as the need arises. For this reason, it is important that a family physician be involved in an assisted care decision in order to match services to current and future needs. It is also important to be aware that this option is not covered by most health insurance or Medicare and costs may be $1,000–$3,000 a month or more.

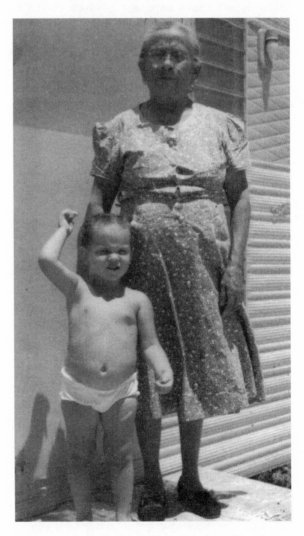

Memories of our grandmothers nourish us throughout our lives.

• Nursing homes. For those needing substantial skilled or long-term care nursing services, a nursing home is an option. Nursing homes provide medical services and monitoring; personal care services such as dressing, grooming, and toileting; meals; and recreational activities. Annual costs average $56,000 and can easily cost more. Medicare only provides short-term coverage and a person will need to "spend-down" their assets to a poverty level to qualify for Medicaid which covers nursing home care for those medically qualified.

2: Discuss the matter with your family. We may think of the apartment we rent or the home we buy as the right size. In the back of our minds we may look forward to the time when the children move out—perhaps we will turn that extra space into an office or study. Or maybe another child is looking forward to finally not having to share a room. And then one day that all has to be put aside as we prepare for a parent or other family member to come and live with us.

For most of us this possibility creates some level of disruption. If it is someone we have always appreciated and who has always been a positive part of the family, we willingly make whatever changes are necessary. But what if it is someone who has not gotten along with you or your partner or the other members of the household? Then what do you do?

The best solution is to talk to a mental health professional so that you and the other members of your household can prepare yourselves for this difficult transition. You should not expect to be able to resolve long-standing problems on your own. Recognizing how each person in the household feels about the parent and coming up with a transition plan together will make it easier for everyone to adapt to the expanded household. Too often we have these discussions with ourselves when in fact they should be shared with other family members.

If we live far away from our parents, it may happen that we have to make arrangements for the parent's care in another city. In some instances we may feel it is necessary to move back home. Whatever choice is made, it is best made by all family members. That way the person who is the primary caretaker will be able to better define his or her responsibilities and the responsibilities of other members of the family.

3: Discuss the matter with your extended family. Once you have agreed that the parent will change their living situation, all the households in the family must be prepared for the changes that will occur. This is never easy. The challenge is twofold: (1) to incorporate the parent's new living situation while maintaining oversight in an unobtrusive manner, and (2) to insure that members of the family who are not primary caregivers still assist in the parent's care. Here are a few key areas that will have to be discussed:

• Household chores. Make sure each person understands his or her responsibility with respect to taking care of the home.

• Care of the parent. It is usually best to make a list of all the things the parent will need and determine which family member will be responsible for each one. For example, the list may include cooking special meals, feeding, bathing, driving, reading, and tracking medication. Striking a fair balance in the responsibilities of different household members will make clear the roles and expectations for everyone.

• Holidays and birthdays. Now that the parent may need to move out of their home, all the other family members have to decide where they will spend the holidays. A parent's home may have been a neutral meeting ground for all the family members, but when the parent moves out, new decisions have to be made about the location of family gatherings.

• Care for the caregiver. Whoever is the main caregiver will face a difficult set of challenges creating new stress in their life. It is important for the family to plan for respite care for the caregiver so they can have free time away from their duties, no matter if your parent lives with the caregiver or in assisted living. It is also important that the caregiver have access to a support group of other caregivers. Such groups can be found through a number of the resources at the end of this chapter.

4: Make adjustments for physical limitations.

Myrna remembered what her father was like when she was growing up. He had worked hard all his life. He had struggled at whatever jobs were necessary to make sure that the family had food, shelter, clothing, and education. He prided himself on being a strong, healthy man and the sole provider for his family. He was a man who commanded respect and love.

Now hours would go by and he would just sit staring out the window. Myrna did not know what he was looking at or what he was waiting for. Not that it really mattered, because one way or the other she had to take care of him. She even had to bathe him.

Myrna was the youngest daughter, and she took care of him because he could no longer take care of himself. It was not easy for him to accept any of this. It was not easy for Myrna to accept it either, but these were the things that had to be done.

Some of our parents may remain physically fit and strong as they get older and retain their mental quickness right to the end. Most of our parents will experience some physical deterioration, however, and it may be increasingly difficult for them to do many of the activities they once enjoyed.

As a daughter, you want to care for and protect your parents. Perhaps the most important way to accomplish this goal is to help them adjust their home to their physical realities. It can be helpful to have your health care provider conduct a formal test and assessment of their level of functioning. This will determine how long they can stand, how many steps they can take before resting, and the degree to which they can bend or stretch. This would also be a good time to have a "mini-mental" test done to assess basic memory skills and detect early signs of memory loss, dementia, or Alzheimer's disease.

In most cases older adults want to maintain as much independence as possible. Many of the concepts behind making a home handicapped-accessible may also be applied to make it easier for older adults to manage their own lives. On the next page are a few changes that may be useful.

5: Review all essential financial and legal records. This is probably one of the most sensitive areas. Parents, like all of us, are usually very private about their financial affairs. Some parents want to "surprise" their children with a secret insurance policy they have been paying. Other parents may be concerned that children just want to take their money. Regardless of where your parents might fall in that continuum, you need to know how to handle their financial affairs should they become unable. Following are some things you can do to facilitate this process while allowing your parents to maintain as much privacy as possible.

• Organize. Set up folders so that papers can be easily found. Some useful categories are residence bills (rent/mortgage, electricity, gas, water, telephone), credit cards, loans, health insurance, life insurance, other assets, and legal documents.

Consejos

To increase physical stability:

- Rearrange furniture so that there are objects that can be leaned on if your parent loses his or her balance.
- Place handrails on walls of long hallways.
- Remove throw rugs, on which an older person may trip or slip.
- Establish clear pathways between rooms by removing furniture that obstructs the passage.
- Put nonskid strips or nonskid paint on sidewalks, porches, and steps in outside areas.

To facilitate daily tasks:

- Buy a "reacher" to help retrieve things that are too high or too low.
- Try to use lighter pots for cooking. Many of your parent's older pots may be too heavy to lift, particularly when full of food.
- Replace manual with electric can openers.
- Replace knobs and faucets that need to be gripped with levers that can be pushed or pulled.
- Make sure clocks have large dials.
- Replace small knobs on lamps with string so that they are easier to turn on and off.
- Put extenders on toilet seats so that the seat is higher and has handrails.
- Get a shower seat so it is possible to sit while showering.
- Make sure there are remote controls for lights and electric equipment wherever possible.
- Add "grab bars" to tub area.

For safety:

- Schedule regular checkups for batteries in smoke detectors, security systems, radios, and flashlights.
- Obtain a phone with an autodialer and an emergency call button.

• Sort. It is best if your parents sort through their own papers, although in some situations you may end up taking over the job when they prove unable or unwilling. As adults, we are all entitled to keep private some areas of our lives. If your parents can do this, it will provide the information that you need and the privacy that they need.

• Develop schedules. Make a payment schedule for any regular bills; include addresses, account numbers, phone numbers, and contact persons. This is especially important with respect to utility companies and insurance companies, which are often quick to cancel services for nonpayment. Also make a schedule of any income that is supposed to be received. This may be particularly sensitive when your parent has been lending money to another person that you may not know about.

• Arrange for signature. Establish who will sign checks and other documents in the event that your parent is unable to do so. While a power of attorney may be advisable, some parents may decide it is easier to add you as an authorized signature for their checking or savings account.

• Plan finances early. Many children and parents are under the impression that assisted living facilities and in-home care services are covered by Medicare. This is NOT true. Neither Medicaid nor Medicare cover assisted living options for those who cannot live independently. Medicare provides only short-term nursing care and it usually must follow a hospitalization. Medicaid will cover nursing home care, but only after spending down to a poverty level to qualify for the program.

Basic Facts—Dementia and Alzheimer's Disease

Dementia is a condition in which a person's intellectual abilities have deteriorated to the point where they cannot think or function. Only 5 to 10 percent of all persons over sixty-five years of age suffer from dementia. Symptoms of dementia may be due to a variety of factors: Alzheimer's disease (57 percent), blood vessel disease in the brain (13 percent), depression (4.5 percent), alcoholism (4.2 percent), reaction to medication (1.5 percent), and numerous others.

Very little is known about Alzheimer's disease, even though it is the most common cause of dementia. What we know is that:

- Hispanics are more likely to have Alzheimer's disease than non-Hispanic whites.
- The average person lives eight to ten years after onset of the disease.
- There are only two known risk factors: (1) family history of dementia and (2) Down syndrome.
- It is often unrecognized or misdiagnosed in its early stages.

Alzheimer's disease is diagnosed based on a series of tests of function and mental status and by elimination of the other causal factors of dementia.

Health Arrangements

Jenny was the nurse on duty when my mom was in intensive care. My mother was in a room by herself, and I had planned to spend the night on the chair by her bed. When evening visiting hours were over, the formerly friendly Jenny came in and sternly said that it was now time for me to leave. I asked why. Her response was that it was hospital policy, and she asked me to leave again. At that point I insisted that I would not leave.

The head nurse on duty came to speak to me to find out why I would not leave. I went through all of the rational reasons: my mother did not speak English very well and the hospital had no bilingual staff; my mother might be frightened to wake up and not see her family; I would be able to help the nurses since they were so understaffed.

The real reasons were not getting me far. So I reminded the nurses of Title IX of the Health Care Antidiscrimination Act, which states that by law hospitals have to have someone always on hand who speaks the language of the patient. On hearing this, the nurses relented and I was allowed to stay.

I confess that I had made these things up—there is neither a Title IX nor a Health Care Antidiscrimination Act.

Very often what goes on in a hospital is for the convenience of the health care providers and not for the good of the patients. For instance, the number of persons allowed to visit a patient is limited because hospital staff wish to minimize the number of caring people who may ask them questions.

Given this situation, it is important that you establish exactly which family members are responsible for communicating your parent's health care decisions. Health care

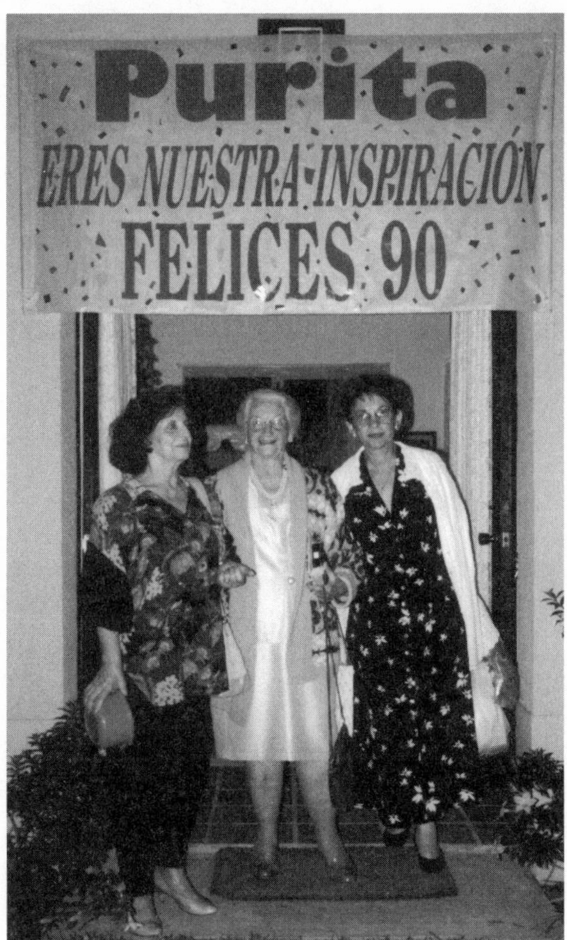

There are many generations that need our special attention.

providers often focus on protecting the patient in ways that go beyond what you know your parent would want. The worst time to establish your role in making these necessary decisions is during an emergency. It is essential that early on you establish a three-way relationship that includes the patient, the health care provider, and you.

Some health care providers are reluctant to do this. Issues of confidentiality and ethics, as well as the litigious nature of society, can make it difficult to establish the communication and lines of authority that genuinely place the patient's interest first. Here are some things you can do to facilitate this process.

1: Make a list of your parent's health care providers. While one health care provider may serve as a gatekeeper, most older patients are under the care of a variety of specialists. You need to know who they are and how they work with one another.

2: Meet the health care provider with your parent. It is very important that you go with your parent to see their health care provider before your parent becomes incapacitated. This will be a first step toward including you in the process of making health care decisions for your parent.

Some health care providers are reluctant to include others in their direct relationship with the patient. To overcome this reluctance, it is critical that you establish a positive relationship with the health care provider. This is the person that your parent trusts, and you need to be part of that trust relationship.

Meeting the provider also makes it possible for you to intervene later should your parent not be pleased with the level of care that they are receiving.

Consejos

Know Your Parents' Health Care Providers

1. Make a list of your parent's health care providers.
2. Meet the health care provider with your parent.
3. Obtain a formal notification from your parent.
4. Visit the nearest hospital.
5. Maintain ongoing communication.

3: Obtain a formal notification from your parent. Obtain and send to each provider a notarized letter signed by your parent stipulating that the health care provider is authorized to share all information with you. In some states it may be necessary to obtain a *medical power of attorney*, in which your parent will designate you as the person who will make all of their health decisions if they are unable to do so themselves. This may also be called a *health care proxy* or *appointment of a health care agent.*

Always keep in mind that if someone is not designated beforehand, it will not be clear who can make decisions when the time comes. This is particularly true if your parent is at the early stages of dementia or Alzheimer's disease.

4: Visit the nearest hospital. The first time we visit the hospital with our parent is too often in an emergency. In their efforts to become more consumer oriented, many hospitals now conduct tours of their facilities. You and your parent should visit your local hospital and become familiar with key units before your parent becomes ill.

5: Maintain ongoing communication. In all likelihood your parent will be seeing a health care provider on a regular basis, and you will be unable to accompany them on each visit. At a minimum you should call the main health care provider once every three months to reestablish contact. Maintaining ongoing positive communication with health care providers demonstrates that you are part of the decision-making process in the health care of your parent.

Getting Adequate Care

Persons sixty-five and older are covered by Medicare and usually by a variety of other private plans for which they have paid. Because some older adults are well insured, they may get too much care. Other older adults who do not have private plans may not get as much care as they need. The ongoing struggle is to get the amount of care that is needed.

1: Review health insurance policies. These policies tend to be rather cumbersome to read, so take your time and read them slowly. Most policies have a consumer information telephone number that you can call with questions. The best time to ask about what is covered is before you need to use the services.

Consejos

How to Get the Care You Pay For

1. Review health insurance policies.
2. Review payment policies of providers.
3. Review Medicare bills.
4. Arrange for home health services.
5. Monitor home health services.
6. Transfer assets early.

2: Review payment policies of providers. Make sure that you and your parent understand what portion of the bill will not be covered by insurance or Medicare. Also find out what type of payment plan your health care provider will accept. Although some may be willing to work out extended no-interest payment plans, others may not be in a position to do so.

3: Review Medicare bills. When you receive a Medicare statement, be sure to review it carefully. If you do not understand what it says (and you may not), call and ask what it means. The statement tells you how much Medicare will pay and how much you have to pay. In some instances your health care provider will have agreed to accept the Medicare payment as full payment.

4: Arrange for home health services. Sometimes it may be more desirable and less expensive for your parent to leave a hospital and obtain the care they need at home. This decision must be made jointly by your parent, the health care provider, and the members of your household. Make sure the services that are necessary will be covered by your health insurance; some insurance covers only hospital care and not at-home nursing.

5: Monitor home health services. You need to check on the quality of the care provided through home health services. Since often these services are contracted out, the attention to detail may not be what you expect. Remember that if services are provided and paid for by Medicare or your supplemental health insurer, you are still paying for the services. You should expect and receive the level of help you need.

You should also let the provider know that you want them to send the same person each time to provide these home services. In this way you and your parent can develop a trusting relationship with them.

6: Transfer assets early. If your parent will need nursing home care, most families can only meet this cost through Medicaid. Nursing home services cost an average of $56,000 annually and can easily cost more. In order to qualify for Medicaid, a person will need to "spend-down" their assets to a poverty level. Transferring assets to a child does not protect these assets, as Medicaid in many states looks back five years or more and has the right to claim those transferred assets before qualifying a person for Medicaid. For this reason, it is often important to plan financially both early and with an accountant who specializes in elder services.

The difficulties of financing assisted living and long-term care should be a lesson for all adult caregivers. It is vital for adults in their forties to obtain long-term care insurance which provides coverage for a wider range of assisted living options in elder years than is available through Medicare or Medicaid.

Making the Final Decisions

The surgery had been successful—or so the surgeon said. Despite this, Nadia kept thinking of the old joke, "The surgery was successful, but the patient died." It didn't seem so funny anymore.

In the room the only sound was the humming and churning of all the high-tech machines that surrounded her mother. One machine pushed air down her throat, another helped her lungs work, another made her heart pump, and another monitored all the other machines.

Nadia looked at her mother. She could only see a head and arms sticking out from the sheets. Her mother had been a tiny woman all her life, like a little doll. She had come out of the surgery looking like a giant, all bloated. Her little hands were puffed up, her tongue was so swollen that she could not close her mouth. She did not look like Nadia's mother. "Is this supposed to be life support?" Nadia thought to herself.

Not long after the surgery, Nadia's mother died.

Regardless of how much we prepare for it, the death of a parent is always hard. Whether our relationship was wonderful or full of conflict, the death of a parent changes who we are and how we see ourselves. It is for this reason that coming to terms with end-of-life decisions is so important.

1: Set up a time for a serious conversation. There is no perfect time to have a discussion about end-of-life decisions. You must gauge how you and your parent feel. The purpose of setting up a time in advance is to give each of you the opportunity to think about the topic and come to the discussion with more emotional control.

Ana had been very close to her mother all her life. She could not bear the thought of her mother's impending death. All the dreams they had had were just starting to be realized, and now they were being cut short by her mother's illness. Ana wanted very much to believe that if she kept her mother alive just a little longer, things would get better.

It did not matter that the doctors had said that her mother was only being kept alive by the machines that did the work for her body. Such is the nature of hope.

*And Ana hoped for more. She wanted more time to make new memories with her mother. But as she looked at her mother, she remembered her words: "*Mi hija, *you have always been a good daughter. When my time comes, do not become a selfish daughter. Just let me go in peace to the Lord."*

Ana turned and faced the doctor. In a voice that sounded as if it came from far away, she heard herself say, "Yes, you can turn off the life support."

2: Discuss end-of-life decisions. Each person tries to live their life as best as they can. The final act of respect and dignity we can offer our parents is to follow their wishes regarding the kind of treatment they want at the end of their life. The faith our parents have practiced or not practiced often guides their decisions. For us the task is to put our beliefs aside and listen to what they want.

3: Develop advance directives. Advance directives are the health care instructions that are to be followed when a person is unconscious or unable to speak and thus cannot state his or her own health decisions. To make certain that the wishes of our parents are followed, it is recommended that they develop their own advance directives. According to the Federal Patient Self-Determination Act, all health care facilities that accept funds from Medicaid or Medicare must let patients know that they have a right to complete advance directives. Some hospitals may have patients fill these out at admission.

Living wills are a category of advance directives. There is great variability in state laws regarding the conditions that may be included in a living will and when a living will goes into effect. In most instances it is easier to have advance directives.

Read everything in the advance directives very carefully. Make sure you understand what each procedure means. If you are not sure, talk to the health care provider and have them discuss it with you and your parent.

Consejos

Know in Advance What Your Parent Wants

1. Set up a time for a serious conversation.
2. Discuss end-of-life decisions.
3. Develop advance directives.
4. Send advance directives to all health care providers and institutions.

Warning

There is great variability by state and local jurisdiction as to the legal requirements for advance directives. Make sure you know what applies in the state where the care will be provided. For more information contact "Partnership for Caring" at (800) 989-9455 or www.partnershipforcaring.org

4: Send advance directives to all health care providers and institutions. Make sure you have sufficient copies of the advance directive for each provider and health care facility. You should also have one with you when you are at the hospital.

Body, Mind, and Spirit

When we take care of our parents we open all the wounds from our childhood—the ones we know we have and the ones buried so deep we have forgotten them. All the issues once handled or hidden seem to surface. The task is to focus on doing the best you can.

It is not easy to become the caregiver to a parent when you have always been the child. Even those of us who may be physically or emotionally distant from our parents feel anguish when they are entering this final phase of life.

There is nothing easy about it, and there is nothing that can prepare us for it, but one thing is certain: we must do whatever we feel is right. For some that means taking over and doing all the caregiving. For others it means stepping back and letting others do the caring. Each one of us will know what is right for us.

For a Latina going through these difficult transitions, here are some truths that can help.

Consejos

Things to Keep in Mind and Heart

1. It is all right to feel guilty.
2. It is all right to get angry.
3. Just because you do more does not mean that you will be loved more.
4. Forgiveness is a good thing.
5. Sometimes we run out of patience.
6. Memories are very important.
7. Some things you never get over.
8. Life goes on.

1: It is all right to feel guilty. No Latina has ever escaped feelings of guilt. We always feel we did not do enough or care enough. But while it is natural to feel guilty, our guilt does not mean we have actually done anything wrong. If we are feeling overcome with guilt, it is important to take a step back and realize that in most instances we did the best we could.

2: It is all right to get angry. Just because someone is sick or even dying does not mean that all of a sudden we can no longer be angry with them. And just because someone is sick does not mean that all of a sudden they will be a kind person.

3: Just because you do more does not mean that you will be loved more. If you do more, you must understand that the only good reason to do it is that you believe it is the right thing to do. Your parent may even seem to show more love to another family member who is less giving. That may be difficult if you have the major responsibility of caring for the parent, but it does not mean that your parent loves you less. Unfortunately, what often happens is that those who do more are usually expected to do even more because they are viewed as more capable than other family members.

4: Forgiveness is a good thing. Many of us seem to believe that forgiveness is only divine. The reality is that we as human beings must learn to forgive each other and most importantly to forgive ourselves. If our relationship with our parent is not what we had hoped, we have to accept that this is the reality of the relationship.

5: Sometimes we run out of patience. Just because someone is sick or dying does not mean that we have to have infinite patience with them. We have to learn to say "enough" and set realistic limits on the extent of our caregiving.

6: Memories are very important. When our parents die, our memories of them are all that remains. So while they are alive it is important to take the opportunity to do the kinds of things with them that we can always treasure. It may be as simple as sitting next to each other on a regular basis and reading or going on walks.

7: Some things you never get over. Losing your parent is not something you just "get over," like a cold or a bad relationship. It is something that lives within us for the rest of our lives.

8: Life goes on. After you have cared for a parent, you come to terms with your own vulnerability. You realize that the spirit does live on. Many of us are blessed with the inner knowledge that somehow our parents are still with us. Often we can look at our own behavior and recognize how we are a reflection of them. For some of us that is comforting; for others it may signal that we have to change. Regardless, there is always pain at the loss.

With time—more time than you may think—you will experience laughter and joy again. And of course you always have your memories.

Summary

As Latinas, it is very likely that we will end up being responsible for the care of a parent or older relative. These are difficult times, which require that we evaluate how we intend to mesh our lives and theirs. When a parent has Alzheimer's disease, some very special concerns are raised.

Caring for your parent in your home may not be the most loving thing you can do. Doing the best thing for your parent is not always clear. Often times, moving a parent into your home disrupts their sense of independence more than an assisted living arrangement would. It also may disrupt their ability for social interaction with people their age. If your parent does move into your home, be mindful of the extra stresses on you and your family. Plan for respite time for you and your parent, join a caregivers support group, and seek adult day care services in your community for your parent.

When we think about how to care for a parent, we must analyze both their housing and health care needs. Often this means that we must discuss topics we have successfully avoided most of our own lives—finances, living arrangements, and even end-of-life decisions.

RESOURCES

General

Organizations

Administration on Aging
U.S. Department of Health and Human Services
330 Independence Avenue SW
Washington, DC 20201
(202) 619-7501
www.aoa.gov

Alliance for Aging Research
2021 K Street NW, Suite 305
Washington, DC 20006
(202) 293-2856
www.agingresearch.org

American Association of Homes and Services for the Aging (AAHSA)
2519 Connecticut Ave. NW
Washington, DC 20008-1520
(202) 783-2242
www.aahsa.org/public/find.htm
Provides information on homes and services for the aging in your community.

American Association of Retired Persons
601 E Street NW
Washington, DC 20049
(202) 434-2277 or (800) 424-3410
www.aarp.org

Asociación Pro-Personas Mayores
234 E. Colorado Blvd., #300
Pasadena, CA 91101
(213) 487-1922

Assisted Living Federation of America
10300 Eaton Place, Suite 400
Fairfax, VA 22030
(703) 691-8100
www.alfa.org
Provides consumer information on how to choose an assisted living facility and lists of facilities.

National Elder Care Institute on Health Promotion
601 E Street NW, 5th Floor
Washington, DC 20049
(202) 434-2200

National Hospice and Palliative Care Organization
1700 Diagonal Rd., Ste 300
Alexandria, VA 22314
(703) 837-1500

National Institute on Aging Information Center
P.O. Box 8057
Gaithersburg, MD 20898-8057
(800) 222-2225
www.nih.gov/nia

Hotlines

Eldercare Locator
(800) 677-1116
Administration on Aging, USDHHS
Eldercare Locator: Will help you identify support services in your community for older adults and their caregivers. Call toll-free 1-800-677-1116 weekdays between the hours of 9:00 a.m. and 8:00 p.m. Eastern Standard Time. Spanish operators are available between 11:30 a.m. and 8:00 p.m. Eastern Standard Time.

Books

Carter, Rosalynn, with Susan K. Golant. *Helping Yourself Help Others—A Book for Caregivers.* New York: Times Books, Random House, 1994.

Publications and Pamphlets

Blackhall, Leslie J., S. I. Murphy, G. Frank, V. Michel, and S. Azen. "Ethnicity and Attitudes toward Patient Autonomy." *Journal of the American Medical Association* 274, no. 10 (September 13, 1995): 820.

"On Being Alone." (Also available in Spanish.) American Association of Retired Persons, Widowed Persons' Service, 601 E Street NW, Washington, DC 20049; (202) 434-2277; (800) 424-3410.

"Thinking about a Nursing Facility: A Consumer's Guide to Long-Term Care." American Health Care Association, 1201 L Street NW, Washington, DC 20005; (202) 842-4444.

Alzheimer's Disease

Organizations

Alzheimer's Association
919 N. Michigan Avenue, Suite 1000
Chicago, IL 60611
(312) 335-8700; (800) 272-3900
www.alz.org

Alzheimer's Disease Education and Referral Center
P.O Box 8250
Silver Spring, MD 20907-8250
(301) 495-3311 or (800) 438-4380
www.alzheimers.org

Books

Gruetzner, Howard. *Alzheimer's: A Caregiver's Guide and Sourcebook.* New York: Wiley, 1992.

Oliver, Rose, and Frances A. Bock. *Coping with Alzheimer's: A Caregiver's Emotional Survival Guide.* North Hollywood, CA: Wilshire, 1989.

Publications and Pamphlets

"Alzheimer's Disease," August 1995. NIH Publication No. 95-3431. A fact sheet on the most common cause of dementia in older people. Alzheimer's Disease Education and Referral Center, P.O. Box 8250, Silver Spring, MD 20907-8250; (800) 438-4380. Other titles include

"Forgetfulness in Old Age: It's Not What You Think," August 1995.

"Multi-Infarct Dementia: Fact Sheet," August 1995.

"Alzheimer's Disease: An Overview," 1994. Pamphlet No. ED 211Z. Alzheimer's Association, 919 North Michigan Avenue, Chicago, IL 60611-1676; (800) 272-3900 or (312) 335-8700. Other titles include:

"Alzheimer's Disease and Related Disorders: A Description of the Dementias." Pamphlet No. ED 206Z.

"Especially for the Alzheimer Caregiver," 1990. Pamphlet No. ED 221Z.

"Is It Alzheimer's? Warning Signs You Should Know," 1996. Pamphlet No. PR/301/Z.

"Steps to Getting a Diagnosis: Finding Out If It's Alzheimer's Disease," 1996. Pamphlet No. ED309Z.

"Memory Loss with Aging: What's Normal, What's Not," 1999. Pamphlet No. 1519. American Academy of Family Physicians, 11400 Tomahawk Creek Pkwy, Leawood, KS 66211-2672; (800) 944-0000.

End-of-Life Decisions

Organizations

Partnership for Caring
1035 30th St. NW
Washington, DC 20007
(800) 989-9455
www.partnershipforcaring.org

Publications and Pamphlets

"Advanced Directives: Living Wills, Durable Power of Attorney for Health Care." Partnership for Caring, Washington, D.C. (800) 989-9455; (410) 962-5454. www.partnershipforcaring.org

American Thoracic Society. "Withholding and Withdrawing Life-sustaining Therapy." Official statement of the American Thoracic Society adopted by the ATS Board of Directors on March 1991. American Review for Respiratory Diseases, September 1991, Vol. 144, Issue 3, Part 1, pp. 726–731.

Annas, George J. "The Health Care Proxy and the Living Will." *New England Journal of Medicine*, April 25, 1991.

Cruzan v. *Director, Missouri Department of Health*, 110 Supreme Court 2841 (1990).

Engelhardt, H. Tristram, Jr. *Freedom vs. Best Interest: A Conflict at the Roots of Health Care*, excerpt, *Dax's Case: Essays in Medical Ethics and Human Meaning*.

In the Matter of Claire C. Conroy, 98 N.J. 321 New Jersey Supreme Court (1985).

Robertson, John A. "Second Thoughts on Living Wills." *Hastings Center Report*, November 1991.

24

Nuestro Mundo . . . Our World

When I look around me I wonder how we ever let things get so out of hand. Once there were trees in this area, and now it is only a vacant lot. I used to love to breathe the morning air and feel the crispness fill my chest. Now I listen to the radio weather report and wonder what I am supposed to do when the air quality is not acceptable. It isn't as if I can just stop breathing for the day.

—*LUISA, 68*

And then there is the water issue. A few times we were told that we had to boil our water before we drank it. I drank bottled water for a few days until the city did whatever had to be done. Later on I heard that the Centers for Disease Control recommends that all persons with HIV/AIDS should only drink bottled water. What happened to the clear water that used to come from my kitchen faucet?

—*PAULA, 41*

When we get together and talk about our health problems, we usually discuss all the topics that filled the previous chapters. We talk about our gynecological problems, the diseases we have, the struggle to have healthy bodies, and about caring for our parents. In all the discussions I have had with Latinas, there has been mention of bioterrorism without discussion of other threats to our environment. Yet nothing is more essential to our health than to have air that is safe to breathe, water that is safe to drink, and food that is safe to eat. Although most of us are concerned about bioterrorism and the impact on our lives, we otherwise go along breathing air, drinking water, and eating food without understanding in what other ways they may be compromised.

Many Latinas comment that we are not encouraged to enter discussions about the environment. The blame for our lack of involvement does not rest solely on our shoulders; it is shared with others. The major environmental organizations have done little to include Latinas in their activities and much to alienate us.

It is not surprising that when Latinas think of the environmental movement in the United States, we think of a movement that consists mainly of men protecting plants rather than people, telling us to have fewer children so that we do not overpopulate the planet, and going to great lengths to save a species we never heard of while many of our families cannot get basic health care. The concerns of environmental activists seem removed from our lives.

Yet we cannot allow ourselves to be as nearsighted in our own way as some environmental groups. These issues are too important for us not to become informed and involved. Without our active voices, the future of our planet will be left to those forces that have spent the last forty years developing action plans that bypassed us and the communities in which we live.

Be certain that environmental issues are about health and about Latinas. Having been historically uninvited or ignored in the discussions of our environment, it is now up to us to become informed.

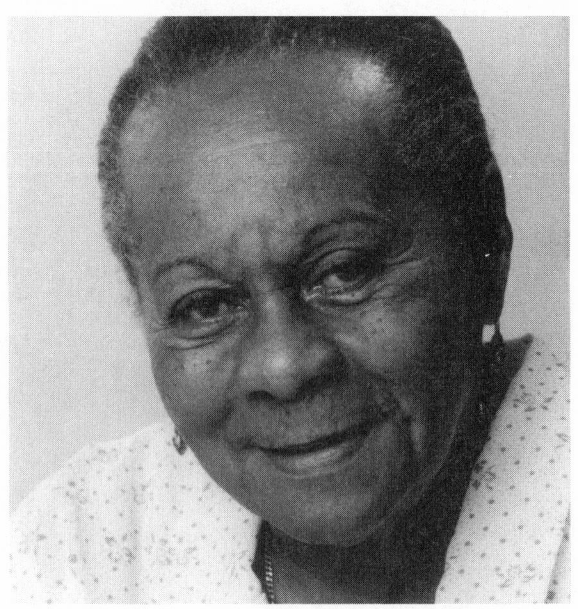

All Latinas can work to have a cleaner environment.

Current Conditions

Air, water, and food are the basics that we need to survive. Yet the quality and the supply of these very essential elements are suffering from the consequences of years of abuse, neglect, and misdirected accommodation to industry. In 1997 the U.S. Environmental Protection Agency (EPA) recognized that:

> One-half of the American people live in an area where, in 1995, the air was too polluted to meet health standards. Thirty-five to forty percent of America's surveyed rivers, lakes, and estuaries are too polluted to fully support uses such as fishing or swimming. One in four Americans lives within four miles of a Superfund site.

For Hispanics the situation was much worse—80 percent lived in an area that did not meet EPA standards for air quality. As a consequence we find rates of asthma increasing among those of us who live in cities, and alarmingly high among Hispanic children.

This abysmal situation exists after decades of regulation by the EPA and advocacy by environmental groups. While the EPA serves as a regulatory agency, its enforcement activities have consistently been weakened by Congress, the President, and the industries it is supposed to oversee. Additionally, the EPA leaves many of its enforcement actions in the hands of regional officials who end up giving fines that amount to little more than parking tickets compared to the profits made by the polluting companies.

Nevertheless, the fact is that the EPA is responsible for establishing standards to protect the health and welfare of the people in the United States. At the same time that the EPA is supposed to accomplish this goal, there is little coordination with local, state, and federal agencies responsible for maintaining the health of communities.

To complicate matters, the scientific research on which the EPA bases its decisions is often isolated from the health research conducted in the National Institutes of Health, Food and Drug Administration, and other government agencies. While research continues on the impact of chemicals on biological processes, too often standards are adopted that support polluting industries rather than erring on the side of protecting people.

Compare what happens with chemicals in medicines to what happens with chemicals and other substances in our air, water, and food. Both the FDA and the EPA are regulatory agencies charged with protecting our health from the effects of harmful substances. The FDA regulates medicines, and the EPA regulates the environment.

Chapter 22 describes the process the FDA imposes on pharmaceutical manufacturers before they are allowed to put a product on the market. The process entails extensive clinical trials to ensure that there are no negative health effects on consumers. And although the manufacturers may think the process is too long and costly, the fact is that it is up to the manufacturers to prove to the FDA that their products are safe and effective.

Warning

Phase out of popular lawn and indoor plant bug killer, diazinon will not be complete till June 2003. This widely used chemical is found in dozens of brand name products and poses unacceptable risks to consumers, especially children. The ban does not extend to agricultural use.

The EPA process is the complete opposite. Manufacturers can do whatever they want until scientific data indicate conclusively that a specific substance has a negative effect on the environment. In the meantime that substance may be in our water, air, and food. It seems that our environmental protection system is similar to our legal system—a substance is innocent until proven guilty. Unfortunately, just as in the legal system, the victim (each and every person who is exposed to hazardous or toxic chemicals) is the one who suffers and is left with the responsibility of proving that something is wrong. Of nearly 70,000 chemicals in use today, fewer than 2 percent have been fully tested for their effects on human and biological health.

Interestingly enough, the EPA has stated as one of its goals that by the year 2005, current, accurate, and easily accessible information on environmental conditions will be available for at least seventy-five of the largest metropolitan areas. But what do we do in the meantime?

At the very least we need a better understanding of our water, air, and food.

Know Your Water

Jane could not believe it. Here she lived in the nation's capital and the radio was advising everyone not to drink the tap water. There were signs in the airport telling all new arrivals that there was a health emergency and the water was not suitable for drinking.

Luckily, Jane only drank filtered water. But she began to wonder what it would mean to shower in water that you could not drink. What if some of the water splashed in your eyes or went up your nose. Then what? They never announced what was wrong with the water—you just could not drink it.

"Water, water everywhere, but not a drop to drink" takes on new meaning when we think of the condition of water in the United States. We should be concerned about both surface water (e.g., lakes, streams, rivers) and ground water (e.g., aquifers, wells). What we know for certain is that every day, surface and

Consejos

If you have lead pipes in your house or in the water lines leading to your house—

1. Do not drink or cook with water that has been in the pipes for more than 6 hours.
2. Let cold water run for 60 seconds before using it.
3. Do not drink or cook with hot water from your pipes.

ground water are being compromised by toxic chemicals, viruses, and other disease-causing organisms. Some of this contamination results from chemicals that are buried and eventually seep through to aquifers, while other contamination is due to pesticides that end up in the soil and enter the ground water system.

The effect of this contamination is major. In 1994 1 out of every 5 persons in the United States who drank from community water systems drank water that violated health standards at least once during the year. This occurred even though in 1986 Congress set mandatory guidelines regulating contaminants in water, banned all future use of lead pipes and lead solder in public drinking water systems, and established programs to protect the ground water sources for drinking water. Remember that tap water is regulated by the EPA, bottled water is regulated by the FDA, and the Centers for Disease Control works closely with state and local health departments to check the water supply for contaminants.

Keeping our water supply clean is a task that involves everybody's cooperation. At the very least we need to make sure that:

- All our drinking water is treated to remove harmful substances.
- We test and monitor the quality of our drinking water on a regular basis. This is especially important for those who drink water from a well or spring.
- We keep informed about what is happening with our water.
- We drink bottled water if we are uncertain about our water quality.

While concerns about drinking water resonate with most people, talk to them about wetlands and their response is uncaring. They may say they are urban dwellers who do not care about "swamps." But insuring our water supply means focusing on more than the water we drink.

A strong connection exists between our wetlands and the water we drink. It seems that wetlands are part of the delicate balance of nature that makes possible water purification, recharging of aquifers, and flood prevention. In the last century we have lost 50 percent of the wetlands in the United States. The wetlands may be far from where we live, but they are still an essential part of having clean water.

Going to the beach is a favorite outdoor activity for many of us, but every year over 7,000 beaches are closed in the United States because of pollution. Thirty-two billion gallons a day of agricultural, urban and industrial pollutants including oil, pesticide and animal waste from big factory farms suffocate our coastal waters, threatening human health and safety.

The EPA has proposed that limits be set on the amount of this "non-point pollution" rivers are allowed to carry to the sea. Some states and industries argue this type of regulation is too expensive. But past regulations that reduced "point source" pollution from

EPA's Safe Drinking Water Hotline
(800) 426-4791

sewage and chemical plants proved highly cost-effective by reducing health care costs when fewer people got sick and also by ensuring increased opportunities for coastal recreation and fishing.

It's important to remember that you also contribute to the problem when you don't take care of the environment. Anything you put down a storm drain, be it used oil from your car, bug spray from your garden or litter swept off your street, will end up in the ocean waters you and your family swim in.

Sometimes it is hard to tell when water is clean since it takes only one microorganism to wreak havoc on our insides. We can look at how other organisms are doing, however, to get a good indication of the water quality. For example, the average mussel feeds itself by filtering up to 50 gallons of water a day through its body. This also makes mussels highly vulnerable to pollution. By monitoring how mussels are doing, we have a way of judging how clean our coastal waters are. As a result of our monitoring efforts, one-third of the shellfish areas are off limits to shell fishermen due to pollution. The pollution is usually a combination of sewage and industrial waste. Unfortunately, current tests of water quality only test for sewage (which may carry hepatitis, cholera, and salmonella) and not for heavy metals or chemicals, which may be a byproduct of industrial waste or agricultural runoff.

Techniques for measuring the presence of chemicals are becoming increasingly sophisticated. Today we can measure one part in a billion parts of water. That is comparable to the first 16 inches of a trip to the moon. And while that amount may seem trivial, remember that that little bit of contamination is all it takes to make us ill. The problem is to determine which substances we should be measuring.

A good example of this problem is the debate on allowable levels of arsenic in drinking waters, where the acceptable amount of arsenic ranged from 50 parts per billion to 5 parts per billion. Small amounts of toxic substances make big differences. Since human beings are 55 to 75 percent water and water is an essential medium for many of the body's key functions, we need to be very careful about the quality of water we drink. We are just at the beginning of learning what it means to our bodies when we accumulate tiny amounts of contaminants or what their long-term effects may be.

Myth: Clear water is pure.

Fact: Clear water may be contaminated with microorganisms that are invisible to the naked eye.

Myth: Rain water is pure.

Fact: The makeup of rain water is a function of the substances it has collected in the sky. If the air is polluted, so is the water that passes through it.

Myth: You can call the EPA and have them tell you whether a stream is polluted.

Fact: You should call your local health department.

Myth: Rushing water is clean.

Fact: The motion of the water does not determine whether it is free of contaminants.

Myth: You can always taste when water is bad.

Fact: Microorganisms are tasteless, while chlorine, which is added to purify water, has an aftertaste.

Know Your Air

The radio announced that the air quality was good, but Denise knew that did not apply to her. She knew it was going to be a bad day for her asthma because she could see the flames burning at the nearby plant.

Outdoor Air

What does it mean when the voice on the radio proclaims it is a good air day? All it means is that for that day the air met the National Ambient Air Quality Standards (NAAQS) for that community. It does not tell us whether or not a local plant is emitting toxic chemicals. The measurement of toxic air pollutants is a different process.

National Ambient Air Quality Standards

The NAAQS relate to ground level ozone (smog), carbon monoxide, sulfur dioxide (SO_2), nitrogen dioxide (NO_2), lead, and particulate matter (very fine dust and soot). Here are some key facts about each of these pollutants.

• Ground level ozone (smog). This should not be confused with the ozone that is in the upper stratosphere and protects us from ultraviolet rays. Ground level ozone is produced when nitrogen oxide and other compounds (volatile organic compounds, or VOCs) combine in the presence of sunlight or heat. VOCs are released by cars, trucks, chemical plants, refineries, factories, paints, solvents, consumer and commercial products, and other industrial sources. The irony is that while some scientists work hard to maintain the protective level of ozone in the stratosphere (to reduce the infamous "hole in the ozone"), at ground level the same substance is a problem.

• Carbon monoxide. This is a by-product of combustion. It has no odor.

• Sulfur dioxide. The source of most sulfur dioxide is power plants and diesel engines. When sulfur dioxide is released in the atmosphere it can change into acidic particles and even into sulfuric acid.

• Nitrogen dioxide. This pollutant is produced by cars, trucks, power plants, and other sources of combustion.

• Lead. The amount of lead in the air has decreased dramatically since leaded gasoline and leaded paint were removed from the market. Most lead in the air is from lead smelters and the burning of lead batteries.

• Particulate matter. This is the term used to refer to very fine dust and soot. Particulate matter can be coarse, such as windblown dust, or fine, such as the product of fuel combustion. Fine particulate matter is so small (less than 2.5 microns) that it would take several thousand to dot this *i*, and it is this very small size that makes it so damaging. Because we can easily inhale the particles, they are apt to accumulate in our lungs. Research has shown that particulate matter is a lot more harmful than originally thought. It poses the greatest risk to older adults, children, and persons with asthma or heart or lung disease.

The cumulative effect of particulate matter is best demonstrated by the way it reduces how far you can see. In the western part of the United States, the visual range would be 140 miles if there were no particulate matter. With particulate matter it is from 33 to 90 miles. In the east the visual range would be 90 miles without particulate matter. With particulate matter it is 14 to 24 miles. Additionally, particulate dust travels easily from one place to another. Today one-third of the haze over the Grand Canyon comes from pollution in Southern California.

Although the NAAQS specify what are acceptable levels of these substances on a daily basis, there are some effects that occur over time. For example, there is long-term damage when small amounts of sulfur dioxide and nitrogen dioxide mix with moisture and fall back to earth as acid rain. The air quality is also tempered by other factors such as the weather and wind.

The two major problems in air quality are (1) smog forming ozone and (2) carbon monoxide produced by emissions from vehicles and some industrial plants. Smog does more than reduce visibility. It also makes it hard for plants to produce food and weakens them over time, kills fish, and creates harmful algae blooms.

And the effects on our bodies are significant too. If you are a healthy person, smog reduces your lung capacity over time by 15 to 20 percent. Smog is also known to have a negative effect on the body's immune system. Just imagine the effect it has on a person who is not healthy.

Toxic Air Pollutants

A toxic air pollutant is a substance in the air that increases the likelihood of a person experiencing a health problem (e.g., benzene found in gasoline is known to increase the risk of cancer) or that has a negative impact on the environment (as when a substance in the air lands on soil or surface water).

When air quality is reported, no data are included about toxic air pollutants. Toxic air pollutants are regulated by requiring use of pollution control devices at the source of the emission rather than by specific air quality standards.

The publicly available National Toxics Inventory (NTI) builds on data from EPA's Toxic Release Inventory (TRI). The TRI reports on emissions from facilities. While these reports are an important way of finding out what toxic chemicals are being released in a community, TRI data cover only 14 percent of total emissions for the nation. Moreover, there is a two-year lag in publication of TRI reports so that by the time the data are available the damage may be beyond repair. For example, the 1994 TRI indicated that Texas had five of the ten most polluted zip code areas in the United States. What happens now? If we are to reduce the release of toxic substances in our communities, Latinas will have to be in the forefront of the campaign for change.

Taking Action

There are several positive steps we can take.

1. Be aware of our own habits that increase pollution.
2. Become familiar with the process government officials and scientists use to assess the risk of exposure to toxic substances in our communities.
3. Inform local EPA and elected officials of our findings.
4. Become active in organizations in our communities that are trying to protect the environment.

1: Be aware of our own habits that increase pollution. This may include not recycling, dumping grease and oil in sewers, and discarding toxic products such as old batteries without regard to safety precautions. It may require us to fix leaky faucets or toilets that waste water, not buy products that contain fluorocarbons, and stop using or overusing commercial fertilizers in our homes and gardens.

2: Become familiar with the process government officials and scientists use to assess the risk of exposure to toxic substances in our communities.

Following are the key steps involved in assessing a community's risk of exposure to toxic substances.

- Step 1. Identify pollutants in your community. Scientists need to know what pollutants are a problem in your community and how they can work with the polluters to make the environment safer. Some common sources of toxic chemicals are:

- Dry cleaners (perchloroethylene)
- Consumer products (paint strippers and degreasers contain methylene chloride)
- Gasoline with benzene
- Metal plating operations (chromium)

• Step 2. Estimate releases from sources. Once scientists have identified the pollutants in your community, they need to estimate the amount of chemicals released. Some toxic releases will be at a specific location (point) such as a plant, mill, or farm, while others may accumulate from several sources in a given area (e.g., emissions from automobiles, dry cleaners, gas stations).

Scientists also need to estimate the pattern of releases. Some releases occur as part of ongoing activities (routine); others are released on a changing schedule (intermittent); and the hardest to calculate are those that occur by accident.

• Step 3. Estimate concentration. The amount of the toxic substance that remains in the community is a function of weather (presence, direction, and speed of wind) and terrain (flat, mountains, valley). Usually the concentrations are milder the farther away you are from the source of the contaminant.

• Step 4. Number of people exposed. When scientists know what is being released and where it is traveling, they can determine how many people are affected.

If the EPA has done a study in your community, you will be able to get a copy of this report from the EPA. This will give you an idea of the situation in your community and help you as you proceed with your role in protecting the environment.

3: Inform local EPA and elected officials of our findings. Inform your elected officials of your concerns (see Appendix C). Short, handwritten notes to your congressional representative and senator are all that is necessary to begin the process. For example, you can write:

I am one of your constituents and I want to live in a healthy, pollution-free environment. Please make sure that we have safe, clean air, water, food, and land. The environment is important to me.

I urge you to ask the EPA to look into the following [add information on a particular problem you see in your community].

4: Become active in organizations in our communities that are trying to protect the environment. There are many organizations that are trying to protect the environment in our communities. Use the names listed in the resource section as a guide. Be aware that the name of an organization may not tell you what they believe. Attend a few meetings to see whether the organization is working on your issues. You may decide to become active in some of their activities.

Indoor Air

Thought it was safe inside? Over the past two decades there has been a deterioration in the quality of indoor air. The EPA lists indoor air as one of the top five environmental risks to public health. Increased exposure to toxic air is due to tightly sealed buildings, reduced ventilation, use of synthetic building materials, and chemicals in pesticides, household cleaners, and personal care products. In some instances a contaminant in indoor air has been measured at a level a hundred times higher than the acceptable level in outdoor air.

Sometimes it is hard to tell if a negative

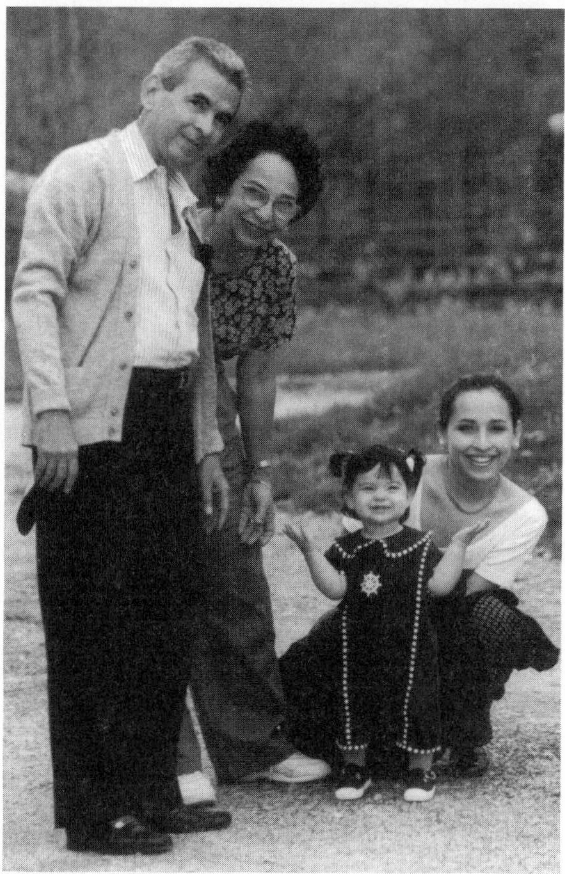

Having a clean environment is good for our families.

effect is due to the quality of indoor air because the immediate effects are similar to those of a cold or other viral disease. Factors such as age and preexisting health conditions determine the impact on each person.

Recently there has been concern about radon. Radon is a radioactive gas that is found in nearly all soils and also in rock and water. As the element decays the gas is released into the ground and seeps into buildings. You cannot smell or see radon, but it can settle in your lungs and cause lung cancer.

Environmental tobacco smoke (ETS), or secondhand smoke, has also been implicated in respiratory illnesses and low-birth-weight babies.

Some people who do not have problems with indoor air seem to develop problems after repeated exposures. It is as if the body at first could process the contaminant but over time it became too much to handle. The best advice is to be attentive to time and place of symptoms. The easiest way to improve indoor air quality is to open windows—as long as the outdoor air quality is acceptable. More costly methods may involve use of air filters and removal of asbestos.

Climate Change

Although it can seem very abstract, climate change, the global warming taking place as the result of burning fossil fuels like coal and oil, poses a real threat to our health. Hotter years, rising seas and more extreme weather can negatively impact our rates of illness and mortality, no matter where we live.

The group Physicians for Social Responsibility, for example, has issued a report on the health impacts of climate change on Michigan. They found that the number of four-day heat waves in Detroit has more than doubled over the past 40 years. As day and nighttime temperatures rise, air quality deteriorates. As ground-level ozone increases with global warming, thousands more people will go to the hospital with respiratory conditions. The 180,000 children in Michigan with asthma are especially at risk.

The number of floods and cases of waterborne diseases are also expected to rise. In addition, more cases of diseases spread by ticks and mosquitoes, such as Lyme disease and encephalitis, could result as warmer temperatures play a role in increasing insect populations.

> **Warning**
>
> In June 2000 EPA negotiated the phaseout of chlorpyrifos, known to many as Dursban. Dursban was the most widely used pesticide in the U.S.

Know Your Food

The FDA, the EPA, and the U.S. Department of Agriculture (USDA) each works to insure the safety of the food supply. For example, the FDA oversees seafood, all imported foods, bottled water, and the use of hormones and medication in animal feed, just to name a few; the USDA regulates meat and poultry; and the EPA regulates the use of pesticides. All are responsible for carrying out timely enforcement action when levels of contaminants exceed established guidelines.

Pesticides

For many of us the agricultural use of pesticides and other chemicals has been a concern with respect to the workers who handle the food. We now know that pesticides and other substances can contaminate food at any point from production to preparation.

Some of the pesticides used in farming are not water-soluble, so that just rinsing the fruit in water does not eliminate the residue. Research is continuing on the effects of eating food with minute residues of pesticides. Moreover, many of us use pesticides on plants in our homes or to kill household pests. When you use these products, remember that their purpose is to disrupt another living organism—plant or animal. They may end up having subtle disruptive effects on humans too. So try to avoid use of pesticides or eating pesticide treated food. Organically grown or raised food may be an expensive but important option.

Fish

Many of us were raised with the belief that fish was healthier than meat. But with increased pollutants entering our waterways, that too has changed.

Recently there has been concern over levels of mercury in fish. Mercury in even minute amounts is a highly toxic substance. According to the FDA, swordfish, shark, and other large predatory fish may contain unhealthy levels of methyl mercury, more than one part per million. While it is safe to eat these fish, the FDA recommends that they be eaten no more than once a week. The FDA adds that cooking does not decrease the level of mercury.

Raw Oysters

Some raw oysters carry a bacterium called *Vibrio vulnificus*, which may be a threat to some people. Particularly vulnerable to this bacterium are persons with liver disease, either from excessive alcohol intake, viral hepatitis, or other causes; hemochromatosis, an iron disorder; diabetes; stomach problems, including previous stomach surgery and low stomach acid (e.g., from antacid use); cancer; and immune disorders, including HIV infection. Long-term steroid use (as for asthma and arthritis) also creates a risk.

This is a serious infection—40 percent of those infected with this bacterium die. The bacteria are found naturally in the waters where the oysters grow and are not due to pollution. This means that you are not safe from exposure just because the oysters are from clean waters or are very fresh. Contrary to popular belief, hot sauce, lemon juice, salt, and drinking alcohol have no effect on the bacteria. The only way to kill the bacteria is to fully cook the oysters.

Looking to the Future

As we look to the future we need to recognize that we have a long way to go with respect to our environment. At the present time the EPA has set some environmental goals for America, with milestones for the year 2005.

1. Clean air
2. Clean waters
3. Healthy terrestrial ecosystems
4. Safe drinking water
5. Safe food
6. Safe homes, schools, and workplaces
7. Toxin-free communities
8. Preventing accidental releases
9. Safe waste management
10. Restoration of contaminated sites
11. Reduction of global and transboundary environmental risks
12. Empowering people with information and education, and expanding their right to know

These goals may seem like things we should already have, but the reality is that we do not. By working together we can make sure that the water, air, and food supply are clean and plentiful for ourselves and the generations to come.

The health of Latinas and our communities depends on it.

RESOURCES

Organizations

Center for Health, Environment, and Justice
P.O. Box 6806
Falls Church, VA 22040
(703) 237-2249
www.chej.org

Clean Water Action
4455 Connecticut Avenue NW,
Suite A300
Washington, DC 20008
(202) 895-0420
www.cleanwater.org

Natural Resources Defense Council
40 West 20th Street
New York, NY 10011
(212) 727-2700
www.nrdc.org

Physicians for Social Responsibility
1101 14th Street NW Suite 700
Washington, D.C. 20005
(202) 667-4260
www.psr.org

Sierra Club
85 Second Street, 2nd Floor
San Francisco, CA 94105-3441
(415) 977-5500
www.sierraclub.org

Hotlines

American Lung Association
(800) LUNG-USA (800-586-4872)

EPA's Safe Drinking Water Hotline
(800) 426-4791

FDA Seafood Hotline
(800) FDA-4010 (800-332-4010)

Proyecto ALFA (Aire Limpio para su Familia)
National Alliance for Hispanic Health
(800) SALUD-1-2 (800-725-8312)

Su-Familia Family Health Helpline
National Alliance for Hispanic Health
866-SuFamilia (783-2645)

Books

Gore, Albert, Jr. *Earth in the Balance.* New York: Penguin, 1992.

Helvarg, David. *Blue Frontier—Saving America's Living Seas.* New York: WH Freeman, 2001.

Helvarg, David. *The War Against the Greens.* San Francisco: Sierra Club Books, 1997.

Publications and Pamphlets

"Access EPA." Printed annually. Office of Information Resources Management, U.S. Environmental Protection Agency, 401 M Street SW, Washington, DC 20460.

"Air Pollution Tips for Exercisers." Order No. 0560. American Lung Association; (800) LUNG-USA (800-586-4872) www.lungusa.org. Other titles include:

"Car Care for Clean Air." Order No. 2111.

"Indoor Air Pollution Fact Sheet."

"Top Ten Tips for a Healthy Home."

"Call Air Quality Trends Report." EPA Office of Air Quality Planning and Standards, U.S. Environmental Agency, OS-120, 401 M Street SW, Washington, DC 20460. Call (800) 490-9198. www.epa.gov. Other titles include:

"Evaluating Exposures to Toxic Air Pollutants: A Citizen's Guide."

"Air Quality Index-A Guide to Air Quality and Your Health."

"Air Quality Trends Report."

"Chemical Risk: A Primer." American Chemical Society, Department of Government Relations and Science Policy, 1155 16th Street NW, Washington, DC 20036.

"El Radon: Guia para Su Protección y la de Su Familia/A Guide to Radon: How to Protect Yourself and Your Family." (Bilingual booklet.) National Alliance for Hispanic Health, 1501 16th Street NW, Washington, DC 20036.

"Toxic Chemicals: What They Are, How They Affect You." Dr. Maria Pavlova, U.S. Environmental Protection Agency, 26 Federal Plaza, Room 737, New York, NY 10278.

APPENDIX A

Latinas Who Influenced This Book

It is important to recognize some of the many Latinas and non-Latinas who have made this book possible and necessary.

Vera Abate
Carmen Abraham
Alice G. Abreu
Christina Abuelo
Raydean M. Acevedo
Yolando Acevedo
Sonia Acobe
Sonja Acosta-Amad
Emily Vargas Adams
María Agostini
María del Carmen Aguad
Magdalena Aguayo
Nina Aguayo-Sorkin
Giselle Aguilar-Hass
Sylvia Aguirre
Marilyn Aguirre-Molina
Adriana Alarcón-Efrach
Rina Alcalay
Leticia Alcantar
Donna M. Alvarado
Elena Alvarado
Matilda Alvarado
Imma Álvarez
María Álvarez
Olga Álvarez
Tensia Alvírez
Eufemia Amabisca
Rose A. Amador
Peggy Amante
Patricia Andreu
Virginia P. Apodaca
Edna Apóstol
Kathy Aquino
María P. Aranda
Bárbara Aranda-Naranjo
Katherine Archuleta
Susanna Arellano
Anna María Arias
Peggy Armante
Annajean Armijo
Elizabeth Arragón
Desiree Arretz
Helen P. Arriola
Judith A. Arroyo
Patricia V. Asip
Susan Ávila
Doris N. Ayala
Iris Ayala
Bettie Baca
Polly Baca
Yvonne Bacarisse
María Eugenia Baeza
María Isabel Báez-Arroyo
Gisela Balcázar
Gloria Baroni
Michelle Barranca
Laura Victoria Barrera
Nancy M. Barrera
Rosita Bauca
Grecia Bautista
Dolores A. Beebe
Graciela Beecher
Rebecca Reza Bejar
Yolanda Beltrán-Halstead
Sofía R. Benson
Jean Bergaust
Jeanette Betancourt
Lourdes Birba
Lydia Blasini
Gloria Bonilla-Santiago
Diana M. Bonta
María Borrero
Joyce Bove
Laura Brainin-Rodríguez
Ana María Branham
Francesca Bravo
Delores Briones
Mary Bundy
Leonor R. Burgos
Leonor Buros
Gloria Burrola
Martha Burruel
Marina J. F. Busatto
María Edelmira Caballero
Lespoldina Cairo
Brenda Calhoun
Lydia Camarillo
Diana Campoamor
Diana M. Campos
Sandra I. Canales
Patricia Canessa
Gloria V. Cantu
Josefina Carbonell
Mimi Carcar
Lucy Cárdenas
Caroline Cardona
Lucy Cardona
Myrta Cardona
Doreen Carey
Roberta Carlin

Rosa María Carranza
Nanci Carvacho
Teresa Casares
Angelina Casillas
Delores Casillas
Rosalva Castañeda
Sara B. Castany
Amelia Castillo
Christa M. Castillo
Ida Castillo
Lilly Castillo
Marie Castillo
Sylvia Castillo
Omayra Castro
Marisela Ceja
Gloria Patlan Cerda
Dorothy Chaconas
Carole Chamberlain
Teresa Chapa
Yolanda Chapa-Gutiérrez
Carla Chávez
Martha R. Chávez
Nelba R. Chávez
Julie Chávez-Bayles
Carmen Chávez-Luján
Priscilla Chávez-Reilly
Isabel Chell
Carole Chrvala
Rosario Cobarrubois
Catalina Cobos
Audrey Cohen
Connie Cole
Molly Collins
Doris I. Flores Colón
Ledia Colón
Margarita H. Colmenares
Kathryn Colson
Carolyn Contreras
Melinda Cordero
Lía M. Cornejo
Silvia G. Corral
Nereida Correa
Lourdes Cortés
Susan L. Costa
Lourdes Cruz
Miriam Cruz
Carolyn Curiel
Lisa Cruz-Avilos
Beth Darmstadler
Isabel Davidoff
Milagros Dávila
Yolanda R. Dávila
Rosamelia de la Rocha
Christine de la Torre
María De Las Alas
Catherine A. de León
Mary Lou de León Siantz
Carmen De Navas
María del Pilar Castro
Claire del Real
Moira Delgado
Christina Delgado-Dayton
Elizabeth Delgado-Dayton
Marti Elizabeth Delgado-Dayton
Debbie Delgado-Vega
Carmen Delgado-Votaw
Consuelo Díaz
Elva Díaz
Eunice Díaz
Xiomara Díaz
Laura Díaz-Baker
Carmen Díaz de León
Carmen Diezcanseco
Rita DiMartino
Dinora C. Domínguez
Charlene Doria-Ortiz
Yolanda Duarte-White
Dory Dubrofsky
Linda Dumas
Ana O. Dumois
Carol Durán
Deborah Guadalupe Durán
Lisa Durán
Rocío Early-González
Lucy Ebel
Sylvia Echave-Stock
Maria Echaveste
Laura Echevarría
Marisel Elías
Maríana Enríquez-Olmos
Sarah Gómez Erlach
María D. Escobar
Iraní Escolano
Yolanda Esparza
Fern R. Espino
Linda Espino
Grace Esquibel-Morales
Eunice Esquivel
Martha Estrella
Myra Evangelista
Becky Fajardo
Patricia Fajardo
Dagmar T. Farr
Carmen Fermín
Carmen L. Fernández
Lillian Fernández
Sandra Ferniza
María Elena A. Flood
Elena Flores
Janet E. Flores
Rosemary Flores
Yvette Flores-Ortiz
Emestina Casas Forman
Myriam Fragoso
G. Aracelis Francis
Gloria Freire
Ángela M. Gaetano
Marcela Gaítan
Anita Gallegos
Martha Galván
Paula M. Gálvez-Fox
Cecilia Galvis
Frances Gámez
Mary Isa Garayua
Hortensia Garcés
Norma Garcés
Alma García
Anna María García
Barbara García
Blanche García
Clara García
Esperanza R. García
Eugene E. García
Eva García
Jane García
Julie E. García
Lorena García
Luz Fátima García
Marcella A. García
Millie García
Nonata García
Nora García
Rosa Elena García
Rosalinda García
Sandra V. García
Sonia García
Tania A. García
Cynthia T. García-Coll
Esperanza García-Walters
Margaret A. Gariota
Antonia M. Garza
Doreen D. Garza
Roxanne Garza
Mercy Gato
Polly Gault
María Elena Girone
Doralba Muñoz Godales
Anamaría Goicoechea-Baobona
Cindy Goldman
Mirtha Gomberg
Cynthia A. Gómez
María S. Gómez
Patricia Gómez
Paula S. Gómez
Irene Gómez-Caro
Polly Gómez-Bustillo
Cathy Gonzales
Dorothy Gonzales
Marta Gonzales
Patrisia Gonzales
Stephanie Gonzales
Virginia Gonzales
Adela N. González
Aída I. González
Belinda González
Carmen Ada González
Guadalupe González

Kathleen González
Leonor González
Lydia González
Martha González
Roberta González
Susan González
Maria Rosa Gonzalez-Carrero
Priscilla González-Leiva
Patricia Guadalupe
Julia A. Guevara
Marga Retama Guillén
Mary Lou Gutiérrez
Sarah Gutiérrez
Penny Guzmán
Rebecca María Guzmán
Rosario Pena Hamilton
Jane Henney
Antonia Hernández
Carmen Hernández
Daisy Hernández
Juanita Hernández
Mary A. Hernández
Sara M. Hernández
Shelley Hernández
Rachel Hernández-Pollack
Olivia Hernández-Sebolt
Delores Herrera
María Herrera
Rafaela Herrera
Melanie Herrera-Bortz
Cecilia Hinojosa
María Hinojosa
Dolores Huerta
Grace Flores Hughes
Cecilia Hunt
Brunella Ibarrola
María Marino Idsinga
Mari-Luci Jaramillo
Sandra Jaramillo
Heather Jeffery
María Jibaja
Kisla M. Jiménez
María Jiménez
Edith M. Jirón
Irma Juardo
Berjouhi Kazanjian
Karen Katen
Yolanda Kizer
Reni Kossow
Carmela G. Lacayo
Onelia G. Lage
Debbie Landesman
Guadalupe G. Lara
Rosa Lara
Magdalena Lewis-Castro
Cristina López
Cynthia López
Diana López
Dominga R. López
Esther López
Gloria A. López
Glorianne Donna López
Laureen López
Lily López
Linda López
Luisa López
Lynda López
Martha L. López
Maxine López
Mónica León López
Virginia Lieras López
Rosemary López-Meder
Eliana Loveluck
Patricia Lozada-Santone
Mónica C. Lozano
Paula Luff
Mirza Lugardo
Elizabeth Luján
Elisa Luna
Consuelo Luz
Caroline A. Macera
Marjorie Macieira
Perena Madrazo
Geraldine Madrid
Sandy Magana
Verónica Majar
Magdalena Malagón
Elena Maciel Manuela
Ruth Manzano
Leila E. Marcial
Cecilia Marques
Debbie Márquez
Nury Márquez
Alba Martínez
Arabella Martínez
Gloria Martínez
Imela C. Martínez
Irena Martínez
Joyce Martínez
Lorraine Martínez
M. Regina Martínez
María Martínez
Olivia Martínez
Rose Marie Martínez
Silvia Martínez
Susana Martínez
Vilma Martínez
Emilia Martínez-Brawley
Isolina Marxuach-Rosario
Pamela Mastrota
Myrian M. Matos
Stephanie Maya
Cheryl Mayo
Mónica A. Medina
Olga Medina
Zashira Medina
Luisa Medrano
Miriam Mejía
Lidia Mena-Hermida
Antoinette Menchaca
Jacqueline Méndez
Nellie J. Méndez
Maritza S. Mendizábal
Lydia Mendoza
Patricia Mendoza
Rosa Inés Merelo
Leonor Merino
Magdalena Miranda
Melissa Miranda-Craig
Vera Mireya
Gloria Molina
Elba Montalvo
Elisa Montalvo
Lori Montenegro
Lorraine Montenegro
Eloisa Montes
Evangelina Montoya
Mary Christine Montoya
Patricia Montoya
Alicia Montoya-Sánchez
Edna Mora
Virginia Morález
Alva A. Moreno
Connie Moreno-Peraza
Hazel Moss
Eva M. Moya
Andrea O'Malley Muñoz
Eliza Muñoz
Helen Muñoz
Sara Murieta
Verónica Murillo
Esther Valles Murray
Ildaura Murrillo-Rhode
Alicia Najera
Evelyn Najera
Diana Naranjo
Gladys Narcisi
Liliana Navarro
Linda Neal
Gisela Negrón
Myriam Luz Neira
Claudia Nenno
Gloria Nieto
Iris Nieves
Antonia Novello
Ana Núñez
Teresa Nuño
Mónica Ochoa
Julia M. Ojeda
Natalia Ojeda del Pozo
Margarita M. Olimpio
Mary Olivieri
Tatiana Olmedo
Norma Olvera-Ezzell
Gabriela Omelas

Concha Orozco
Graciela Orozco-Moreno
Deborah L. Ortega
Karen Ortega
Cathy Ortiz
Christine Ortiz
Elvira Ortiz
Gloria Ortiz
Lydia Ortiz
María D. Ortiz
Marion C. Ortiz
Myrna Ortiz
Francy Otero
Regina Otero-Sabogal
Natalie Padilla
Sandy Padilla-Salzman
Leticia Pae
María Palacios
Jessica Palomino
Norma Pando
Rosanna Pardo
Asela Paredes
Beatriz Parga
Carmen I. Paris
Mara Patermaster
Marsha B. Peláez
Celeste Pena
Janet Perales
Ana Pereira
Delta E. Pereira
Christina Pérez
María Pérez
Marybelle Pérez
Patricia Pérez
Sallie Pérez
Sandra Pérez
Mirta Roses Periago
Julia Perilla
Gini Pineda
Alicia M. Pitarque
Eileen Polidoro
Luisa del Carmen Pollard
Guillermina Porras
Jessica Porras
Sandra G. Posada
Lydia Prado
Agnes Priscaro
Irene Queiro-Tajalli
Caroline Quijada
Lorelei Quintana
Regina Quintana
Rosario Quintanilla-Vior
Jessica Quiroz
Amelie G. Ramírez
Rochelle Ramírez
Annette Ramírez de Arellano
Sharon Ramírez-Good
Faustina Ramírez-Knoll
Claudia Ramos
Rebeca Ramos
Theresa Ramos
Carmen Ramos-Kalsow
Rosario Rangel
Sheila Raviv
Aida Redondo
Gesele Rey
Lupita Reyes
Naomi Reyes
Anna Ríos
Isabel Rivera
Lillian Rivera
Mayda I. Rivera
Migdalia Rivera
Norma Rivera
Ana Rivera-Tovar
Sally Robles
Sylvia Robles
Azalia Rodríguez
Casimara R. Rodríguez
Gloria M. Rodríguez
Jessica Rodríguez
Rosalinda Rodríguez
Magaly Rodríguez de Bittner
Helen Rodríguez-Trias
Delia M. Rojas
Diane Rojas
María D. Rojas
Rebecca Rojas
Elizabeth Rojas-Colville
Miriam Román
Socorro M. Román
Josie T. Romero
Eunice Romero-Gwynn
Elizabeth Romo
Araceli Rosales
Marta Rosenblatt
Ila Roy
Arecely Ruano
Wanda Rubianes
Carmen Ruiz
Delores J. Ruiz
Teresa Rupp
Elva Saavedra
Anita Salas
Margarita F. Salas
Patricia Salas
Irene Salazar
Theresa Salazar
Yolanda Salazar
Alina Salganicoff
Doris Salomon
Sara Salvide
María E. Samperio
Celeste Sánchez
Corinne Sánchez
Digna Sánchez
Dolores Sánchez
Elisa Marie Sánchez
Elizabeth Sánchez
Flora Sánchez
Marisabel Sánchez
Mary Sánchez
Sylvia Sánchez
Ruth Sánchez-Way
Gladys Sandlin
Arlene Sandoval-Guerra
Madeline Santiago
Aída Santory
Silvia Santos
Yolanda Santos
Sylvia Sapien
Oliva Saracho
Nadia Schomer
Ninfa Segarra
Janet Serenio
Imma Serrano
Ligia Serrano
Laura Sheppard
Marta Siberio
Karen Silver
Lucia Rojas Smith
Catalina Sol
Ana Soler
Elena Soler
Rita Soler-Ossolinski
Dora Solís
Faustina Solís
Hilda L. Solís
Patty Solís
Ana Solorzano
Lydia M. Sosa
Mary Sosa
Gloria Sotelo
Nélida Sousa
Valerie Suares
Lourdes Suárez
Lucina Suárez
Melissa Talamantes
Delfina Telles
Trinidad Téllez
Barbara Terrazas
Nohemy Terrazas
Mary Thorngren
Marta Tienda
Margarita Toraya
Maríanne Toro
Ivette A. Torres
Myriam Torres
Ramona Torres
Rosario Torres
Sara Torres
Alicia Torruella
María D. Tovar
Luz Towns-Miranda
Karen Ulloa
Roxana Ulloa
Aída de León Uribe
Vilma Valdés
Cecilia Valdez
Guillermina G. Valdez
Suzanna Valdez

Lina T. Valdivia
Angela G. Valencia
Lydia Valencia
Sandra L. Valenzuela
Palma Valverde
Vivian Varella
Zulma Vargas
Olga Vásquez
Lisa Vázquez
Myrna Karena Vázquez
Judith Vega
Marta Vega
Mayra L. Vega
Yvonne Martínez Vega
Irma Vega-Zadeh
María E. Vegega
Carmen Velásquez
Evelyn Vélez
Norma Vélez
Faustina M. Vigil
Lucretia Vigil
Rebecca Vigil-Giron
Catalina Villalpando
Leticia Villarreal
Sylvia Villarreal
Louise Villejo
Edna Viruell
Mary C. Wallace
Enriqueta Wallace
Esther Coto Wallach
Esperanza García Walters
Diane Weissman
Valerie Williams
Esther Valladolid Wolf
Elva Yáñez
Leticia Zamarripa
Myra Zambrano
Ruth Zambrano
Geraldine Zapata
Mitra Zehtab
Linda Zuba
Deborah A. Zuloaga
María Luisa Zúñiga de Nuncio

APPENDIX B

Health Journal, Visit Summary, and Chart of Basal Body Temperature

Health Journal

Date ________________

Body

1	2	3	4	5	6	7
Extremely Negative	Moderately Negative	Slightly Negative	Neutral	Slightly Positive	Moderately Positive	Extremely Positive

Comments (symptoms, changes, medications)________________

Mind

1	2	3	4	5	6	7
Extremely Negative	Moderately Negative	Slightly Negative	Neutral	Slightly Positive	Moderately Positive	Extremely Positive

Comments (symptoms, changes, medications)________________

Spirit

1	2	3	4	5	6	7
Extremely Negative	Moderately Negative	Slightly Negative	Neutral	Slightly Positive	Moderately Positive	Extremely Positive

Comments (symptoms, changes)________________

Visit Summary

Date ____________

Health Care Provider____

Address____

Telephone____

Symptoms, changes, medications____

____

____

Diagnosis____

____

____

Treatment

What to do____

____

____

What to take

Name	Dose	When	Purpose (other comments)

Follow-up

____

____

____

Other comments

____

____

Chart of Basal Body Temperature

Month and year

Day of cycle	1	2	3	4	5	6	7	8	9	10	11	12	13	14	15	16	17	18	19	20	21	22	23	24	25	26	27	28	29	30	31	32	33	34	35	36	37	38	39	40
Day of month																																								
Menstruation																																								
Coitus																																								
Mucus																																								
Temp																																								
99.0																																								
98.8																																								
98.6																																								
98.4																																								
98.2																																								
98.0																																								
97.8																																								
97.6																																								
97.4																																								
97.2																																								
97.0																																								

Month and year

Day of cycle	1	2	3	4	5	6	7	8	9	10	11	12	13	14	15	16	17	18	19	20	21	22	23	24	25	26	27	28	29	30	31	32	33	34	35	36	37	38	39	40
Day of month																																								
Menstruation																																								
Coitus																																								
Mucus																																								
Temp																																								
99.0																																								
98.8																																								
98.6																																								
98.4																																								
98.2																																								
98.0																																								
97.8																																								
97.6																																								
97.4																																								
97.2																																								
97.0																																								

APPENDIX C

Making Our Voices Heard

Key Things to Do

1: Write.

All elected officials respond to letters written by their constituents. If you have a concern, they must know about it. Your letter can be short and handwritten. You can even use a postcard. As long as you write, your opinion is noted and counts toward influencing your elected official.

2: Call.

All elected officials keep logs of how many calls they get and how their constituents feel about key issues.

3: Visit.

All elected officials have offices in their home districts where you can visit them or their staffs. If you are in your state capital or in Washington, DC, you should stop by their offices. Although you may not meet them, your visit will be noted. In most instances the staffs of elected officials are responsible for conveying your concerns to them.

4: Be active.

If there is an issue that you feel needs your attention, you may want to become a volunteer or donor to a political campaign.

How to Reach:

The President

Write to:
The White House
1600 Pennsylvania Avenue NW
Washington, DC 20500
Dear Mr. President:
call: (202) 456-1414

The Vice President

Write to:
The White House
1600 Pennsylvania Avenue NW
Washington, DC 20500
Dear Mr. Vice President:
call: (202) 224-2424

WHITE HOUSE COMMENTS

To register your opinion on an issue
(202) 456-1111

To learn whether a bill has been signed or vetoed
(202) 456-2226

Congress

U.S. CAPITOL SWITCHBOARD

To locate all persons in Congress including staff on Capitol Hill

(202) 224-3121

YOUR SENATOR

Write to:

The Honorable [full name]
U.S. Senate
Washington, DC 20510

Dear Senator [last name]:

SENATE RECORDED INFORMATION

Running accounts on floor proceedings:
Democrat: (202) 224-8541
Republican: (202) 224-8601

TO OBTAIN A BILL OR COMMITTEE REPORT

Senate Document Room: (202) 224-7860

YOUR REPRESENTATIVE

Write to:

The Honorable [full name]
U.S. House of Representatives
Washington, DC 20515

Dear Representative [last name]:

HOUSE RECORDED INFORMATION

Running accounts of floor proceedings:
Democrat: (202) 225-7400
Republican: (202) 225-7430

TO OBTAIN A BILL OR COMMITTEE REPORT

House Document Room: (202) 225-3456

State Legislatures

Main telephone numbers and home pages

ALABAMA
(334) 242-8000
www.archives.state.al.us./legislat

ALASKA
(907) 465-2111
www.legis.state.ak.us

ARIZONA
(602) 542-4900
www.azleg.state.az.us

ARKANSAS
(501) 682-3000
www.arkleg.state.ar.us

CALIFORNIA
(916) 322-9900
www.assembly.ca.gov/

COLORADO
(303) 866-5000
www.state.co.us/gov_dir/stateleg.html

CONNECTICUT
(860) 566-2211
www.cga.state.ct

DELAWARE
(302) 739-4000
www.state.de.us/research/assembly

FLORIDA
(850) 488-1234
www.leg.state.fl.us

GEORGIA
(404) 656-2000
www.ganet.state.ga.us/services/

HAWAII
(808) 586-2211
www.capitol.hawaii.gov

IDAHO
(208) 334-2411
www.state.id.us/legislat.html

ILLINOIS
(217) 782-2000
www.state.il.us/state/legis

INDIANA
(317) 232-3140
www.state.in.us/legislative

IOWA
(515) 281-5011
www.legis.state.ia.us/

Kansas
(785) 296-0111

Kentucky
(502) 564-2500
www.lrc.state.ky.us

Louisiana
(225) 342-6600
www.house.state.la.us

Maine
(207) 624-9494
www.janus.state.me.us/legis/

Maryland
(410) 841-3000
mlis.state.md.us

Massachusetts
(617) 727-2121
www.state.ma.us/legis/

Michigan
(517) 373-1837
www.michiganlegislature.org

Minnesota
(651) 296-6013
www.leg.state.mn.us/

Mississippi
(601) 359-1000
www.ls.state.ms.us

Missouri
(573) 751-2000
www.moga.state.mo.us

Montana
(406) 444-2511
www.leg.state.mt.us

Nebraska
(402) 471-2311
www.unicam.state.ne.us/index.htm

Nevada
(775) 687-5000
www.leg.state.nv.us

New Hampshire
(603) 271-1110
www.state.nh.us/gencourt/iegencourt

New Jersey
(609) 292-2121
www.njleg.state.nj.us

New Mexico
(505) 827-9632
www.legis.state.nm.us

New York
(518) 474-2121
www.senate.state.ny.us/
www.assembly.state.ny.us

North Carolina
(919) 733-1110
www.ncga.state.nc.us

North Dakota
(701) 328-2000
www.state.nd.us/lr

Ohio
(614) 466-2000
www.legislature.state.oh.us

Oklahoma
(405) 521-2011
www.lsb.state.ok.us/

Oregon
(503) 986-1180
www.leg.state.or.us/

Pennsylvania
(717) 787-2121
www.legis.state.pa.us

Rhode Island
(401) 222-2466
www.rilin.state.ri.us/

SOUTH CAROLINA
(803) 734-1000
www.state.sc.us/legislature.htm

SOUTH DAKOTA
(605) 773-3011
www.legis.state.sd.us

TENNESSEE
(615) 741-3011
www.legislature.state.tn.us

TEXAS
(512) 463-4630
www.senate.state.tx.us/
www.house.state.tx.us/

UTAH
(801) 538-3000
www.state.ut.us/government/legislative

VERMONT
(802) 828-1110
www.leg.state.vt.us/

VIRGINIA
(804) 786-0000
www.vipnet.org/vipnet/government/legislativebranch

WASHINGTON
(360) 753-5000
www.leg.wa.gov/wsladm

WEST VIRGINIA
(304) 558-3456
www.legis.state.wv.us

WISCONSIN
(608) 266-2211
www.legis.state.wi.us

WYOMING
(307) 777-7011
legisweb.state.wy.us/

AMERICAN SAMOA
(684) 633-1372
www.government.as/legislative.htm

DISTRICT OF COLUMBIA
(202) 783-5065, Congressional Representative's Office
(202) 727-1000 City Wide Call Center
www.house.gov/norton

GUAM
(671) 477-4272
www.guam.net/gov/senate

PUERTO RICO
(787) 723-6333, (787) 841-3209
www.house.gov/acevedo-vila

VIRGIN ISLANDS
(809) 774-4408, (809) 778-5900
www.gov.vi/html/leg.html

Environmental Protection Agency Regional Offices

REGION 1
Connecticut, Maine, Massachusetts New Hampshire, Rhode Island
EPA Region 1
John F. Kennedy Federal Building
1 Congress Street
Boston, MA 02114-2023
(888) 372-7341 or (617) 918-1111

REGION 2
New Jersey, New York, Puerto Rico, Virgin Islands
EPA Region 2
290 Broadway
New York, NY 10007
(212) 637-3000

REGION 3
Delaware, District of Columbia, Maryland, Pennsylvania, Virginia, West Virginia
EPA Region 3
1650 Arch Street
Philadelphia, PA 19103-2029
(215) 814-5000 or (800) 438-2474

REGION 4
Alabama, Florida, Georgia, Kentucky, Mississippi, North Carolina, South Carolina, Tennessee

EPA Region 4
Atlanta Federal Center
61 Forsyth St. SW
Atlanta, GA 30303-3104
(404) 562-9900 or (800) 241-1754

REGION 5

Illinois, Indiana, Michigan, Minnesota, Ohio, Wisconsin
EPA Region 5
77 West Jackson Boulevard
Chicago, IL 60604-3507
(312) 353-2000 or (800) 621-8431

REGION 6

Arkansas, Louisiana, New Mexico, Oklahoma, Texas
EPA Region 6
1st Interstate Bank Tower at Fountain Place
1445 Ross Avenue, Suite 1200
Dallas, TX 75202-2733
(214) 655-2200 or (800) 887-6063

REGION 7

Iowa, Kansas, Missouri, Nebraska
EPA Region 7
901 North 5th St.
Kansas City, KS 66101
(913) 551-7003 or (800) 223-0425

REGION 8

Colorado, Montana, North Dakota, South Dakota, Utah, Wyoming
EPA Region 8
999 18th Street, Suite 500
Denver, CO 80202-2466
(303) 312-6312 or (800) 227-8917

REGION 9

American Samoa, Arizona, California, Guam, Hawaii, Nevada
EPA Region 9
75 Hawthorne Street
San Francisco, CA 94105
(415) 744-1305

REGION 10

Alaska, Idaho, Oregon, Washington
EPA Region 10
1200 Sixth Avenue
Seattle, WA 98101
(206) 553-1200 or (800) 424-4372

APPENDIX D

National Health Information Clearinghouses

Cancer Information Service

National Cancer Institute

(800) 4-CANCER (800-4-226-237)

Provides cancer information to the public. Distributes National Cancer Institute publications.

Clearinghouse on Child Abuse and Neglect Information

(703) 385-7565 or (800) 394-3366

Collects, processes, and disseminates information on child abuse and neglect. Responds to information requests.

Clearinghouse on Disability Information

(202) 205-8241

Responds to inquiries by referral to organizations that supply information to handicapped individuals relating to their disabilities. Provides information on federal benefits, funding, and legislation for the handicapped.

Clearinghouse on Health Indices

National Center for Health Statistics

Office of Analysis and Epidemiology Program

(301) 436-8500

Provides information to assist in the development of health and quality of life measures for health researchers, administrators, and planners.

Clearinghouse for Occupational Safety and Health Information

(800) 35-NIOSH (356-4674), (513) 533-8326

Provides technical support for National Institute for Occupational Safety and Health research programs and supplies information to others on request.

Environmental Protection Agency Public Information Center

(202) 260-5922

Provides public information materials, offers information on the agency and its programs and actions.

Office of Population Affairs

(301) 654-6190

Collects, produces, and distributes materials on family planning, adolescent pregnancy, and adoption; also makes referrals to other information centers.

Food and Drug Administration Office of Consumer Affairs

(888) Info FDA (463-6332)

Answers consumer inquiries and serves as a clearinghouse for the FDA's consumer publications.

Food and Nutrition Information Center

(301) 504-5719

Serves the information needs of professionals, students, and consumers interested in nutrition education, nutrition science, food service management, food science, and food technology.

HUD User Housing Data

(800) 245-2691; (301) 251-5154 (Maryland residents only)

Disseminates the results of research sponsored by the U.S. Department of Housing and Urban Development. Health-related topics included in the database are housing safety, housing for the elderly and handicapped, and hazards of lead-based paint. There is a fee for publications.

CDC National Prevention Information Network

(800) 458-5231

Provides referrals and information on AIDS-related organizations and their services, as well as educational materials. Also supplies publications from the U.S. Public Health Service.

National Alliance for Hispanic Health

866-SuFamilia (783-2645) (Bilingual)

Provides information and referral to 16,000 local providers and fact sheets on over 30 health topics.

National Arthritis and Musculoskeletal and Skin Disease Information Clearinghouse

(301) 495-4484

Distributes information to health providers and consumers. Serves as an information exchange for educational materials. Refers requests from patients to the Arthritis Foundation.

National Center for Education in Maternal and Child Health

(703) 524-7802

Answers requests from health care professionals and the public in all areas relating to maternal and child health. Produces bibliographies, resource guides, and directories. Maintains a resource center that is open to the public by appointment.

National Cholesterol Education Program-Information Center

(301) 496-1051

Provides information on cholesterol to health providers and the public.

National Clearinghouse for Alcohol and Drug Information

(301) 468-2600; (800) 729-6686

Gathers and disseminates current information on drug- and alcohol-related subjects. Responds to information requests and prepares bibliographies on topics related to alcohol. Distributes publications about alcohol and drug abuse.

National Clearinghouse for Primary Care Information

(703) 821-8955 ext. 248

Provides information services to support the planning, development, and delivery of ambulatory health care to urban and rural areas where there are shortages of medical personnel and services. Although the clearinghouse will respond to public inquiries, its primary audience is health care providers who work in community health centers.

National Diabetes Information Clearinghouse

(301) 654-3327

Collects and disseminates information on diabetes and its complications. Maintains an automated file of educational materials on the Combined Health Information Database.

National Digestive Disease Information Clearinghouse

(301) 654-3810

Provides information on digestive diseases to health professionals, patients, and their families.

National High Blood Pressure Education Program Information Center

(301) 592-8573

Provides information on the detection, diagnosis, and management of high blood pressure to consumers and health professionals.

National Highway Traffic Safety Administration Information Center

NES-11 HL, U.S. Department of Transportation
(800) 424-9393 (Auto Hotline);
(202) 366-0123 (DC Metro area)

Publishes a variety of safety information brochures, conducts public education programs that promote the use of safety belts and child safety seats, and informs the public of the hazards of drunk driving. Maintains a toll-free hotline for consumer complaints.

National Information Center for Children and Youth with Disabilities

(800) 695-0285

Helps parents of handicapped children, disabled adults, and professionals locate services for the handicapped and information on disabling conditions.

National Information Center for Orphan Drugs and Rare Diseases

(800) 300-7469; (301) 656-4167 (MDs only)

Gathers and disseminates information on products for rare diseases. Responds to inquiries from patients, health professionals, and the general public.

National Injury Information Clearinghouse

(301) 504-0424

Collects and disseminates injury data and information relating to the causes and prevention of death, injury, and illness associated with consumer products.

National Institute of Mental Health Public Inquiries Branch

(301) 443-4513

Distributes institute publications and provides information and publications on the Depression/Awareness, Recognition, and Treatment (D/ART) program. This is a national program to educate the public, primary care physicians, and mental health specialists about depressive disorders and their symptoms and treatments.

National Kidney and Urologic Diseases Information Clearinghouse

(301) 654-4415

Collects and disseminates information on patient education materials. Maintains kidney and urologic diseases subfile of the Combined Health Information Database. Responds to public inquiries from consumers and health professionals.

National Library Service for the Blind and Physically Handicapped

(202) 707-5100; (800) 424-8567

Works through local and regional libraries to provide service to persons unable to use standard printed materials because of blindness or physical impairment. Provides information on blindness and list of participating libraries on request.

National Maternal and Child Health Clearinghouse

(703) 356-1964

Distributes publications on maternal and child health to consumers and health professionals.

National Rehabilitation Information Center

(800) 346-2742 (voice & TDD); (301) 562-2400 (MDs only)

Provides information on disability-related research, resources, and products for independent living. Provides fact sheets, resource aides, and research and technical publications.

Office of Disease Prevention and Health Prevention National Health Information Center

(800) 336-4797; (301) 565-4167 (MDs only)

Helps the public locate health information through identification of health information resources and an inquiry referral system. Refers questions to appropriate resources. Prepares and distributes publications and directories on health promotion and disease prevention topics.

Office of Minority Health Resource Center

(800) 444-6472; (301) 230-7198

Responds to consumer and professional inquiries on minority health-related topics by distributing materials, providing referrals to appropriate sources, and identifying sources of technical assistance. Operates a toll-free number.

Office on Smoking and Health Technical Information Center

(404) 488-5705

Offers bibliographic and reference services to researchers and others and publishes and distributes a number of publications in the field of smoking.

President's Council on Physical Fitness and Sports

(202) 690-9000

Produces informational materials on exercise, school physical education programs, sports, and physical fitness for youth, adults, and the elderly.

INDEX

Note: **Bold** page numbers indicate contact information for specific organizations.